P9-CFP-828

INTRODUCTION TO ADDICTIVE BEHAVIORS

The Guilford Substance Abuse Series

Howard T. Blane and Thomas R. Kosten, Editors

RECENT VOLUMES

Introduction to Addictive Behaviors, Third Edition
Dennis L. Thombs

Clinical Work with Substance-Abusing Clients, Second Edition
Shulamith Lala Ashenberg Straussner, Editor

Treating Substance Abuse: Theory and Technique, Second Edition
Frederick Rotgers, Jon Morgenstern, and Scott T. Walters, Editors

Addiction and Change: How Addictions Develop and Addicted People Recover
Carlo C. DiClemente

Seeking Safety: A Treatment Manual for PTSD and Substance Abuse
Lisa M. Najavits

Substance Abuse Treatment and the Stages of Change:
Selecting and Planning Interventions
Gerard J. Connors, Dennis M. Donovan, and Carlo C. DiClemente

Psychological Theories of Drinking and Alcoholism, Second Edition
Kenneth E. Leonard and Howard T. Blane, Editors

New Treatments for Opiate Dependence
Susan M. Stine and Thomas R. Kosten, Editors

Couple Therapy for Alcoholism: A Cognitive-Behavioral Treatment Manual
*Phylis J. Wakefield, Rebecca E. Williams, Elizabeth B. Yost,
and Kathleen M. Patterson*

Clinical Guide to Alcohol Treatment: The Community Reinforcement Approach
Robert K. Meyers and Jane Ellen Smith

Psychotherapy and Substance Abuse: A Practitioner's Handbook
Arnold M. Washton, Editor

Introduction to Addictive Behaviors

THIRD EDITION

DENNIS L. THOMBS

THE GUILFORD PRESS
New York   London

© 2006 The Guilford Press
A Division of Guilford Publications, Inc.
72 Spring Street, New York, NY 10012
www.guilford.com

All rights reserved

No part of this book may be reproduced, translated, stored in a retrieval system,
or transmitted, in any form or by any means, electronic, mechanical,
photocopying, microfilming, recording, or otherwise, without written permission
from the Publisher.

Printed in the United States of America

This book is printed on acid-free paper.

Last digit is print number: 9 8 7 6 5 4 3 2 1

Library of Congress Cataloging-in-Publication Data
Thombs, Dennis L.
  Introduction to addictive behaviors / Dennis L. Thombs.—3rd ed.
  p. cm. — (The Guilford substance abuse series)
  Includes bibliographical references and index.
  ISBN-10 1-59385-278-9 ISBN-13 978-1-59385-278-8 (cloth)
  1. Substance abuse—Etiology. 2. Substance abuse—
Treatment. I. Title. II. Series.
  [DNLM: 1. Substance-Related Disorders—etiology. 2. Substance-Related
Disorders—therapy.   WM 270 T465i 2006]
  RC564.T55 2006
  616.86—dc22
                                                          2005030211

About the Author

Dennis L. Thombs, PhD, FAAHB, is Associate Professor in the Department of Health Education and Behavior at the University of Florida. The focus of his scholarship is addictive behavior, with special interests in the epistemology of addiction and in alcohol and drug use during the period of emerging adulthood. Dr. Thombs's research has been supported by the National Institute on Alcohol Abuse and Alcoholism. He is a Fellow in the American Academy of Health Behavior.

Acknowledgments

The following publishers have generously given permission to use extended quotations or paraphrases, and/or to reprint or adapt tables or figures, from published works:

Beyond Freedom and Dignity by B. F. Skinner, 1975, New York: Bantam. Copyright 1975 by B. F. Skinner. Used by permission of Random House, Inc.

"Theory in the Practice of Psychotherapy" by M. Bowen, 1976, in P. J. Guerin (Ed.), *Family Therapy: Theory and Practice*, New York: Gardner Press. Copyright 1976 by Gardner Press, Inc.

"Principles of Alcoholism Psychotherapy" by S. Zimberg, 1978, in S. Zimberg, J. Wallace, and S. Blume (Eds.), *Practical Approaches to Alcoholism Psychotherapy*, New York: Plenum Press. Copyright 1978 by Springer Science and Business Media.

"What Motivates People to Change?" by W. R. Miller and S. Rollnick, 1991, in *Motivational Interviewing: Preparing People to Change Addictive Behavior*, New York: Guilford Press. Copyright 1991 by The Guilford Press.

"Drugs of Abuse: Anatomy, Pharmacology and Function of Reward Pathways" by G. F. Koob, 1992, *Trends in Pharmacological Sciences, 13*, 177–184. Copyright 1992 by Elsevier Science Ltd.

"Sex and Age Effects on the Inheritance of Alcohol Problems: A Twin Study" by M. McGue, R. W. Pickens, and D. S. Svikis, 1992, *Journal of Abnormal Psychology, 101*, 3–17. Copyright 1992 by the American Psychological Association.

"Dual Diagnosis: A Review of Etiological Theories" by K. T. Mueser, R. E. Drake, and M. A. Wallach, 1998, *Addictive Behaviors, 23*, 717–734. Copyright 1998 by Elsevier.

Diagnostic and Statistical Manual of Mental Disorders, Fourth Edition, Text Revision, by the American Psychiatric Association, 2000, Washington, DC: American Psychiatric Association. Copyright 2000 by the American Psychiatric Association.

"Rates of Psychiatric Comorbidity among U.S. Residents with Lifetime Cannabis Dependence" by V. Agosti, E. Nunes, and F. Levin, 2002, *American Journal of Drug and Alcohol Dependence, 28,* 643–652. Copyright 2002 by the Taylor and Francis Group.

"Nicotine Dependence and Psychiatric Disorders in the United States: Results from the National Epidemiologic Survey on Alcohol and Related Conditions" by B. F. Grant, D. S. Hasin, S. P. Chou, F. S. Stinson, and D. A. Dawson, 2004, *Archives of General Psychiatry, 61,* 1107–1115; "Prevalence and Co-Occurrence of Substance Use Disorders and Independent Mood and Anxiety Disorders: Results from the National Epidemiologic Survey on Alcohol and Related Conditions" by B. F. Grant, F. S. Stinson, D. A. Dawson, S. P. Chou, M. C. Dufour, W. Compton, R. P. Pickering, and K. Kaplan, 2004, *Archives of General Psychiatry, 61,* 807–816; and "Co-Occurrence of 12-Month Alcohol and Drug Use Disorders and Personality Disorders in the United States: Results from the National Epidemiologic Survey on Alcohol and Related Conditions" by B. F. Grant, F. S. Stinson, D. A. Dawson, S. P. Chou, W. J. Ruan, and R. P. Pickering, 2004, *Archives of General Psychiatry, 61,* 361–368. Copyright 2004 by the American Medical Association.

Preface

This book was written for practicing health and human services profession-als with no formal training in substance abuse prevention and treatment, and for undergraduate and graduate courses on addictive behavior. The book has two primary goals. The first is to challenge and strengthen the reader's understanding of addiction by exploring how others in the field have come to know it. I hope that this will enable the reader to create a clear and logically consistent perspective on addiction. The second goal is to show the reader how theory and research are important to both the pre-vention and the treatment of substance abuse. This should provide the reader with an array of strategies for addressing substance abuse problems, and help make him or her an effective practitioner.

There are a number of good books currently available on substance abuse and dependence. For the most part, however, these books either are written at an advanced level for the sophisticated practitioner or researcher or focus on a limited set of theoretical orientations. The present text is unique in that it attempts to present a comprehensive and thoughtful review of theory and research with the front-line practitioner and student in mind. Exposure to complex and divergent theories of addictive behavior has often been neglected in the preparation and training of health and human services professionals, including substance abuse counselors, pre-vention specialists, social workers, psychologists, nurses, and so forth. Some of these practitioners are familiar with one or more of the disease models, but even here they often have not had the opportunity to examine its propositions critically. This book assumes virtually no preexisting knowledge in the biological and behavioral sciences, medicine, or public health. In each chapter, a careful attempt has been made to explain the con-ceptual underpinnings of the theories and approaches described herein, as well as the research supporting these frameworks.

The third edition of *Introduction to Addictive Behaviors* has been revised to appeal to a broader audience of practitioners and students. The primary focus of the first two editions was to provide a multidisciplinary foundation for addiction treatment. The third edition has been revised to include a theoretical and research foundation for substance abuse *prevention* as well. The third edition also includes two new chapters. Each presents cutting-edge knowledge in two very different but important areas in the study of addictive behavior. The new chapters are titled "Public Health and Prevention Approaches" and "Toward an Understanding of Comorbidity." All the chapters from the second edition have been updated and included in the third edition.

Special thanks are in order to those who helped me complete the third edition. I am grateful to The Guilford Press, and especially to Jim Nageotte and Jane Keislar, for their encouragement and assistance in preparing the third edition. A number of anonymous reviewers provided feedback that also was extremely helpful in steering the direction of the book.

DENNIS L. THOMBS
University of Florida

Contents

CHAPTER 1

The Multiple Conceptions of Addictive Behavior and Professional Practice Today

CONCEPTIONS OF ADDICTION IN U.S. HISTORY

For most of U.S. history, habitual drunkenness and drug use have been viewed as both sinful conduct and disease. In recent decades, they also have been considered maladaptive behavior (i.e., debilitative behavior that is "overlearned"). Today, some insist that addiction evolves from all three sources—namely, that it is a *disease* in which people *learn* to act in *immoral* ways. This incongruent vision of addiction has a long history. In the United States, the conception of addiction to alcohol has been evolving since the colonial period. At that time, alcohol consumption in the populace was high (by today's standards) and inebriety was quite common (Goode, 1993); there was little concern about excessive drinking and drunkenness. Americans generally had a high tolerance for social deviance, and thus they were mostly indifferent to the problems caused by heavy drinking. Alcohol was used as a beverage, as medicine, and as a social lubricant. The town tavern was at the center of social and political life. Workers often drank throughout the day, and some employers actually supplied them with free liquor.

During the 17th century and for most of the 18th, alcohol was not seen as an addictive substance and habitual drunkenness was not viewed as a disease (Levine, 1978). Moreover, frequent, heavy drinking was not understood to be a compulsion involving "loss of control," nor was it considered a progressive, deteriorative disorder. Though most Americans considered excessive drinking to be of little importance, some prominent figures did warn and chastise about drunkenness. In these instances, it often was defined as immoral behavior. In sermons, Puritan ministers warned that drunkards faced eternal suffering in hell, and though Cotton Mather referred to alcohol as the "good creature of God," he also described drunkenness as "this engine of the Devil" (Mather, 1708). In the 1760s, John Adams proposed restrictions on taverns and Benjamin Franklin described these establishments as "pests to society" (Rorabaugh, 1976).

The first American to clearly articulate the modern conception of alcoholism as a disease state was Dr. Benjamin Rush. He was a Philadelphia physician, signer of the Declaration of Independence, and surgeon general of the Continental Army who, in 1784, authored a pamphlet titled *An Inquiry into the Effects of Ardent Spirits on the Human Mind and Body*. In this work, Rush challenged the conventional view that habitual drunkenness was an innocuous activity. He did not condemn alcohol use per se but, rather, excessive consumption and drunkenness. Throughout his writings on alcohol, he made an attempt to alert Americans to the dangers of unrestrained drinking. He emphasized that alcohol misuse was contributing to an array of social problems: disease, poverty, crime, insanity, and broken homes.

Rush's writings greatly contributed to a paradigm shift that redefined the problem of "habitual drunkenness." According to Levine (1978), Rush's new construction was based on four propositions that are still relied on today to explain problematic alcohol and drug use:

1. Hard liquor is an addictive substance.
2. There exists a compulsion to drink that arises from a loss of control.
3. Frequent drunkenness is a disease.
4. Total abstinence from alcohol is the only way to cure the drunkard.

Though Rush was not optimistic about reform in the United States, his writings laid the groundwork for the temperance movement. The first temperance society was formed in 1808. Three years later a number of independent groups united, and in 1826 the American Society for the Promotion of Temperance (later renamed the American Temperance Society) was founded. Consistent with the views of Dr. Rush, the initial objective of the Society was to promote moderation—not prohibition. To accomplish this goal, the Society organized itself into local units that sent lecturers out into the field, distributed information, and served as a clearinghouse for movement information.

By the mid-1830s, more than 500,000 Americans had joined the temperance movement *and* had pledged to abstain from all alcoholic beverages (Levine, 1978). The emphasis on moderation gave way to a commitment to the necessity of abstinence for all citizens. Thus, the "temperance" movement became a "prohibitionist" movement, and increasingly inebriety was seen as immoral conduct. After the Civil War, this view was applied to opium and morphine, which also came to be seen as inherently addicting poisons.

Those in the Temperance Society worked hard to proselytize others, and to an extent they were successful. Employers stopped supplying alcohol to their employees on the job. Politicians were more restrained in their relations with alcohol producers and distributors. In many areas, local legislation was passed to regulate taverns—an outcome of lobbying by the Society. Goode (1993) reports that between 1830 and 1840, annual alcohol use dropped from 7.1 gallons per person (age 15 or older) to 3.1 gallons.

Leaders in the temperance movement held assumptions about the "disease" of alcoholism that are quite similar to those espoused today in Alcoholics Anonymous (AA). Levine's (1978) historical review found that habitual drunkards were described as having the following disease symptoms and features:

1. Loss of control.
2. Intense cravings when not drinking.
3. A physical compulsion to drink because of the power of alcohol.
4. A vulnerability to excessive drinking determined by hereditary characteristics.
5. Complete abstinence as the only cure.

John B. Gough (1881), a prominent temperance lecturer, said that he considered "drunkenness as sin, but I consider it also disease. It is a physical as well as moral evil" (p. 443). Levine (1978) found the following passage from a 1873 annual report of the Society: "The Temperance press has always regarded drunkenness as a sin and a disease—a sin first, then a disease; we rejoice that the Inebriate Association are now substantially on the same platform (p. 157)."

Thus, much of the modern, post-Prohibition thinking about alcoholism can be traced back through the temperance movement and to Benjamin Rush's early conceptualization in the late 1700s. This construction of substance abuse combines notions of sin and disease without much concern for the inconsistencies and inevitable questions that it generates. For instance, are we free to choose disease? Are we free to avoid it? Such questions were not addressed by temperance leaders.

Yalisove (1998) has noted that AA is largely responsible for the adoption of the disease concept in most treatment settings in the United States. The only significant difference between temperance ideology and the views promoted by AA, beginning in the late 1930s, is the emphasis placed on the *source of alcohol addiction.* Prior to national Prohibition, temperance leaders blamed both the agent (alcohol) and the drinker. Later, AA shifted the focus to characteristics within the drinker, chiefly "loss of control," a problem sometimes responsive to mutual social support, and one certainly not requiring the social activism embedded in temperance ideology. This modification of the conception of alcoholism was in line with the post-Prohibition climate in the nation. After its repeal in 1933, national Prohibition was perceived to have been a failure and public policies shifted to alcohol control. There was little interest in sharply curtailing the alcohol supply—the intervention of choice in an "agent-focused" conceptualization.

It should be noted that the mixed "disease–moral model," cultivated by the temperance movement, still guides alcohol and drug control policies today. For instance, drug courts "sentence" offenders to "treatment," DWI (driving while intoxicated) offenders are required to participate in treatment and/or attend AA meetings, employers make workers' continued employment contingent upon seeking treatment, and so on. Peele (1996) describes this as the "disease law enforcement model" and states:

> When public figures in the United States discuss drug policy, they generally veer between these two models, as in the debate over whether we should imprison or treat drug addicts. In fact, the contemporary U.S. system has already taken this synthesis of the law enforcement approach to drug abuse and the disease approach almost as far as it can go. (p. 204)

This brief historical review shows that the conception of addiction, particularly alcoholism, in the United States has long been defined by incongruous assumptions involving morality and disease. Neither perspective has entirely supplanted the other. Thus, there remains much disagreement and confusion about the nature of addiction, which tends to impede progress toward developing widely shared social norms about acceptable and unacceptable substance use and spurs acrimonious debates about public drug control policy.

Perspectives on addiction can be classified into three distinct sets of beliefs. Each set points to different strategies for controlling the problem of addiction in our society. Let us examine each in greater detail.

ADDICTION AS IMMORAL CONDUCT

The first set of beliefs maintains that addiction represents a refusal to abide by some ethical or moral code of conduct. Excessive drinking or drug use is considered freely chosen behavior that is at best irresponsible and at worst evil. By identifying addiction as sin, one does not necessarily ascribe the same level of "evilness" to it as one would to rape, larceny, or murder. Nevertheless, in this view it remains a transgression, a wrong.

Note that this position assumes that alcohol and drug abuse are freely chosen—in other words, that in regard to this sphere of human conduct, people are free agents. Alcoholics and addicts are not considered "out of control"; they choose to use substances in such a way that they create suffering for others (e.g., family members) and for themselves. Thus, they can be justifiably blamed for having the alcohol/drug problem.

Because addiction results from a freely chosen and morally wrong course of action, the logical way to "treat" the problem is to punish the alcoholic or addict. Thus, from this perspective, legal sanctions such as jail sentences, fines, and other punitive actions are seen as most appropriate. The addict is not thought to be deserving of care or help. Rather, punishment is relied on to rectify past misdeeds and to prevent further chemical use. Relapse is considered evidence of lingering evil in the addict; again, then, punishment is believed needed to correct "slipping" or backsliding.

In our society today, this perspective on alcohol and other drug abuse is typically advocated by politically conservative groups, law enforcement organizations, zealous religious factions, and groups of individuals who have been personally harmed by a substance abuser (e.g., Mothers Against Drunk Driving). During political campaigns, candidates frequently appeal to this sentiment by proposing tougher legal penalties for possession and distribution of illicit drugs and for drunken driving. U.S. history is marked by repeated (and failed) government efforts to eliminate addiction with such legal sanctions. The crackdown on Chinese opium smokers in the 1800s and the enactment of Prohibition in the early 20th century stand as two noteworthy examples.

The "addiction as sin" position has several advantages as well as disadvantages. One advantage is that it is straightforward and clear. There is little ambiguity or murkiness associated with this stance. Furthermore, it is absolute; there is no need for theorizing or philosophizing about the nature of addiction. It is simply misbehavior and as such needs to be confronted and hence punished. Scientific investigation of the problem is believed to be unnecessary, because that which must be done to correct it (i.e., application of sanctions) is already well understood. In this view, our society's inability to adequately address the problems of alcoholism and addiction reflects widespread moral decay. Proponents of the addiction-as-sin model typically call for a return to "traditional" or "family" values as the way to ameliorate the problem.

There are at least three disadvantages to the addiction-as-sin model as well. First, science suggests that alcoholism and addiction are anything but simple phenomena. They appear to be multifactorial in origin, stemming from pharmacological, biological, psychological, and social factors. The apparent complexity of addiction is underscored by the variety of diverse theories seeking to explain it (many of which are described in this volume). Moreover, as science has begun to shed light on various aspects of compulsive chemical use, it has become clearer that much still remains to be learned. The genetic vulnerability hypothesis, alcohol expectancy theory, and the purported stabilizing effects of alcoholism on family structure are all cases in point.

Another disadvantage with the moral point of view is that it is not at all clear that drug and alcohol dependence are freely chosen. In fact, the disease models (see Chapter 2) maintain that exactly the opposite is the case. That is, excessive drinking or drugging represents being out of control, or a loss of control exists; in either case, the individual does not freely choose substance abuse. A further point of departure is offered by the behavioral sciences, where, at least in several theoretical perspectives, a high rate of drug self-administration is understood to be under the control of social or environmental contingencies. These contingencies are usually external to alcoholics or addicts and not under their personal control. Thus, both the disease models and the behavioral sciences challenge the notion that addiction is willful misconduct.

A third disadvantage with the addiction-as-sin position is that history suggests that punishment is an ineffective means of reducing the prevalence of addictive problems in the population. Aside from the issue of inhumane sanctions (a real possibility if a political majority adopts the moral view of addiction), a reasonably strong case can be made, based on historical precedents, that striking back at substance abusers via governmental authority simply does not work over an extended period. In fact, law enforcement crackdowns often have the unintended effects of being an impetus for strengthening organized crime networks, creating underground markets, bolstering disrespect for the law, clogging court dockets, and overloading prisons (at substantial cost to the taxpayer).

ADDICTION AS DISEASE

In the second view, excessive consumption of alcohol or drugs is the result of an underlying disease process. The disease process is thought to cause compulsive use; in other words, the high rate and volume of use are merely the manifest symptoms of an illness. The exact nature of the illness is not fully understood at this point, but many proponents of the disease models believe that the illness has genetic origins. For these reasons, it is hypothesized that individuals cannot drink or drug themselves into alcoholism or drug addiction. If the disease (possibly arising from a genetic vulnerability) is not present, then dependencies cannot develop, no matter how much of the substance is ingested.

The addiction-as-a-disease conception maintains that the alcoholic and the addict are victims of an illness. The afflicted individual is not evil or irresponsible, just sick. Thus, the chemical abuse is not freely chosen; rather, the excessive drinking or drugging is seen to be beyond the control of the sufferer. In fact, a common feature of the disease conceptions is the loss of control over substance use. It is hypothesized that once an addict has consumed a small amount of a drug, intense cravings are triggered via unknown physiological mechanisms, and these cravings lead to compulsive overuse. This mechanism is beyond the personal control of the addict.

Because alcoholics and addicts are seen as suffering from an illness, the logical conclusion is that they deserve compassionate care, help, and treatment. Because the condition is considered a disease, medical treatment is appropriate. Competent treatment, then, especially on an inpatient basis, should be supervised by physicians. Traditionally, treatment based on the disease models emphasized the management of medical complications (e.g., liver disease, stomach ulcer, and anemia), as well as patient education about the disease models and recovery.

Disease models are strongly advocated by at least three groups in our society today. One of these is the profession of medicine. Critics have indicated that physicians have a vested interest in convincing society that addiction is a disease. As long as it is considered such, they can admit patients to hospitals, bill insurance companies, and collect fees. However, in today's health care system, the pressure of "managed care" has greatly reduced physician authority, making such criticism seem less relevant. Another group that has strongly advocated the disease conception is the alcohol industry (i.e., brewers, distillers, and winemakers), which also has a vested interest in viewing alcoholism, specifically, as a disease. As long as it is a disease suffered by only 10% of all drinkers, then our society (i.e., our government) will not take serious steps to restrict the manufacture, distribution, sale, and consumption of alcoholic beverages. In other words, the alcohol industry wants us to believe that the problem lies within the "host" (i.e., the alcoholic), and not with the "agent" (i.e., alcohol). A third group that strongly advocates the disease notion is the "recovery movement," which is made up of individuals and families recovering from chemical dependencies. This group can also be considered to have a vested interest in identifying alcoholism and addiction as diseases. First, calling alcoholism or addiction a disease makes it more respectable than labeling it a moral problem or a mental disorder. Second, maintaining that it is a disease can serve to reduce possible guilt or shame about past misdeeds. This may allow recovering individuals to focus on the work that they need to do to maintain a drug-free life.

There are a number of advantages to the disease models. Most important, addiction is taken out of the moral realm, and its victims are helped rather than scorned and punished. In addition, society is more willing to allocate resources to help persons who have a disease than to help individuals who are merely wicked. It is also clear that the disease models have helped hundreds of thousands of alcoholics and addicts to return to healthful living. Thus, its utility in assisting at least a large subset of addicts is beyond question.

There are also a number of disadvantages to the disease models; only a few are discussed here. (Chapter 2 includes a more extensive discussion of these disadvantages.) Briefly, several of the key concepts of the disease models have not held up under scientific scrutiny. For example, the loss-of-control hypothesis, the supposedly progressive course of alcoholism, and the belief that a return to controlled drinking is impossible are all propositions that have been seriously challenged by scientific investigations. Within the scientific community, it is acknowledged that these assumptions are not well supported by empirical evidence. Unfortunately, a large segment of the treatment community appears to be unaware of this literature, or perhaps chooses to ignore it.

ADDICTION AS MALADAPTIVE BEHAVIOR

The third position holds that addiction is a behavioral disorder; as such, it is shaped by the same laws that shape all human behavior. Essentially, then, addiction is learned. It is neither sinful (as the moral model purports) nor out of control (as the disease models purport). Instead, it is seen as a problem behavior that is clearly under the control of environmental, family, social, and/or even cognitive contingencies. As in the disease models, the person with an addiction problem is seen as a victim—not a victim of a disease but a victim of destructive learning conditions. For the most part, addictive behavior is not freely chosen, although some behavioral science theories (e.g., social learning theory) do assert that addicts retain some degree of control over their drinking or drug use.

It is important to understand the value placed on objectivity in the behavioral sciences. When alcoholism (or addiction) is described as a "maladaptive behavior," it is very different from describing the condition as "misbehavior" (a moral perspective). Behavioral scientists avoid passing judgment on the "rightness" or "wrongness" of substance abuse. By "maladaptive," the behavioral scientist means that the behavior pattern has destructive consequences for addicts and/or their families (and possibly society). It does not imply that the addicts are bad or irresponsible.

In the behavioral science view, the most appropriate interventions are based on learning principles. Specifically, "clients" (this term is preferred over "patients") are taught skills to prevent relapse. The medical aspects of treatment are attended to when necessary, but they are generally deemphasized. The emphasis instead is placed on changing the environment, teaching clients skills, and experimenting with these procedures. Professionals in the behavioral sciences and public health are most heavily involved in these approaches to substance abuse prevention and treatment.

Interventions attempting to influence the social environment and behavior of individuals are labor intensive and evaluation focused. Thus, professional practice ideally should be "data driven" and subject to frequent modification. Though these characteristics are consistent with today's emphases on efficiency and accountability, many prevention and treatment programs are slow to adopt this kind of empirical approach (Lamb, Greenlick, & McCarty, 1998). This reluctance is part of the problem known as "technology transfer," which is discussed later in this chapter.

At present, the strong advocacy groups for this approach to treatment tend to be found in the field of psychology. Division 50 (the Addictions) of the American Psychological Association is one example. This group, as well as others like it (e.g., the American Public Health Association and the International Coalition for Addictions Studies Education), do not wield significant political power and thus have not had a major impact on public policy toward substance abuse prevention and treatment.

THE NEED FOR THEORY

Why a book on theories of addictive behavior? As the discussion up to this point has outlined, three broad perspectives (i.e., sin, disease, and maladaptive behavior) on the nature of addiction exist today. The first, the moral model, is not a theory, at least as the term "theory" is understood in science. The disease models are the theoretical base from which most treatment providers operate in the United States today. Behavioral science perspectives, though sharing an emphasis on faulty learning, are represented by an array of distinctive theoretical positions.

It is my own belief that the addiction-as-sin position is the only perspective that is clearly understood by the majority of professionals working in the alcohol and drug abuse field today. This is not to say that they rely on it; indeed, the moral model is almost universally rejected by competent practitioners (with good reason, as has been mentioned earlier). Unfortunately, it appears that critical examination of the disease models and the various behavioral science theories has been largely ignored by many in the alcohol and drug abuse field. All too often, practitioners rigidly cling to their favorite theory, in many cases without fully understanding all its concepts and implications. At the same time, other theories may be callously disregarded. Stefflre and Burks (1979) maintain that because all practitioners necessarily operate from a theory (it may be informal or personal but nevertheless exists), it is essential that they hold the theory "explicitly"— that is, that they understand it with great clarity.

The nearly dogmatic stance that some organizations and practitioners have taken regarding the disease models has slowed the development of the substance abuse prevention and treatment fields. Clearly, the disease models have helped a large number of substance abuse clients. However, as judged by the very large number of substance abusers who avoid or refuse treatment, drop out of treatment, and/or relapse, it can be reasonably asserted that these particular models are not a "good fit" for many (perhaps most) persons. It is imperative that practitioners consider alternative prevention and treatment models, especially for populations and individual clients who cannot work within a disease model. All too often, objections to an alternative prevention or treatment approach are characterized as "denial" about the substance abuse problem, which may obscure the possibility that the problem rests within the model or the approach rather than in the population, community, or individual. As professionals, we should possess the flexibility to work with different communities and clients and tailor our approaches to their needs. The theories and models outlined in detail in this volume will inform and assist in identifying appropriate intervention options.

WHAT EXACTLY IS A THEORY?

The popular understanding of the term "theory" is usually "a belief that stands in opposition to fact." Many of us have heard someone retort, "Oh, that's just a theory." In other words, theories are commonly thought to be unsubstantiated hypotheses or speculation. Furthermore, there is a tendency to equate theory with things that are impractical or devoid of common sense. However, as Monette, Sullivan, and DeJong (1990) note, all of us necessarily rely on theories to function in our relationships with family members, friends, professional colleagues, and others. In most cases, these theories are crude and not explicit; nonetheless, they exist, if only in our minds. Thus, to dismiss theory as useless is to fail to recognize its universal application, both in science and in everyday life.

In the behavioral sciences, the term "model" is often used in place of "theory." When a paradigm is not well developed or it attempts to only explain a narrow aspect of some behavior, we often refer to it as a model. In this volume, both terms are used and attempts to distinguish between them are not made.

Hall and Lindzey (1978) define the term "theory" as a "set of conventions created by the theorist" (p. 10). This straightforward definition underscores that theories are not predetermined by nature or data, or any other orderly process. It rests largely on the theorist's prior knowledge and creativity. The function of theory is to organize and impose order and meaning on a collection of isolated observations or data (Monette et al., 1990). Thus, theories attempt to make sense of dissimilar findings and to explain relationships among variables of interest. In the study of addictive behavior, theory helps us understand the etiology of substance abuse and points to ways to prevent and treat it.

Because a theory is provisional (i.e., it does not explain in absolute or final terms), it is inappropriate to characterize it as "true" or "false." Instead, it is best described as "useful" or "not useful" (Hall & Lindzey, 1978). A theory's utility, then, can be assessed by its ability to predict events, or by how closely the data generated in research support hypothesized relationships.

ATTRIBUTES OF A GOOD THEORY

Stefflre and Burks (1979) have identified five attributes of a good theory, described in the following paragraphs.

1. *Clarity.* A good theory must exhibit clarity in a number of ways. First, there should be agreement among its general assumptions (i.e., its philosophical foundation), as well as agreement between its consequences and generated data or observations (i.e., its scientific foundation). Second, the propositions of a good theory should be clearly described and easily communicated. Third, a good theory should serve as "an easily read map" (Stefflre & Burks, 1979, p. 9).

2. *Comprehensiveness.* A good theory can be applied to many individuals in many different situations. Its ability to explain events should extend across a variety of time periods, geographic areas, sociocultural contexts, and sociodemographic variables (gender, race, religion, etc.).

3. *Explicitness.* Precision is a chief characteristic of a good theory. Important theoretical concepts must be capable of being defined operationally. That is, concepts must be measurable with a high degree of reliability. Theories that rely on vague, ill-defined, or difficult-to-measure concepts cannot be checked against clear referents in the real world (Stefflre & Burks, 1979).

4. *Parsimony.* A good theory explains phenomena in a relatively simple and straightforward manner. A theory that can explain behavioral events in innumerable ways is suspect. A theory that "overexplains" something may be creative, but it may also be fiction. That is, it may not accurately reflect reality.

5. *Generation of useful research findings.* A good theory has a history of generating research findings (i.e., data) that support its concepts. Theories that have little or no empirical support are less useful than those that have considerable data driving further investigation of its propositions. Stefflre and Burks (1979) summarize these attributes by stating the following: "A theory is always a map that is in the process of being filled in with greater detail. We do not so much ask whether it is true, but whether it is helpful" (p. 9).

THE DISSEMINATION OF EVIDENCE-BASED PRACTICE

Across a broad range of human endeavors (business, agriculture, government, education, human services, etc.), it has been recognized that people often find it difficult to adopt new practices or products in their occupations. This is particularly the case when the rationale for change is based on information generated from behavioral science research where the effectiveness of the new "technology" or "best practice" may be established, but it is based on abstract concepts considered "soft" (Tenkasi & Mohrman, 1995). This situation often exists in programs that seek to prevent and treat substance abuse. Many reasons have been given for why employees and organizations resist change and innovation, despite the evidence supporting a new practice. As Diamond (1995) notes, at a deep level, change is experienced as an emotional and cognitive loss. Typically, it evokes anxiety, insecurity, and fear in the practitioner.

The issues related to the dissemination, adoption, and implementation of evidence-based practice are commonly referred to as problems in "technology transfer" or the "adoption of innovation." In the substance abuse prevention and treatment fields, the diffusion of innovation has not followed the expanding knowledge base (B. S. Brown, 1995; Rogers, 1995a). Thus, interest in these problems has grown in recent years. Backer, David, and Soucy (1995) have identified the following six strategies to optimize adoption of innovation in substance abuse settings.

1. *Interpersonal contact.* To get an innovation used in new settings, there needs to be direct, personal contact between those who will be adopting the innovation and its developers or others with knowledge about the innovation.

2. *Planning and conceptual foresight.* A well-developed strategic plan for how an innovation will be adopted in a new setting . . . is essential to meet the challenges of innovation adoption and sustained change.
3. *Outside consultation on the change process.* Consultation can provide conceptual and practical assistance in designing the adoption or change effort efficiently and can offer useful objectivity about the likelihood of success, cost, possible side effects, and so forth.
4. User-oriented transformation of information. What is known about an innovation needs to be translated into language that potential users can readily understand. Materials must be abbreviated so that attention spans are not exceeded, and it is important that the focus remain on two key issues: "Does it work?" and "How can it be replicated?" Attempts in recent years to address these questions have led to the increasing reliance on manual-driven prevention and treatment programs.
5. Individual and organizational championship. An innovation's chances for successful adoption are much greater if influential potential adopters (opinion leaders) and organizational or community leaders express enthusiasm for its adoption.
6. Potential user involvement. Everyone who will have to live with the results of the innovation needs to be involved in planning for innovation adoption, both to get suggestions for how to undertake the adoption effectively and to facilitate ownership of the new program or activity (thus decreasing resistance to change). (pp. 4–5)

The National Institute on Drug Abuse (NIDA) has provided leadership in stimulating technology transfer in the substance abuse prevention and treatment communities. NIDA's Technology Transfer Program was officially formed in 1989. The goals of the program are twofold: (1) reduce demand for drugs by improving prevention and treatment practices, and (2) enhance drug abuse-related HIV/AIDS risk reduction. The program's objective is not simply to disseminate research findings but to assist practitioners with actually implementing new treatment protocols in their programs. The products of the program include conferences, a videotape series, technology transfer packages (protocol materials), and clinical reports.

Despite efforts such as these, it is my view that insufficient resources are being directed to technology transfer for the front-line practitioner. To enhance the quality and consistency of service delivery, there is a need for new innovation adoption initiatives. Unfortunately, significant resources to support such activity probably will not be forthcoming until there is a shift in federal drug control policy *away* from drug interdiction/user criminalization and *toward* prevention and treatment. Drug interdiction and mandatory minimum prison sentences have been costly practices to carry out, their effectiveness as public policies is questionable, and they have been challenged by critics holding diverse political views (Messing & Hazelwood, 2005; Caulkins, Rydell, Schwabe, & Chiesa, 1997; Transnational Institute, 2005). Furthermore, there is a strong need to educate the public that substance abuse prevention and treatment do "work." A number of public policy groups have been pushing for fundamental changes in our drug control policies for some time (e.g., Join Together, 1996). However, to date, their efforts have not seen much success.

EFFECTIVE PREVENTION AND TREATMENT PROGRAMS

Successful advocacy in the drug control policy arena depends on evidence of positive program outcomes. It is a bit of a paradox then that the major problem in U.S. drug control policy today is the lack of awareness among both the general public and political leaders that competently administered prevention programming and addiction treatment are effective approaches to dealing with the problem of substance abuse; that is, prevention and treatment do "work" (Center for Substance Abuse Treatment, 1997; Substance Abuse and Mental Health Services Administration, 2004). Nevertheless, public funding to control drug use remains heavily invested in law enforcement first, followed by treatment and prevention (U.S. Office of National Drug Control Policy, 2004).

Why advocate for drug abuse prevention? Since 1989, a number of well-controlled preventive interventions have identified effective approaches to deterring tobacco, alcohol, and illegal drug use among youth (seminal studies include Botvin, Baker, Dusenburg, Botvin, & Diaz, 1995; Ellickson, Bell, & McGuigan, 1993; Hansen & Graham, 1991; Pentz et al., 1989; Perry et al., 1996). Some of these approaches are school based (e.g., Botvin et al., 1995; Ellickson et al., 1993), whereas others have been community based with parent and school components (e.g., Pentz et al., 1989; Perry et al., 1996). Among the lessons learned from these trials was that positive program outcomes decay over time and as a result, ongoing "booster sessions" are essential to maintain gains (Botvin et al., 1995; Ellickson et al., 1993). Of course, this requires resources and commitment and collaboration among communities, schools, and parents. Another finding of these studies was that perceived social norms are an important mediator between program activities and outcomes (Hansen & Graham, 1991; Pentz et al., 1989; Perry et al., 1996). Prevention programming appeared to be effective to the extent that it could instill conservative norms about substance use. In other words, if youth were influenced to perceive that substance use was uncommon (not prevalent) and socially unacceptable among their peers, then they were less likely to initiate or continue substance use. Interestingly, normative education may be more effective than peer pressure resistance training in deterring use in children and teens (Hansen & Graham, 1991). This also may be part of the explanation for the failure of

Drug Abuse Resistance Education (DARE) to demonstrate much in the way of positive program outcomes (Ennett, Tobler, Ringwalt, & Flewelling, 1994).

Existing research also provides a strong rationale for greater public support of addiction treatment programs (Center for Substance Abuse Treatment, 1997; Mueller & Wyman, 1997; Project MATCH Research Group, 1997). The National Treatment Improvement Evaluation Study (NTIES) assessed 4,411 clients of treatment programs from across the United States. One year after treatment, clients' use of their primary drug of choice was 48.2% lower than in the 12 months before entering treatment (Center for Substance Abuse Treatment, 1997). During the same period, cocaine use dropped by 54.9%, followed by reductions in crack cocaine (50.8%) and heroin (46.6%). NTIES also found that addiction treatment reduces crime. Among the sample, shoplifting decreased by 81.6%, with reductions also observed for selling drugs, 78.3%; assault and battery, 77.7%; and arrests for any crime, 64.3%. NTIES also revealed that addiction treatment has a positive impact on job income, homelessness, mental and physical health, and involvement in high-risk sexual behavior (Center for Substance Abuse Treatment, 1997).

Another recent nationwide study, the Drug Abuse Treatment Outcomes Study (DATOS), yielded results similar to those of NTIES. The DATOS sample consisted of 10,010 clients from nearly 100 treatment programs in 11 U.S. cities (Mueller & Wyman, 1997). In a subsample of 3,000 randomly selected clients, investigators compared clients' weekly and daily drug use in the year before entering treatment to that 12 months after treatment ended. The clients came from four types of treatment programs: methadone maintenance, outpatient, short-term inpatient, and long-term residential. Regardless of the type of program in which clients participated, it was observed that drug use declined substantially after treatment (Mueller & Wyman, 1997). For example, among clients who participated in outpatient treatment, cocaine, alcohol, and marijuana use were each reduced by at least 50%, at the 12-month follow-up. In addition, all types of treatment had a positive effect on illegal conduct, employment, and suicide thoughts and attempts.

Project MATCH was a major study of alcoholism treatment in which the benefits of matching clients to three different forms of therapy (Project MATCH Research Group, 1997) were compared. In both aftercare and outpatient settings, 1,726 alcoholic clients were randomly assigned to one of three 12-week, individually delivered treatments: cognitive-behavioral coping skills therapy, motivation enhancement therapy, or Twelve-Step facilitation therapy. Clients were assessed 15 months after completing treatment. Though there was little difference in outcomes by type of treatment, Project MATCH significantly reduced drinking in alcoholic clients (Project

MATCH Research Group, 1997). The investigators found that at follow-up, inpatient clients were abstinent on almost 90% of the days, compared to 20% before treatment. Outpatient clients were abstinent on almost 80% of days. Among the inpatient sample, 35% were continuously abstinent during the 15-month follow-up period, compared to 19% of the outpatients. Furthermore, 60% of the inpatients never had 3 consecutive days of drinking during follow-up, compared to 46% of outpatients.

Treatment not only produces positive outcomes but is cost-effective as well. For example, the Rand Corporation (1994) found that for every dollar spent on treatment, $7 is saved on crime-related costs and lost workplace productivity. Another Rand study has found that treatment is more cost-effective than either conventional law enforcement or mandatory minimum drug sentences in reducing both cocaine consumption and related violence (Caulkins et al., 1997). Furthermore, it appears that publicly funded substance abuse treatment can reduce Medicaid medical expenses among the poor by as much as 50% over a 5-year period (Washington State Department of Social and Health Services, 1997).

The outcomes of the major prevention and treatment studies described here indicate that competently administered interventions are effective in deterring youth from beginning to use drugs and in helping those persons with addiction problems. Though much remains to be learned, it appears that the quality of service delivery makes a difference across a variety of approaches. Still, there is a continuing need for research, especially when the products are reports that are accessible to front-line practitioners, the public, and policymakers (Join Together, 1998). A major challenge facing the substance abuse field is developing the educational and training programs needed to prepare the next generation of competent practitioners.

PURPOSE OF THE BOOK

This book should be of great assistance to the reader in developing the multidisciplinary foundation that is unique to the substance abuse prevention and treatment fields. Though idealistic, I do hope that at least in a small way, the book helps to bridge the gap that exists between theory and research, on one side, and practice, on the other. I also hope that students and in-service professionals find the review of theory and research to be provocative enough to cause them to reconsider their conceptions of alcohol and drug abuse. The text should serve to strengthen understanding of diverse theoretical perspectives on substance use and abuse and assist readers in helping communities and individuals effectively address these problems.

REVIEW QUESTIONS

1. What are the three fundamentally different views of addiction? How has the conception of addiction changed during U.S. history?

2. What are the characteristics of these three views that make them distinctive and logically exclusive of one another?

3. What are the advantages and disadvantages of each view?

4. According to the author of this book, which view is best understood? Which is most used in the alcohol and drug abuse field?

5. What are the characteristics of theory?

6. What are the attributes of a good theory?

7. Why is the dissemination of evidence-based practices a challenge in the substance abuse prevention and treatment fields?

8. How do we know that prevention and treatment services are effective in addressing substance abuse problems?

CHAPTER 2

The Disease Models

In the United States today, the predominant model for understanding alcoholism and other addictions is the view that these disorders are diseases (Yalisove, 1998). This view is particularly strong within the treatment community and within self-help fellowships such as Alcoholics Anonymous (AA) or Narcotics Anonymous (NA). The vast majority of treatment programs rely on the disease (or medical) models for a conceptual base; it shapes selection of treatment options and focuses the content of patient and family education. Thus, most treatment programs in this country employ a supervising physician, require AA or NA attendance, advocate abstinence, teach that the disorder is a chronic condition, and so forth. To the credit of the treatment community, these efforts have lessened the stigma associated with alcohol and drug dependence. Compared to 50 years ago, alcoholics and addicts today are less likely to be scorned and more likely to be offered help.

However, it should be recognized that controversy continues to surround the disease concept of addiction. Some legal experts and criminologists insist that the use and abuse of drugs and alcohol are intentional acts that deserve punishment (Wilbanks, 1989). In such a view, substance abuse results from a lack of self-restraint and self-discipline. Herbert Fingarette (1988), a philosopher, maintains that the disease models are a myth that endures because it fulfills economic or personal needs of some groups (i.e., the medical community and recovery groups, respectively). Fingarette (1988) strongly supports helping alcoholics or addicts but believes that the "disease myth" limits treatment options for many needy individuals. Behavioral science researchers have questioned the validity of the models (Peele, 1985), and for some time, others have described such models as patently unscientific (e.g., Alexander, 1988).

Such disparate views are not likely to be resolved in the near future. To evaluate these arguments and counterarguments knowledgeably, it is essential to understand exactly what is meant by addiction as a disease. Only then can the advantages and disadvantages of this model (i.e., its utility) be intelligently weighed.

DIFFERENT DISEASE CONCEPTIONS

Before the core concepts of the disease models are reviewed, it should be noted that there is not just one disease model. A number of proponents of the models, though not necessarily in disagreement, have emphasized different elements. The differences can be striking. For instance, V. E. Johnson's (1980) description of the dynamics of alcoholism progression is different from that described by Milam and Ketcham (1983), and Vaillant (1990) provides yet another perspective. The models differ with respect to the importance of physical, psychological, and spiritual factors in the etiology of alcoholism. These different emphases are probably related to the authors' personal experience with alcoholism (i.e., whether or not they are recovering alcoholics) and their professional training (i.e., whether they are physicians, psychiatrists, or psychologists).

Peele (1996) provides a useful distinction for thinking about the different disease models. He suggests that there are relatively distinct *susceptibility* and *exposure* constructions. The susceptibility variant emphasizes that genetic factors play an important role in the development of substance dependence. These factors influence the individual's vulnerability to the disorders. In contrast, the exposure position holds that chemicals and their actions on the brain are the primary causes of addiction. Here, risk for these disorders is determined by the extent to which the individual is exposed to drugs of abuse. These two disease models are not in conflict with one another. They simply represent different emphases. Each is discussed in detail in this chapter.

The disease model of AA differs somewhat from that espoused by the medical community. The disease model as emphasized by AA stresses the importance of spirituality in the etiology of, and recovery from, alcoholism. Indeed, many AA members report that they are recovering from a "spiritual disease." Though many outsiders to AA consider "spiritual disease" an oxymoron (i.e., a figure of speech that is a contradiction in terms), many recovering persons feel that it accurately describes their drinking problems. AA encourages its members to find a "Higher Power" and to turn their will and life over to a supernatural being. These spiritual conversions are considered crucial to recovery.

In contrast, the medical community tends to point to the significance of biological factors in alcoholism. Physicians often emphasize the role of genetic susceptibilities, increasing tolerance, withdrawal symptoms, liver disease, brain abnormalities, and so forth. Of course, this biomedical approach is consistent with their training. It is not that they ignore spiritual elements; rather, they tend to give such factors less weight than, for example, laboratory test results.

There is another difference between the disease model of AA and that of the medical community. It is a subtle difference, and it is closely related to the dichotomy of spirituality versus science. In AA, members often use the disease concept in a metaphoric sense; that is, they describe their alcohol problems as being "like" a disease. In many cases, recovering individuals do not intend (or perhaps even care) to convey that they literally have a disease. They simply are attempting to express that the experience of compulsive chemical use feels like having a disease. It is characterized by feelings of loss of control and hopelessness, conditions familiar to the victims of other diseases (cancer, heart disease, emphysema, etc.).

Most often, physicians do not use the term "disease" as a metaphor. They tend to use the term in a literal sense—that is, "Alcoholism *is* disease." Consider the following statement by a physician who directed a chemical dependency rehabilitation program:

> Whether you become an alcoholic or not depends on genetic predisposition. We know the reason the compulsivity exists is because of a change in the endorphin and cephalin systems in a primitive portion of the brain. The reason for this disturbance in the biochemistry of the primitive brain is a predisposition. Nobody talks any longer about becoming an alcoholic. You don't become an alcoholic—you are born an alcoholic. (Talbott, 1989, p. 57)

As this discussion illustrates, the disease models are not a unitary framework for understanding addiction. However, despite nuances and ambiguities, certain concepts exist that have traditionally represented the disease model of addiction. Let us examine these concepts in light of the current scientific literature.

TOLERANCE AND WITHDRAWAL

The two clinical features of substance dependence or addiction that are commonly viewed as disease symptoms are tolerance and withdrawal. Drug tolerance is the need to use increasingly greater amounts of a substance to obtain the desired effect. With regular use, tolerance develops to most of the commonly abused psychoactive drugs, including alcohol, cocaine, heroin, LSD, and so on. Though some substance users may initially take pride in their ability to consume large amounts of a drug, increasing tolerance is regarded as an early symptom of dependence (Milam & Ketcham, 1983).

Acute drug withdrawal results when blood or body tissue concentrations of a substance decline following a period of prolonged heavy use (American Psychiatric Association, 2000). The duration, symptoms, and severity of withdrawal vary across drugs and according to the amount of the substance being consumed prior to cessation. Alcohol withdrawal, in particular, varies significantly in both its symptoms and severity (Saitz, 1998). Clinical manifestations in alcohol withdrawal can range from insomnia to severe conditions such as delirium tremens (DTs) and possibly even death.

Prolonged use of most psychoactive drugs can produce a withdrawal syndrome. These include opiates, heroin, barbiturates, cocaine, and a variety of other substances. The exceptions are several of the commonly abused hallucinogens (LSD, psilocybin, mescaline). The unpleasant symptoms of withdrawal provide motivation for the person to self-administer more of the drug to relieve or even to avoid discomfort.

It is important to note that the contemporary view of drug dependence does not require the presence of either tolerance or withdrawal. According to the diagnostic criteria that appear in the current *Diagnostic and Statistical Manual of Mental Disorders* (DSM-IV-TR), there are seven major symptoms of "substance dependence" (American Psychiatric Association, 2000). As can be seen in Table 2.1, the presence of any three symptoms justifies the dependence diagnosis.

ADDICTION AS A PRIMARY DISEASE

Addiction, especially alcoholism, is often described as a "primary disease"; that is, it is not the result of another condition. This is usually taken to mean that the disease is not caused by heavy drinking or drug use, stress, or psychiatric disorders; rather, it is thought to be the cause of these very conditions. In other words, heavy drinking/drug use, stress, psychiatric disorders, and so forth are secondary symptoms or manifestations of an underlying disease process known as addiction. If the drinking or drug use is stopped, it is believed that the symptoms will, for the most part, disappear (Milam & Ketcham, 1983; Talbott, 1989).

This is contrary to popular conceptions of addiction, especially alcoholism. To take alcoholism as an example, many laypeople (even those who view alcoholism as a disease) feel that alcoholism results from abusive drinking, which in turn stems from irresponsibility, stress, or emotional problems. The disease models, properly understood, dispute these ideas (Milam & Ketcham, 1983). The models propose that alcoholics are not responsible for contracting their disease; the disease itself causes or drives the heavy drinking. Furthermore, it is maintained that those drinkers who

TABLE 2.1. DSM-IV-TR Criteria for Substance Dependence

A maladaptive pattern of substance use, leading to clinically significant impairment or distress, as manifested by three (or more) of the following, occurring at any time in the same 12-month period:

(1) tolerance, as defined by either of the following:
   (a) a need for markedly increased amounts of the substance to achieve intoxication or desired effect
   (b) markedly diminished effect with continued use of the same amount of the substance
(2) withdrawal, as manifested by either of the following:
   (a) the characteristic withdrawal syndrome for the substance
   (b) the same (or closely related) substance is taken to relieve or avoid withdrawal symptoms
(3) the substance is often taken in larger amounts or over a longer period than was intended
(4) there is a persistent desire or unsuccessful efforts to cut down or control substance use
(5) a great deal of time is spent in activities necessary to obtain the substance (e.g., visiting multiple doctors or driving long distances), use the substance (e.g., chain-smoking), or recover from its effects
(6) important social, occupational, or recreational activities are given up or reduced because of substance use
(7) the substance use is continued despite knowledge of having a persistent or recurrent physical or psychological problem that is likely to have been caused or exacerbated by the substance (e.g., current cocaine use despite recognition of cocaine-induced depression, or continued drinking despite recognition that an ulcer was made worse by alcohol consumption)

Specify if:
   With Physiological Dependence: evidence of tolerance or withdrawal (i.e., either Item 1 or 2 is present)
   Without Physiological Dependence: no evidence or tolerance or withdrawal (i.e., neither Item 1 nor 2 is present)

Note. From American Psychiatric Association (2000). Copyright 2000 by the American Psychiatric Association. Reprinted by permission.

lack genetic susceptibility to the disease cannot drink themselves into alcoholism (Milam & Ketcham, 1983).

However, various lines of research have developed data that contradict the primary-disease concept for all alcoholics. For example, researchers note that there may be multiple types of alcoholism (National Institute on Alcohol Abuse and Alcoholism [NIAAA], 1990). Some forms may be more sensitive to genetic factors, while others are influenced by environmental conditions (Cloninger, 1987). Environmental factors (stress, marital and family problems, depression, anxiety, etc.) may cause some forms of alcoholism. Schuckit (1989) has reported that a proportion of alcoholics "fulfill criteria for a clearly preexisting antisocial personality disorder (ASPD)"

(p. 2). This suggests that severe antisocial life problems may cause alcoholism in some. Cox (1985) has noted that certain psychological traits predispose individuals to substance abuse in general:

> Specifically, future substance abusers are characterized by disregard for social mores, independence, impulsivity, and affinity for adventure. These are enduring personality characteristics that appear to be biologically mediated (Eysenck, 1981; Zuckerman, 1983). Persons exhibiting these personality characteristics are able to satisfy their psychological needs through substance use, and they appear to be especially susceptible to environmental influences promoting substance use. (p. 233)

This passage cogently describes how genetics and environment interact to promote alcohol and drug abuse. It also suggests that a "sensation-seeking" alcoholic personality will not disappear on cessation of alcohol use. Successful recovery may often depend on the alcoholic's finding alternative (i.e., nonchemical) ways to fulfill psychological needs for excitement and risk taking.

Findings such as these suggest that the causes of alcoholism (and probably other addictions as well) are multiple and mediated by both genetic and environmental factors. For each alcoholic, there is probably a relatively unique combination of forces that led to the development of his or her drinking problem. Some cases may be strongly influenced by genetic factors; others may be mediated solely by environmental ones. In the future, the concept of "primary" alcoholism is likely to be further restricted as various types of the disorder continue to be identified and its comorbidity with other psychiatric disorders is recognized to be a common phenomenon (see Chapter 4).

GENETIC ORIGINS OF ADDICTION:
THE SUSCEPTIBILITY MODEL

There is compelling evidence of the familial transmission of substance use disorders (e.g., Bierut et al., 1998; Merikangas et al., 1998). This familial transmission is thought to occur via both genetic and psychosocial pathways. The genetic factors may involve individual differences in drug metabolism, tolerance, sensitivity, and/or side effects (Merikangas et al., 1998). The accompanying psychosocial (or environmental) pathways are numerous and may include inadequate parental monitoring and supervision, child–parent modeling processes, marital discord, family stress, child abuse, and so on (Patterson, 1996). Thus, the clustering of substance use in families is determined by the confluence of genetic and environmental variables.

As noted in Chapter 1, the idea that alcoholism, in particular, has genetic origins can be traced back to 19th century (Levine, 1978). More recently, scientists also have examined the role of genetic influence on other drugs of abuse. Interest in the general field of behavioral genetics has grown for three reasons (Mann, 1994). First, there is a large body of research showing hereditary influence on animal behavior. Second, the methodologically sound twin studies conducted since the 1980s have consistently found that genes contribute to the development of complex disorders, such as alcoholism. Third, and perhaps of greatest importance, there is an increasing awareness that genes and the environment *jointly* determine human behavior—particularly addictive behavior.

Genotype and Phenotype

The study of genetics deals with characteristics that are transmitted from parents to their offspring via biological mechanisms. These characteristics are not acquired as a result of learning, modeling, socialization, or other postnatal experiences; they are hereditary or inborn. Such human characteristics as eye color and blood type are determined by genetic factors.

"Genes" are the basic structural units of heredity. Each person shares 50% of the genes of each parent in a unique arrangement that is different from both parents. This assemblage of genes is the person's "genotype." During both pre- and postnatal development, the individual is exposed to a variety of environmental influences. This interaction between genotype and environment generates an enormous number of individual traits and characteristics, which are referred to as the person's "phenotype." The phenotype, then, is the outcome of the interaction between genes and environment. It should be noted that fetal exposure to alcohol or other drugs is an environmental influence on the phenotype; fetal alcohol syndrome and related conditions among newborns are not genetic disorders.

During the last 15 years, advances made in the field of behavioral genetics have generated evidence to support claims that heredity plays a role in a wide range of human behavior. The popular press sometimes distorts these findings with superficial reports describing an "intelligence gene" and a "violence gene" (Mann, 1994). Too often, the magnitude of the genetic influence is exaggerated or relevant environmental factors are unduly minimized, often as a result of ignorance about the interactive nature of each. This lack of understanding also has fueled the mistaken belief in "genetic determinism." Clearly, for complex human traits, genes are not destiny but parameters of risk as well as protection. According to Kenneth Kendler, a behavioral genetics researcher, "genes and environment loop out into each other and feed back on each other in a complex way that we have just begun to understand" (Mann, 1994, p. 1687). The important point is that genes operate in a probabilistic manner in addictive behavior (Goldman & Bergen, 1998). They are not deterministic factors.

Researchers acknowledge that genetic factors play a role in the development of the substance use disorders. However, today considerable disagreement remains about the relative contribution of "nature" and "nuture" (Walters, 2002). Lester (1988), Searles (1988), and others have been highly critical of heritability measures that genetic researchers use to claim, for instance, that a trait is "60% inherited." According to Lester (1988), "For concepts like intelligence, or schizophrenia, or alcoholism, there is no evidence that simple relationships exist; indeed, there is every reason to believe that the highest levels of organismic function are involved, embracing the most complex developing and evolving relationships of humans as social beings" (p. 2). Yet, heritability measures are typically based on the assumption that the relationship between inherited characteristics and environmental variables is additive—when it is not. These two sets of influence are most likely reciprocal or interactive in influencing addiction. In a related point, Searles (1988) notes that a serious flaw in the genetic research on the addictions is the inadequate measurement of environmental variables. He states: "What is termed 'environment' in most studies is usually not the complex, multifaceted construct that the word implies. It often is simply what is left after genetic factors are removed, or it reflects overly broad influences of crudely measured variables" (p. 164).

In a meta-analysis of 50 family, twin, and adoption studies, Walters (2002) concluded that the genetic foundations of problem drinking and alcoholism are "modest and heterogeneous" (p. 557). In contrast to estimates from single studies often reported in the research literature, Walters (2002) found that overall the heritability of alcohol misuse was in the range of only 20–26%. In studies restricted to males with severe forms of alcohol dependence, he found that heritability was somewhat higher (30–36%) but still below levels commonly reported in some individual studies. Given the inadequacy of current research methods to accurately assess "nature versus nurture," and varying ways to interpret genetic data, we should view as tentative those findings that assign values to the respective contributions of genetic factors and the environment. The following discussion reviews some of what is known about the roles of genetics and the environment in shaping alcohol and drug dependence.

Twin Studies

Before findings from twin studies are examined, let us examine the logic, design, and limitations of a twin study. There are two types of twins: "monozygotic" (MZ) and "dizygotic" (DZ). MZ twins develop from a single ovum and sperm, whereas DZ twins develop from separate ova and sperm. MZ twins share identical genotypes; however, DZ twins share only one-half of their genes. MZ twins are usually referred to as "identical" twins, whereas DZ twins are often known as "fraternal" twins. Of course, MZ twins are always of the same gender. DZ twins may be of different genders, and are no more alike (in terms of genetic makeup) than any two siblings.

In twin studies, concordance rates are determined for a specific characteristic or trait. A "concordance rate" is the degree of similarity between the twins in each pair in a series on any given characteristic. The greater concordance between MZ twins, as compared to DZ twins, is taken as evidence of the degree of genetic determination for a characteristic. Stated in another way, the concordance rate of the DZ twins serves as a baseline representing environmental input on a characteristic. The greater the degree to which the MZ twins' concordance rate exceeds that of the DZ twins, the greater the role heredity plays in determining that characteristic.

Lester (1988) points out that twin studies are based on a set of assumptions. Though these problems do not discredit well-designed twin studies, we should be aware that the following problems may exist:

1. Twin studies assume that mating of the parents is random or "non-assortative." More specifically, it is assumed that the selection of a mate is not influenced by drinking or drug use habits.
2. [It is assumed that] no dominance or other genetic effects are involved in the particular disorder (alcohol or other drug use).
3. The within-pair environmental variance is the same in DZ twins as in MZ twins. That is, the post-natal experience of the identical twin pairs is roughly equivalent to that of fraternal twins. It is assumed that fraternal twins have the same degree of social contact with each other as do identical twins. (p. 6)

The first assumption involving random mating is particularly problematic and could lead to inflated estimates of the genetic contribution to alcoholism or other drug dependencies. In regard to the third assumption, recent twin studies have used statistical controls to adjust for MZ/DZ differences in social environment.

Findings from Alcohol-Specific Twin Studies

Twin studies conducted since the late 1980s have established that both environmental and genetic factors play a role in the development of alcoholism. Kaprio et al. (1987) conducted a twin study involving 2,800 male pairs from Finland. The subjects responded to a questionnaire that assessed quantity and frequency of drinking, density of drinking (i.e., regularity of drinking at particular times, such as weekends), frequency of passing out from drinking, and frequency of social contact between twins (including cohabitation). Kaprio et al. (1987) found that (1) identical twins had more social contact with each other (as adults) than did fraternal twins, (2) frequent social contact between twins was significantly correlated with concordance rates in drinking patterns, (3) the concordance rate among the identical twins was somewhat higher than that for the fraternal twins, and (4) the higher concordance rate among the identical twins was explained by both social contact (an environmental factor) and genetic variables. Kaprio et al. (1987) estimated that for measures of quantity, frequency, and density of drinking, "environment" accounted for 60–64% of the variance in these three variables. Frequency of drinking to unconsciousness was completely explained by environmental factors.

Insight into how genetic and environmental factors interact has emerged from a twin study conducted by Heath, Jardine, and Martin (1989). This is one of the few studies that relied on female twins. The sample was obtained through the Australian National Twin Register; it consisted of 1,200 identical twin pairs and 750 fraternal twin pairs (all twins were female). The most important finding of this study was that marital status was a major modifier of genetically influenced drinking patterns. Among both younger and older adult women, being married (or living with a man but not actually being married) suppressed the emergence of genetically influenced drinking patterns. Women who were not married (or not in a similar relationship) tended to drink more heavily (Heath et al., 1989). This supports the notion that both environment and genetics are important, and that they interact in a variety of complex ways to spur the development of alcoholism. In other words, genetics sets the stage for vulnerability to later environmental influences.

Further support for the interactive influence of both genetics and environment comes from a twin study conducted by McGue, Pickens, and Svikis (1992). The investigation located co-twins of probands (i.e., patients) from alcohol and drug abuse treatment programs in Minnesota. About 57% of the same-sex twin pairs had their zygosity (MZ vs. DZ status) determined by blood test, whereas the remainder were determined by self-report questionnaire administered to both the probands and their co-twins. Approximately 8% of the pairs were eliminated from the data analyses because the questionnaire method could not confirm their zygosity. The sample of twin pairs was then broken down by gender and age of first symptom of alcoholism. Within each gender, "early-onset" twin pairs were identified as those in whom the probands reported a symptom of alcoholism prior to the age of 20. Otherwise, the pairs were classified as "late onset" (McGue et al., 1992).

As shown in Table 2.2, 0.725 (or 73%) of the variance in alcoholism among the male early-onset twin pairs could be accounted for by genetic factors. This compared to about 30% of the variance in the male late-onset pairs, and to about 54% of the variance among the total number of male twin pairs. In contrast, the data provided no evidence of genetic influence in female alcoholism for either age group (McGue et al., 1992). These data suggest that genetic factors play a strong role in male alcoholism that appears prior to the age of 20. Genetic variables seem to have only a moderate influence on male alcoholism that begins later in life, and inheritance may play no role in the development of female alcoholism (McGue et al., 1992).

Areas of scientific inquiry that are in formative stages, such as the role of genetics in alcoholism, often include investigations that yield inconsistent or contradictory results. Another twin study from the same year is a case in point. Directly contradicting the work of McGue et al. (1992), an investigation by Kendler, Heath, Neale, Kessler, and Eaves (1992) found evidence supporting a genetic basis for female alcoholism. In this study, data analyses used 1,030 female–female twin pairs of known zygosity from the Virginia Twin Registry. The data were collected from structured psychiatric interviews. The interviewer was "blinded" as to the psychopathological status of each co-twin.

The feature of this study that distinguishes it from the McGue et al. (1992) study is that it did not use a co-twin's admission to an alcoholism treatment facility as the basis for selecting the twin pair for the study. The

TABLE 2.2. Sex and Age Effects on the Inheritance of Alcohol Problems: A Twin Study

| | Monozygotic | | Dizygotic | | Proportion of variance | | |
Group	Number of pairs	Concordance rate	Number of pairs	Concordance rate	Genetic	Shared environmental	Unshared environmental
			Males				
Early onset	52	.865	44	.568	.725	.232	.043
Late onset	33	.606	52	.509	.295	.372	.333
Total	85	.765	96	.536	.543	.331	.126
			Females				
Early onset	20	.500	22	.500	.000	.732	.268
Late onset	24	.292	21	.333	.000	.525	.475
Total	44	.386	43	.419	.000	.635	.367

Note. Adapted from McGue, Pickens, and Svikis (1992). Copyright 1992 by the American Psychological Association. Adapted by permission.

Kendler et al. (1992) study was a population-based study in which twin pairs were identified through a registry. The proportion of the twins who had received treatment for a drinking problem was not reported.

Kendler et al. (1992) used four different definitions of alcoholism. They found that genetics accounts for 50–60% of the variance in female alcoholism. However, these estimates assumed that the environmental experiences of the MZ and DZ twins were equal. When this factor was controlled for, the heritability of liability to alcoholism in women was in the range of 40–50% (Kendler et al., 1992).

Why are the findings of McGue et al. (1992) and Kendler et al. (1992) so contradictory with respect to the role of genetics in female alcoholism? The authors of the second study state it best: "One plausible hypothesis is that the genetic loading for alcoholism in the modest proportion of women who seek treatment may not be typical of that found in the entire population of women with alcoholism. It is possible, for example, that patients seen in treatment settings may have been particularly influenced by social or environmental factors" (Kendler et al., 1992, p. 1881). Thus, it is entirely possible that studies conducted to date have been limited by small nonrepresentative samples of women. In a review of this literature, Prescott (2002) suggests that women and men may be at approximately the same genetic risk for alcoholism. Further research is needed before firm conclusions can be reached about sex differences in the etiology of alcoholism.

Twin Studies of Other Drug Use

Initial twin study research reported that there were modest genetic influences on cigarette smoking (Carmelli, Swan, Robinette, & Fabsitz, 1992) and illicit drug use in general (Jang, Livesley, & Vernon, 1995). These findings were then replicated in a more rigorous investigation conducted by Tsuang et al. (1998). The investigators studied 3,373 male twin pairs from the Vietnam Era Twin Registry. The population-based sample represented 65% of the pairs in the registry. In addition to finding that the use of different drugs tend to co-occur in individuals, Tsuang et al. (1998) developed statistical models indicating the presence of a latent or an underlying *vulnerability* to substance abuse. This vulnerability was influenced jointly by (1) genetic factors, (2) family environmental factors, and (3) nonfamily environmental factors. The respective contributions of each of these three factors varied by drug of abuse. Table 2.3 shows these additive influences.

The data from the Tsuang et al. (1998) study suggest that genetic factors play the greatest role in heroin abuse. Marijuana abuse appears to be influenced substantially by all three sources of influence. In contrast, nonfamily environmental variables appear to be the predominant influ-

TABLE 2.3. Additive Influences of Genetic, Family Environmental, and Nonfamily Environmental Factors on Substance Abuse

Drug	Genetic influence	Family environmental	Nonfamily environmental
Heroin	54%	13%	33%
Marijuana	33%	29%	38%
Stimulants	33%	19%	48%
Sedatives	27%	17%	56%
Psychedelics	26%	21%	53%

Note. Data from Tsuang et al. (1998).

ences on stimulants, sedatives, and psychedelics. The reader should note that these estimates of additive influence were based on data collected from males only and that for particular individuals the contribution of genotype and environment will vary (Goldman & Bergen, 1998). Nevertheless, the data are evidence that a genetic susceptibility to drug abuse exists.

Genetic Regulation of Nicotine Metabolism

Research also has identified genes that influence smoking initiation, nicotine dependence, and smoking cessation. Pianezza, Sellers, and Tyndale (1998) found that individuals who lack a genetically variable enzyme known as CYP2A6 have impaired nicotine metabolism. Persons with the CYP2A6 deficiency smoked significantly fewer cigarettes than did those with normal metabolism. As a result, these individuals appear to be somewhat "protected" from developing tobacco dependence (Pianezza et al., 1998).

Other studies have examined the relationship between smoking and dopamine regulation. In a case control study of 289 smokers and 233 nonsmoking controls, Lerman et al. (1999) found that individuals with a specific genotype known as SLC6A3-9 were significantly less likely to be smokers. Sabol et al. (1999) extended the findings of Lerman et al. (1999) by discovering that the effect of SLC6A3-9 was on smoking cessation rather than on smoking inititation. Sabol et al. (1999) also found that the SLC6A3-9 gentotype was correlated with low scores on the personality trait known as novelty seeking. The correlation suggests that individuals carrying the SLC6A3-9 sequence have altered dopamine transmission and thereby less need for reward from external stimuli, including that provided by cigarettes. Although these findings await replication, the relationship between SLC6A3-9, novelty seeking, and tobacco use may represent a possible mechanism by which genotype exerts influence on smoking behavior.

Alcohol Metabolism: The Genetic Regulation of Liver Enzymes

A variety of processes are involved in the metabolism of drugs. These processes break down or inactivate drugs so that they can be eliminated from the body. For some time, researchers have been interested in alcohol metabolism because of speculation that alcoholics may suffer from an inherited "error in metabolism." Indeed, research has demonstrated that genetic factors are involved in the metabolism of alcohol (Li, 2000), and there is ethnic variation in the liver enzymes that break down alcohol (NIAAA, 2003). This section provides an overview of work in this area.

Alcohol is absorbed from the stomach and the small intestine into the circulatory system and transported to the liver for metabolism. The first step in alcohol metabolism involves the conversion of alcohol to acetaldehyde by a liver enzyme known as alcohol dehydrogenase or "ADH" (see Figure 2.1). Acetaldehyde, in turn, is converted to acetic acid by another liver enzyme: aldehyde dehydrogenase (ALDH). Acetic acid is metabolized further into carbon dioxide and water, which is eliminated from the body (NIAAA, 1994).

In the 1970s, medical researchers began publishing studies purporting to show that alcoholics and relatives of alcoholics tend to metabolize (i.e., to break down) alcohol in abnormal ways. In most of these studies, the alcohol metabolite of concern was acetaldehyde. Acetaldehyde is a rather toxic breakdown product; it was postulated to be responsible for the increasing tolerance and physical dependency that are sometimes part of alcoholism. Some studies that measured blood levels of acetaldehyde found higher levels in alcoholics and relatives of alcoholics than in individuals with no positive family history of alcoholism (Schuckit, 1984). However, as

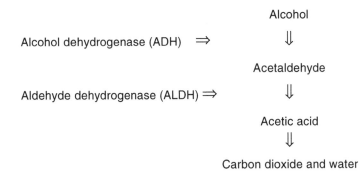

Alcohol dehydrogenase (ADH)   ⇒

Alcohol
⇓
Acetaldehyde

Aldehyde dehydrogenase (ALDH) ⇒

⇓
Acetic acid
⇓
Carbon dioxide and water

FIGURE 2.1. Metabolism of alcohol via the ADH pathway. From National Institute on Alcohol Abuse and Alcoholism (1994).

the NIAAA has observed, the hypothesis that acetaldehyde is a genetic marker for alcoholism predisposition is not well supported by evidence. In 1987, the NIAAA concluded:

> On balance, these studies suggest a probable increase in acetaldehyde in alco-
> holics, but the measurement of acetaldehyde in biological fluids is fraught with
> technical difficulties and is subject to significant errors. In any case, the posi-
> tive studies provide no information as to whether this tendency is antecedent
> to the development of alcoholism or is a consequence of it. (p. 36)

This highlights two serious problems with this line of research—that is, measurement of acetaldehyde in body fluids and uncertainty about whether acetaldehyde is a cause or a consequence of years of heavy drinking. For a technical review of the problems with these studies, readers should see Lester (1988).

Another set of studies has examined alcohol elimination in certain eth-nic groups (e.g., Japanese and Native Americans), (Okada & Mizoi, 1982; Tsukamoto, Sudo, Karasawa, Kajiwara, & Endo, 1982). The hypothesis here is that rates of alcoholism among an ethnic group are determined by an inborn reaction to ethanol, called a "flushing response." Members of some groups tend to flush (reddening of the face, warm sensations, dizzi-ness) when they drink because they are relatively deficient in ALDH. As a result of this deficiency, acetaldehyde is metabolized more slowly, allowing the toxic substance to accumulate in body fluids (and cause flushing).

Here, the hypothesis becomes contradictory, or at the very least it branches into two inconsistent ones. One hypothesis is that ethnic groups that eliminate alcohol slowly and tend to flush (e.g., East Asians) will have lower rates of alcoholism, because the flushing is an aversive consequence that discourages heavy drinking. As a result, members of these groups will not abuse alcohol because of this uncomfortable reaction when ethanol is consumed. However, others put forth the hypothesis that those groups that eliminate alcohol slowly and tend to flush (e.g., Native Americans) will be very susceptible to alcoholism, because the high levels of acetaldehyde cause tolerance to alcohol to increase. Clearly, alcohol elimination cannot be used to explain alcoholism etiology in opposite directions. Schwitters, Johnson, McClearn, and Wilson (1982) comment on these studies: "Once persons drink at all, whether flushing occurs following the use of alcohol has only a trivial effect on drinking behavior" (p. 1262).

Findings from a cross-cultural study of Asian and North American populations support this view. Though East Asian populations have been identified as having an ALDH deficiency, which presumably would protect them from alcoholism, Helzer et al. (1990) found that a Korean sample had the highest rate of alcohol abuse and alcohol dependence among five studied groups. The samples were from St. Louis, Missouri; Taiwan; Puerto Rico; and Canada. About 43% of the Koreans met criteria for alcohol abuse or alcohol dependence. Again, this suggests that social influences that promote abusive drinking can override alcohol metabolism deficits.

It is important to note that these studies ignore important differences among ethnic subgroups. This is particularly true of such ethnic groups as "Asians" (who include Chinese, Japanese, Koreans, Vietnamese, etc.) and "Native Americans" (who come from dozens of different clans), (NIAAA, 1990). For example, Christian, Dufour, and Bertolucci (1989) found that among 11 Native American tribal groups in Oklahoma, the alcohol-related death rate ranged from less than 1% to 24%. Such a finding suggests that abuse of alcohol among Native Americans is much more closely related to the norms and customs of specific tribal groups than it is to possible metabolic abnormalities of genetic origin.

Overall, the research in this area indicates that there is genetic variation in the metabolism of alcohol. However, within the matrix of multiple risk factors, there is considerable uncertainty about how much unique impact these genetic factors might have on the development of alcoholism. More research is needed in this area.

Event-Related Potentials: The P3 Brain Wave Studies

Event-related potentials (ERPs) are brain electrical signals that are generated in response to a specific stimulus, such as a light or a sound (National Institutes of Health, 1998). These electrical signals of the brain provide sensitive measure of cognitive activity. ERPs are measured at the scalp of the head with standard electroencephalography (EEG) technology, and displayed as wave-like lines. They are assessed according to their height (or amplitude) and elapsed time following a stimulus. The P3 (or P300) component of ERP peaks between 300 and 500 milliseconds after a stimulus. P3 amplitude is higher for significant stimuli than for insignificant stimuli.

The brain wave is thought to be associated with information processing, decision making, and memory (Donchin & Coles, 1988). Individuals with low P3 amplitude are thought to have difficulty distinguishing between significant and insignificant stimuli. Research has established that low P3 voltage is found in persons suffering from alcoholism (Cohen, Wang, Porjesj, & Begleiter, 1995), schizophrenia (Ford, White, Lim, & Pfefferbaum, 1994), and attention-deficit disorder (Klorman, Salzman, Pass, Borgstedt, & Dainer, 1979).

Interest in the P3 deficit in alcoholism began in the mid-1980s. In a seminal study, Begleiter, Porjesz, Bihari, and Kissin (1984) reported that in a sample of preadolescent sons of alcoholics who had never themselves consumed alcohol or illicit drugs, the P3 wave amplitude was greatly reduced compared to a control group of similar-age sons of nonalcoholic fathers. This was a remarkable finding because previously it had been assumed that the P3 deficit was a consequence of the deleterious effects of alcohol on the brain (Porjesz & Begleiter, 1985). Instead, it appeared that the P3 deficit may precede the development of alcoholism; that is, it may be a biological marker for susceptibility to the disorder.

During the next few years, several laboratories replicated the findings of Begleiter et al. (1984). One rigorous study found that the amplitude of the P3 wave in abstinent alcoholics was not associated with avoiding alcohol but was significantly related to the number of problem drinkers in their family (Pfefferbaum, Ford, White, & Mathalon, 1991). However, some studies failed to observe the expected differences in P3 wave amplitude between high-risk and low-risk subjects (e.g., Polich & Bloom, 1988). These inconsistencies were addressed in a meta-analysis of the P3 literature, where it was concluded that the expected differences can be observed with the application of difficult visual tasks (Polich, Pollock, & Bloom, 1994). Today, among neurophysiology researchers, there is consensus that reduced P3 wave amplitude is associated with alcoholism susceptibility (NIAAA, 1997).

Begleiter et al. (1998) reported preliminary findings on the "hunt" for the genes associated with P3 wave abnormalities in alcoholism. Genetic analysis of 103 "dense alcoholic" and random control families has revealed a number of candidate genetic loci. The strongest linkages were found on chromosomes 2 and 6, with suggestive evidence on chromosomes 5 and 13 (Begleiter et al., 1998). Each chromosomal region contains several hundred genes that will require high-resolution mapping to determine whether they are actually associated with P3 wave abnormalities.

Collaborative Study on the Genetics of Alcoholism

The $60 million project known as the Collaborative Study on the Genetics of Alcoholism (COGA) is mapping the human DNA sequence (Begleiter et al., 1995). Funded by the NIAAA, this project is a component of the larger Human Genome Project (Collins & Fink, 1995). COGA seeks to identify the specific genes that increase alcoholism susceptibility through one or more channels including neuron communication and alcohol metabolism.

Preliminary COGA findings indicate that alcoholism susceptibility is probably linked to several genes (Reich et al., 1998). In other words, the disorder is likely "polygenic" and not the result of a mutation in a single gene. This may point toward alcoholism subtypes, which may vary with respect to gene–environment contributions. Interestingly, COGA has found that there may be "protective genes" against alcoholism (Reich et al., 1998). Thus, genetic characteristics may decrease, as well as increase an individual's risk for alcoholism.

The Social Impact of Genetic Research

The information and technology gained as a result of the Human Genome Project (and COGA) are expected to have a profound social impact. Stigmatization and discrimination based on hereditary characteristics and other misuses and misinterpretations of genetic information are significant social and public policy concerns (Khoury & Genetics Work Group, 1996). Predictive genetic screening of complex traits, such as alcoholism susceptibility, raises conceptual and philosophical questions about personal responsibility for one's conduct, future reproductive decisions, genetic determinism and one's health, and the definition of "normal" and "abnormal" drinking practices. Furthermore, multiple, and often contradictory, values and belief systems influence public and personal views about the morality of genetic technologies. Therefore, the psychosocial aspects of genetic technology in disease prevention and treatment will require evaluation before testing should be introduced into medical practice (Khoury & Genetics Work Group, 1996).

The translation of genetic technologies into patient care brings with it special concerns about how these tools will be applied, and thus the Human Genome Project has committed research money to study the ethical, legal, and social implications of emerging genetic testing technology (Collins & Fink, 1995). Results of genetic studies can be interpreted in such a way that the causes of disease, disability, and behavioral characteristics (traits) are reduced to the expression of particular genes, thereby excluding the contribution of psychosocial and environmental factors (Croyle & Lerman, 1995). An important and challenging role for health and human services practitioners will be to educate clients and their families about genetic test technology so that they make informed decisions about testing.

In general, relatively little is known about whether at-risk individuals will want to know their risk status based on their personal genetic profile. The process involved in arriving at a decision for or against testing is complex and not well understood at this time. Also, compared to other disorders, utilization of screening for alcoholism susceptibility may have unique features in that persons at highest risk for developing a drinking problem may be those least likely to seek testing (Thombs, Mahoney, & Olds, 1998).

Genetic Risk Summary

There are six essential points that the substance abuse practitioner should understand about the genetics of addictive behavior.

1. *Genes and the environment jointly determine alcohol and drug addictions.* Mann (1994) quotes research scientist Robert Plomin as saying, "Research into heritability is the best demonstration I know of the importance of the environment" (p. 1689).

2. *The inherited characteristic is not a disease but a predisposition or susceptibility.* In other words, addiction is not an inherited disease caused by a variant in a single gene, such as in the cases of cystic fibrosis or Huntington's disease. Rather, addiction is a complex disorder caused by a variety of genetic and environmental variables. Genetic risk factors either increase or decrease risk for developing the disorder. It may be found that some gene mutations actually provide protection against alcoholism and some drug addictions.

3. *Among persons with addiction problems, there is heterogeneity to the contribution of genes and environment that influences individual patterns of substance use.* In the future, it may be discovered that there are subtypes of alcoholism, for example, ranging from those that are largely genetic in origin, on one extreme, to those determined entirely by the environment, on the other end of the spectrum. Alcoholism subtypes also may be based on the presence or absence of antisocial personality traits and age of onset (Anthenelli & Tabakoff, 1995).

4. *Recognizing the role of genetic risk factors does not require that alcoholism and other drug dependencies be defined as disease states.* A wide range of human traits are influenced by genes, including physical endurance (Montgomery et al., 1998) and perceived social support (Kendler, 1997), that by social convention are not considered diseases.

5. *Research on the genetics of addiction is important because it may lead to more effective ways to prevent and treat the problem of addiction.* According to research scientist Xandra Breakefield, "The purpose of behavioral genetics is not to push people into trouble but to pull them out" (Mann, 1994, p. 1687). For example, a genetic test for alcoholism could identify children who are at risk for developing the disorder in the future. Such a test also could be used in the assessment and diagnosis of alcoholic clients and as motivation enhancement for ambivalent clients.

6. *In the future, genetic testing will likely gain acceptance in the general population. Individuals will increasingly need assistance with genetic testing decisions and how to interpret test results.* Individuals may respond differently to positive test results depending on their perceived capability to change their drinking or drug use behaviors. For instance, a positive test

result could exacerbate a person's alcohol problems by inducing a sense of futility and hopelessness. On the other hand, some might interpret a negative test result to mean that they can continue to drink with impunity. Other client responses probably exist as well. At this point, we can only speculate on how the results of a genetic test for susceptibility to alcohol or drug dependence will be used by individuals.

EFFECTS OF DRUGS ON BRAIN STRUCTURE AND FUNCTION: THE EXPOSURE MODEL

Cell Activity of the Brain

Cells of the brain are known as "neurons." Figure 2.2 illustrates the structural features of a presynaptic and postsynaptic neuron. It should be noted that this figure depicts only two neurons and thus is quite simplistic. In the brain, each neuron forms synapses with many other neurons and, in turn, receives synaptic connections from an equally large number of neurons.

The brain's signaling functions are primarily conducted by the neurons of the brain. There are approximately 1 trillion neurons in the brain (NIAAA, 1997). They provide the capacity for sensation, movement, language, thought, and emotion. Though neurons in different parts of the brain vary in size, shape, and electrical properties, most share the common features that appear in Figure 2.2. The cell body containing the nucleus

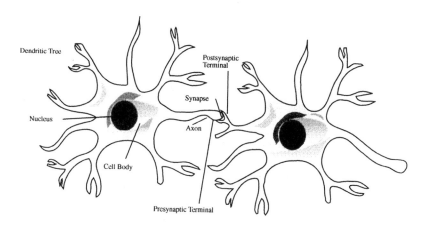

FIGURE 2.2. Structural features of a presynaptic and postsynaptic neuron. This schematic drawing depicts the major components of neuronal structure, including the cell body, nucleus, dendritic trees, and synaptic connections. From National Institute on Alcohol Abuse and Alcoholism (1997).

holds the cell's genetic information. Dendrites are the tree-like projections that integrate information from other neurons. Many neurons have a single axon that conducts electrical signals away from the cell body. At the end of each axon, branches terminate at a microscopic gap known as the synapse. Thus, neurons do not physically connect with one another but are separated by a very small fluid-filled gap (see Figure 2.3).

The presynaptic axon terminals release brain chemicals, known as neurotransmitters, into the synapse in response to electrical stimuli. There are homeostatic mechanisms in operation that attempt to maintain the appropriate concentration or balance of neurotransmitter in the synapse. One mechanism involves the action of enzymes that break down available neurotransmitters. (Enzymes are specialized proteins that serve as a catalyst

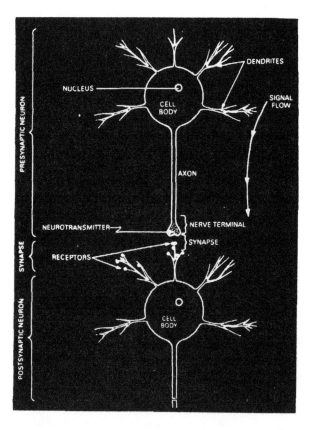

FIGURE 2.3. Typical nerve cell. Provided by Dr. Boris Tabakoff. From National Institute on Alcohol Abuse and Alcoholism (1997).

for a specific chemical reaction.) When the concentration of a neurotransmitter becomes too great, enzymatic activity in the synapse increases to reduce it. A second mechanism is known as "reuptake." Here, presynaptic "pumps" draw neurotransmitter molecules back into the presynaptic terminal. This reabsorption process intensifies when the concentration of neurotransmitter in the synapse becomes too great. In tandem, the processes of enzymatic activity and reuptake work to maintain optimal neurotransmitter concentration. (Some of the ways that drugs of abuse alter normal brain chemistry are described later.)

Postsynaptic dendritic terminals (see Figure 2.3) receive and respond to the particular neurotransmitter they are designed to operate. At the postsynaptic terminals, there are target areas for the neurotransmitter molecule. These target areas are known as "receptor sites" or just "receptors." Typically, each neurotransmitter has an affinity for a specific type of receptor, and their relationship has often been described as akin to that of a key (the neurotransmitter) to its lock (the receptor). In some cases, a receptor may recognize more than one chemical. Nevertheless, the design of the receptor is such that it usually responds only to the specific molecular structure of its neurotransmitter. The postsynaptic terminals respond to the presence of a neurotransmitter by sending an electrical signal toward its cell body. In this way, the neurons relay information to one another in a rapid manner.

Mesolimbic Dopamine Pathway: The Brain's Reward Center

One characteristic that all commonly abused drugs share is their ability to stimulate reward centers in the brain. Many drugs stimulate a chemical circuit in the brain known as the mesolimbic dopamine pathway (Gardner, 1992). This pathway is a system of neurons that operates primarily on dopamine and extends through several regions of the brain. Other chemical pathways, using serotonin and glutamate, also are implicated in the reinforcing effects of particular drugs, but these are not reviewed here in an extensive manner.

As can be seen in Figure 2.4, the mesolimbic system consists of the medial forebrain bundle, the ventral tegmental area, and the nucleus accumbens, with projections to the limbic system and the frontal cortex (Julien, 1998). The medial forebrain bundle, sometimes known as the brain's "seat of pleasure," links the ventral tegmental area with the nucleus accumbens. When activated by drugs, the medial forebrain bundle scatters impulses to a number of reward centers throughout the mesolimbic system (Palfai & Jankiewicz, 1997). Of particular importance is the nucleus accumbens; when stimulated, it provides pleasure and thus serves as a strong reinforcer. Humans and animals will repeat any behavior that

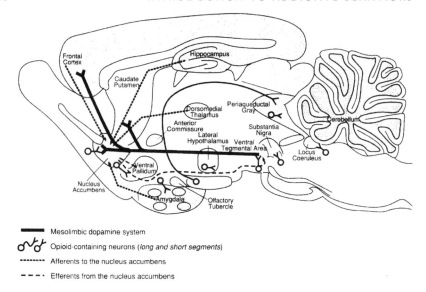

Mesolimbic dopamine system

Opioid-containing neurons (*long and short segments*)

Afferents to the nucleus accumbens

Efferents from the nucleus accumbens

FIGURE 2.4. Section of the rat brain illustrating several neurochemical systems prominently implicated in the rewarding and dependence-inducing effects of alcohol and other drugs of abuse. Adapted from Koob (1992) by National Institute on Alcohol Abuse and Alcoholism (1997). Copyright 1992 by Elsevier Science Ltd. Adapted by permission.

evokes stimulation from this part of the brain, even if it requires a great deal of effort.

Drugs stimulate the reward centers of the mesolimbic system by rapidly intensifying the actions of the neurotransmitter knoiwn as dopamine (Koob, 1992). High levels of dopamine make the mesolimbic reward pathway more sensitive, whereas low levels decrease its sensitivity. These changes in the mesolimbic system may be the neurobiological basis for "wanting," but not necessarily "liking," the effects of a drug (White, 1998).

Drugs of abuse alter the cellular activity of neurons that use dopamine and other neurotransmitters. For instance, cocaine blocks the "reuptake" or reabsorption of dopamine by the neurons (brain cells) that release it (Leshner, 1996). This reduction in neuronal reuptake of dopamine increases the neurotransmitter's concentration in the extracellular spaces known as "synapses." When dopamine levels are elevated, activation of the reward pathway occurs, thereby reinforcing the behavior associated with it (e.g., smoking crack cocaine). It is interesting to note that even nondrug behaviors, such as playing video games, stimulate dopaminergic neurotransmission (Koepp et al., 1998). Though it is not clear that this is the basis for "nondrug addictions," such as gambling, advances in neuroscience will continue to encourage such speculation.

Recent rat research suggests that serotonin, another neurotransmitter, also may be implicated in cocaine's activation of the mesolimbic system. The absence of a particular type of serotonin receptor—1B—appears to potentiate the rewarding effects of cocaine (Rocha et al., 1998). Rats without serotonin-1B receptors were found to be much more willing than control rats to "work" for cocaine. The lack of modulation from this serotonin receptor subtype may increase stimulation of the mesolimbic dopamine system. Thus, serotonin may play a role in susceptibility to cocaine addiction. This discovery may eventually lead to a clearer understanding of the individual variation in cocaine abuse and dependence.

Other stimulants, such as amphetamine, cause an excessive release or "leaking" of dopamine into the synapse. The increased concentration sensitizes the mesolimbic system. The presence of nicotine in the brain prompts a series of chemical changes that somewhat elevate dopamine levels by slowing the breakdown of its molecules in the synapse. However, it is known from animal research that nicotine is less effective as a positive reinforcer than other commonly abused drugs (Risner & Goldberg, 1983). It appears that nicotine dependence is motivated more by negative reinforcement (relief from withdrawal) than by stimulation of reward pathways. Epping-Jordan, Watkins, Koob, and Markou (1998) found that the decrease in brain reward function during nicotine withdrawal is "comparable in magnitude and duration to that of other major drugs of abuse" (p. 76).

Other commonly abused drugs initiate their action on the mesolimbic system through a "second stage" of dopamine neurons found in the ventral tegmental area (Julien, 1998). Opiates, such as heroin and morphine, act on an endogenous opioid circuitry that loops into the mesolimbic pathway. Alcohol was demonstrated to activate this reward pathway as well (Ingvar et al., 1998). Alcohol also stimulates release of glutamate, an excitatory neurotransmitter, and some opiate receptors. Furthermore, alcohol, barbiturates, and the benzodiazepine tranquilizers increase the release of gamma-aminobutyric acid (GABA), an inhibitory neurotransmitter found in many areas of the brain. The $GABA_A$ subtype of receptors is thought to contribute to the depressant effects of alcohol (NIAAA, 1997).

The biological purpose of the mesolimbic system probably is to mediate reward and pleasure and to create motivation to engage in life-sustaining tasks (e.g., eating and reproduction). However, it should be noted that motivation has both cognitive and emotional dimensions. Cognitive expectations in the form of anticipated reinforcement arise from previous life experiences and influence motivation. It is likely not an accident that our expectations of future events are formed in the prefrontal cortex, which is linked to the nucleus accumbens. Previous drug "highs" may be preserved as memories, and they may motivate the user to engage in repeated self-administration of a euphoric substance. Furthermore, as this region of the brain becomes increasingly exposed to excess dopamine during a period of substance abuse, its natural production may decline, resulting in fewer and less sensitive receptors for the neurotransmitter. This is one mechanism for the development of drug tolerance.

As a result of these changes to the brain, the addicted person gradually relies more and more on the drug as the source of gratification and pleasure. In this process, addicts tend to develop the perception that they have an inability to regulate their desire for the drug (i.e., perceived loss of control). As interest in nondrug activities diminishes, involvement in drug-related behaviors increases. Drug seeking, intoxication, and recovering from the deleterious effects (e.g., hangover) typically become the central activities in the addict's life.

LOSS OF CONTROL

Loss of control is a central premise of the traditional disease model of alcoholism. Indeed, Step One of AA's "Twelve Steps" is an admission that alcoholics are "powerless over alcohol" (AA, 1981). It is asserted that the alcoholic's loss of control stems from some unknown defect or abnormality. This abnormality is described as a compulsion or an intense craving (Milkman & Sunderwirth, 1987). More rigorous examinations of drug urges and cravings have been conducted in cognitive psychology (e.g., Tiffany, 1990) and these appear in Chapter 7.

In the traditional disease model, the exact nature of the abnormal craving for alcohol is not claimed to be well understood, but the "Big Book" of AA teaches as follows: "We are equally positive that once he takes any alcohol whatever into his system, something happens, both in the bodily and mental sense, which makes it virtually impossible for him to stop. The experience of any alcoholic will abundantly confirm this" (AA, 1976, pp. 22–23). As this passage indicates, the notion of loss of control is consistent with the subjective experience of many alcoholics. Why, then, do so many of the leading alcoholism researchers reject the concept?

Logical Inconsistency

Fingarette (1988), a philosopher, has pointed out that the classical loss-of-control concept is illogical. It maintains that after a minimal amount of alcohol enters the body, all ability to control drinking disappears. If this were actually the case, an alcoholic would have no desire, cravings, or compulsion to drink when sober. Abstention from drinking and recovery from alcoholism would actually by quite easy. Fingarette (1988) observes:

> If the loss of control is triggered by the first drink, then the only hope for an alcoholic is to refrain from that first drink, that is, total abstention. But if loss of control is triggered only after the first drink, and not before, why should the alcoholic have any special difficulty mustering the self-control to simply avoid that first drink? Why should abstinence pose any special problem? (p. 34)

Long ago, practitioners recognized that many alcoholics would terminate use of disulfram (Antabuse) in order to resume drinking several days later (Merry, 1966). Behavior of this type suggests that the loss-of-control construct is invalid because at least among some alcoholics, the intention to drink is formed prior to any consumption. In such situations, binge drinking may not be impulsive at all but actually planned for a future point in time.

Why is the hypothesis maintained that control is lost after consumption has begun? One can only speculate, but it may be related to the alcoholic's need to blame the drug (alcohol) or some unknown biological mechanism. If the hypothesis did not first require alcohol to be introduced into the body, the only possible explanations would be psychological or behavioral in nature. Proponents of the traditional disease model typically prefer to avoid nonbiological explanations.

Laboratory Experiments

Conclusive evidence exists that chronic alcoholics (including those who have previously experienced alcohol withdrawal sickness) can drink in a controlled manner in laboratory settings (Pattison, Sobell, & Sobell, 1977). A 1977 review of the alcoholism research literature found that in almost 60 laboratory studies, some involving experiments lasting as long as 2 months, alcoholics demonstrated no loss of control (Pattison et al., 1977). Fingarette (1988) points out that the amount of alcohol consumed by alcoholics is a function of the "costs and benefits perceived by the drinker—an observation that radically contradicts the idea of some overpowering inner drive that completely overwhelms all reason or choice" (p. 36). The contingencies (i.e., rewards and punishers) attached to drinking (as perceived by the drinker) appear to control the amount consumed. The arrangement of contingencies in three different studies involving alcoholics (Cohen, Liebson, Fallace, & Speers, 1971b; Bigelow & Liebson, 1972; Cohen, Liebson, Fallace, & Allen, 1971a) is summarized by Fingarette (1988):

One research team was able, by offering small payments, to get alcoholics to voluntarily abstain from drink even though drink was available, or to moderate their drinking voluntarily even after an initial "priming dose" of liquor had been consumed. (The larger the "priming dose," the less moderate the subsequent drinking, until a modest increase in the amount of payment offered prompted a resumption of moderation.) In another experiment, drinkers were willing to do a limited amount of boring work (pushing a lever) in order to earn a drink, but when the "cost" of a drink rose (that is, more lever pushing was asked of them) they were unwilling to "pay" the higher price. Still another experiment allowed alcoholic patients access to up to a fifth of liquor, but subjects were told that if they drank more than five ounces they would be removed from the pleasant social environment they were in. Result: Most of the time subjects limited themselves to moderate drinking. (p. 36)

A common counterargument to these findings is that the drinking occurred in artificial or unnatural drinking environments (i.e., hospital units or laboratories), and thus the data have little relevance for understanding typical alcoholic drinking. In other words, drinking in a clinic under the observation of investigators radically affects an alcoholic's self-control and drinking behavior. This counterargument is faulty and does not adequately address deficiencies in the loss-of-control hypothesis. If it is argued that the social setting and/or observation by others affects alcoholic drinking, it cannot be argued that loss of control stems from the effects of alcohol or some biological abnormality. Thus, even though the experimental settings may have been anomalous, the findings indicate that frequency and quantity of drinking among alcoholics are not determined solely, or even in a significant way, by ethanol or endogenous mechanisms.

ADDICTION AS A PROGRESSIVE DISEASE

In the classic disease model, addiction is believed to follow a "progressive" course (Talbott, 1989). That is, if alcoholics or addicts continue to abuse chemicals, their condition will deteriorate further and further. Marital, family, work, and medical problems only worsen over time; they do not get better with continued use. Life becomes increasingly unmanageable.

V. E. Johnson (1980) has described the progression of alcoholism in terms of the alcoholic's emotional relationship to the drug. His scheme has four phases. The first two phases represent "normal" drinking, while the third and fourth are typical of alcoholic drinking. Johnson identifies these four phases as (1) learning the mood swing, (2) seeking the mood swing, (3) harmful dependence, and (4) drinking to feel normal.

In phase 1, learning the mood swing, the drinker is initiated into the use of alcohol. In our culture, it usually occurs at a relatively young age.

The drinking is associated with pleasant feelings. There are no emotional "costs" as a result of the consumption. In phase 2, seeking the mood swing, the drinker purposely drinks to obtain euphoria. The amount of alcohol increases as intoxication becomes desired; however, in this phase, there are still no significant emotional costs or adverse consequences. In phase 3, harmful dependence, an "invisible line" is crossed (V. E. Johnson, 1980, p. 15). In this first stage of alcoholic drinking, the individual still finds euphoria in excessive consumption, but there is a price to pay. Following each drinking episode, there are consequences (e.g., hangovers, damaged relationships, and arrests for driving while intoxicated). Despite such problems, the alcoholic continues to drink excessively. In the last phase, the alcoholic's condition has deteriorated to the point that he/she must drink just to feel "normal." When the alcoholic is sober, he/she is overwhelmed by feelings of remorse, guilt, shame, and anxiety (V. E. Johnson, 1980); the natural tendency is to drink to block out these feelings. V. E. Johnson (1980) describes the alcoholic in this last phase as at risk for premature death.

Milam and Ketcham (1983) describe the progression of alcoholism in somewhat different terms. Their scheme focuses more on physiological deterioration than on the emotional relationship with the chemical. It consists of three stages: (1) the adaptive stage, (2) the dependent stage, and (3) deterioration.

In the adaptive stage, the chief characteristic is increasing tolerance to the drug. Alcoholics believe they are blessed by having such a capacity for alcohol because they experience no negative symptoms. They typically do not appear to others to be grossly intoxicated; thus, there is no apparent behavioral impairment. However, physiological changes associated with increasing tolerance are occurring. The drinker is not aware of these changes (Milam & Ketcham, 1983).

The chief characteristic of the dependent stage is physical withdrawal. These symptoms build gradually during this stage. Initially, they are not recognized as withdrawal symptoms but are confused with symptoms of a hangover. To manage these symptoms "effectively," many alcoholics fall into a "maintenance drinking" pattern in which they drink relatively small amounts at frequent intervals to avoid withdrawal sickness. They usually avoid gross intoxication out of a fear of having their problem exposed to others (Milam & Ketcham, 1983).

The last stage, deterioration, is characterized by major medical problems. Various organs are damaged as a result of long-term heavy drinking. In addition to the liver, the brain, the gastrointestinal tract, the pancreas, and even the heart may be affected. These pathological organ changes will cause death if an alcoholic does not receive treatment (Milam & Ketcham, 1983).

V. E. Johnson's (1980) and Milam and Ketcham's (1983) cogent descriptions of the progression of alcoholism (and possibly other addictions) are not consistent with epidemiological findings, however. Studies that examine large populations, rather than just those alcoholics who present themselves for treatment, indicate that alcoholism and other addictions do not follow a predictable sequence of stages in which the user inevitably deteriorates (NIAAA, 1990). On the contrary, so-called natural remission (disappearance of an alcohol problem without treatment) is not uncommon among men as they move into older age categories (Fillmore, 1987a). Furthermore, it appears that among males there is a relationship between dependence problems and alcohol-related social problems on the one hand and age on the other. Generally, by the time men reach their 40s, alcohol problems have declined; in many cases, such men still drink, but more moderately (Fillmore & Midanik, 1984). In women, alcohol problems appear to peak in the 30s (compared to the 20s for men). Also, women are more likely than men to display considerably higher rates of remission across all decades of life (Fillmore, 1987b).

Even among clinical populations (treated alcoholics and problem drinkers), there is evidence to dispute the conception of alcoholism as a progressive disorder. For example, in Norway, Skog and Duckert (1993) tracked the drinking behavior of 182 alcoholics (men and women) over a 4½-year period following inpatient treatment, and that of 135 problem drinkers (men and women) over a 2¼-year period following outpatient treatment. All clients were assessed by a standardized alcoholism assessment instrument and by a personal interview that focused on patterns of drinking during the previous year. In the outpatient group, blood samples were collected and analyzed for a liver enzyme (GT) that is responsive to the presence of alcohol. This was done to determine whether self-reported light drinking was actually the result of consistent underreporting (i.e., minimizing alcohol intake). The data analyses included calculating one-step transition matrices that estimated the likelihood that a participant would move from one level of drinking to another between two successive follow-up assessments.

Skog and Duckert (1993) found that 1 year following treatment, only 11% of the inpatients and 5% of the outpatients were abstinent. However, treatment appeared to have a substantial positive impact on the drinking practices of both client groups. At each follow-up, self-reported alcohol intake was considerably lower than at admission to treatment. This was true for both groups of clients. Among the outpatient group, liver enzyme levels were consistent with self-report intake—making it unlikely the results (at least for this group) were biased by underreporting.

Though there was a good deal of change in the drinking patterns of individuals from one assessment interval to the next, the investigators could find no strong or clear trends for the groups as a whole (Skog & Duckert, 1993). Some participants were increasing their drinking, while a nearly equal number were consuming less. When change did occur, it most likely was to a neighbor consumption category (e.g., abstinence to moderation). According to the investigators, "Very large and dramatic jumps are, in effect, unlikely. Hence, the data suggest that processes of change are reasonably smooth" (Skog & Duckert, 1993, p. 183). Futhermore, there was no evidence of "loss of control" or heavy consumption following periods of abstinence or light drinking, and heavy drinkers tended to gradually decrease their intake rather than quit abruptly. None of these findings fit with the conception of a "progressive disease." Skog and Duckert (1993) conclude that among treated clients, "the observed pattern of change more resembles an indeterministic (or stochastic) process than a systematic natural history of a disease" (p. 178).

Peele (1985) has advanced a concept known as "maturing out" to explain how many alcoholics and addicts give up substance abuse without the benefit of treatment or self-help programs. The term was coined earlier by Winick (1962), who sought to explain the process by which many heroin addicts cease using the drug as they grow older. Today, the concept has been applied more broadly to include alcohol and other drugs.

This natural remission is believed related to developmental issues. Peele (1985) suggests that addiction is a maladaptive method of coping with the challenges and problems of young adulthood. Such challenges may include establishing intimate relationships, learning to manage one's emotions, finding rewarding work, and separating from one's family of origin. Abuse of alcohol or drugs is a way to evade or postpone dealing with these challenges. Peele (1985) contends that as addicts tire of the "night life" and the "fast lane" and become more confident in their ability to take on life challenges (i.e., responsibilities), they will gradually (in most cases) give up substance abuse.

In a series of empirical studies, the process of maturing out was examined among a group of heroin addicts who had been admitted to the California Civil Addict Program during the years 1962–1964 (see Anglin, Brecht, Woodward, & Bonett, 1986). In 1974–1975, the investigators conducted a follow-up assessment of the original sample using a longitudinal retrospective procedure. The studies revealed that maturing out was prevalent in this population, but it was conditional on a number of factors. For example, 75% of "older addicts" and 50% of "younger addicts" had ceased heroin use if they lacked antisocial characteristics and were not involved in crime/drug dealing (Anglin et al., 1986). However, among those still involved in crime/drug dealing to some degree, there was no relationship between maturing out and age. Furthermore, younger addicts assessed as high in "personal resources," an aggregate measure combining educational status, post-high school vocational training, employment history, and parents' socioeconomic status, were found to cease heroin use at a somewhat earlier point in their addiction careers (Brecht, Anglin, Woodward, & Bonett, 1987). Finally, participation in methadone maintenance facilitated maturing out in older addicts more than in younger addicts, but legal supervision had no differential effect across age categories (Brecht & Anglin, 1990).

Evidence also shows that the alcohol consumption of young adults tends to follow the process of maturing out. Similar to heroin, the process seems to be conditional on a number of individual characteristics and social variables. Gotham, Sher, and Wood (1997) assessed 284 college students, most of whom were seniors. Three years later, after all had earned a bachelor's degree, they were assessed a second time. At this follow-up, the cohort's frequency of weekly intoxication had dropped substantially. Three variables were associated with decreased college drinking: a full-time job, being male, and being less "open to experience." Individuals who scored relatively high on a measure of extraversion were most likely to have continued a pattern of frequent intoxication during the 3-year period. In another study, Miller-Tutzauer, Leonard, and Windle (1991) conducted a 3-year longitudinal study of 10,594 persons, ages 18–28. The purpose of their investigation was to examine the impact of marriage on alcohol use. They found that individuals tended to moderate their alcohol use prior to actually becoming married and that drinking continued to decline into the first year of marriage. This decline in alcohol use appeared to stabilize by the end of the first year. Miller-Tutzauer et al. (1991) conclude that the transition to marriage is often associated with a maturation in drinking behavior.

How is it that the disease models have emphasized that the course of addiction is invariably progressive (a notion supported by many in recovery) and yet empirical data indicate that natural remission increases with age? This discrepancy can probably be traced to the fact that the disease models emerged from recovering alcoholics' first-person accounts and from clinical anecdotes. All these were given by alcoholics who recovered through AA or presented themselves for treatment. Such individuals probably represent just a subgroup of all those persons with addiction problems. Thus, although the concept of addiction as a progressive disease may fit some alcoholics and addicts, it does not apply to most with these problems.

ADDICTION AS A CHRONIC DISEASE

Questions about the "chronicity" of addiction constitute one of the most controversial issues in the field and are a source of tension between the treatment and research communities (Marion & Coleman, 1990; Peele, 1985). The disease models maintain that addiction is a chronic disorder, meaning that it never disappears (e.g., "Once an alcoholic, always an alcoholic"). The disease can be readily treated with sustained abstinence and growth within AA or NA, but it is never "cured." For this reason, most individuals in AA or NA refer to themselves as "recovering," rather than "recovered." In this way, substance dependence is likened to other chronic diseases, such as cancer, diabetes, or heart disease.

Abstinence from all mood-altering substances, then, is the goal of virtually all treatment programs in the United States (it should be noted, however, that caffeine and nicotine are not prohibited). Marion and Coleman (1990) admit that the basis for this treatment goal is not based on science but, rather, on folklore. They write: "Abstinence in recovery is supported by the knowledge gained by the experience of drug addicts and alcoholics in their attempts to recover. Through A.A./N.A. 'leads' and testimonials, alcoholics and drug abusers daily report their inability to recover while using any mood- and mind-altering chemicals" (p. 103).

In contrast, the research community has produced a relatively large body of data indicating that controlled drinking is a viable treatment strategy for many alcoholics, particularly those of younger ages (Heather & Robertson, 1983; Miller, 1982). In addition, it appears that it may produce better posttreatment outcomes than abstinence-oriented treatment (Sobell & Sobell, 1976). However, more comparative research is needed.

DENIAL

Denial is another central feature of the traditional disease model. According to Massella (1990), it is the "primary symptom of chemical dependence" (p. 79). Denial is best characterized as an inability to perceive an unacceptable reality; the unacceptable reality is being an "alcoholic" or an "addict." Denial is not lying. It is actually a perceptual incapacity—the most primitive of the psychological defenses. Denial protects the ego from the threat of inadequacy. George (1990) recognizes that it also "protects the option to continue to use, which for the addicted individual is the essence of life" (p. 36). Further discussion of denial and other defense mechanisms is reviewed in Chapter 5.

Stories of alcoholic denial are legendary. I have personally consulted with so-called end-stage alcoholics, who were gravely ill (e.g., pancreatitis, gastrointestinal bleeding, and liver cirrhosis) and hospitalized and have heard them deny that alcohol had any role in causing the medical crises. Certainly, denial is a common aspect of alcoholism and other addictions. However, instead of narrowly defining it as a symptom of a disease, it is useful to take a broader view and to consider how other forces, in combination, foster its use. For instance, the general social stigma attached to addiction is responsible in part for the frequent emergence of the defense. There are few labels today worse than that of "alcoholic" or "addict." With this moral condemnation, it is no wonder that individuals unconsciously react the way they do when initially offered help. Another contributing factor is the coercive methods that are sometimes used to force clients into treatment. The use of confrontative procedures (e.g., family interventions, employee assistance program efforts, and group confrontation) to break down the denial may in many situations have the unintended effect of actually strengthening it.

This is not to say that substance abuse should be ignored or "enabled." However, it should be kept in mind that at least in some cases, denial is a product of well-intentioned coercion by "concerned others" or treatment personnel. To describe denial as a disease symptom is to ignore its social origins and the universality of its use by almost all humans, addicted as well as nonaddicted.

STRENGTHS OF THE DISEASE MODELS

The enduring value of the disease models is that they remove alcohol and other drug addictions from the moral realm. It proposes that addiction sufferers should be treated and helped rather than scorned and ridiculed. Though the moral model of addiction has by no means disappeared in the United States, today more resources are directed toward rehabilitation rather than just toward punishment. The emergence of the disease models is largely responsible for this shift in resources. Increasingly, it is being recognized that harsh penal sentences do little to curb substance abuse in our society.

The contributions of molecular genetics and neuroscience in recent years have begun to elucidate the genetic parameters of addiction. These developments will likely solidify the treatment community's conception of addiction as a disease state. If technological advances lead to implementation of genetic screening as a diagnostic tool, the credibility of the disease view may increase among the general public. From a public policy perspective, the more addiction can be attributed to genetic factors (as opposed to willful misconduct), the greater the likelihood of public support for increased resources being directed to treatment.

Putting science aside, another strength of the *classical* disease model is its simplicity. Recall from Chapter 1 that a good theory is one that is parsimonious. This applies to the traditional disease model: It can be taught to clients in a relatively simple and straightforward manner. Clients, in turn, are often comfortable with the disease conception because it is familiar. Most clients have known someone with a disease (heart disease, diabetes, etc.), so it is not a foreign notion.

The disease models provide the individual who is new to recovery with a mechanism for coping with any guilt and shame stemming from past misdeeds. This framework teaches that problem behaviors are symptoms of the disease process. The alcoholic or addict is not to blame; the fault rests with the disease process. As one alcoholic with many years in recovery shared with me, "Calling it [alcoholism] a disease allows us to put the guilt aside so that we can do the work that we need to do."

The unwavering commitment to abstinence as the goal of treatment and sobriety as a way of is a principle promoted by the disease models and a source of their strength as well. Clearly, the large majority of clients who appear for treatment would benefit most by complete abstinence from psychoactive drugs (other than prescribed medications). Hundreds of thousands, if not millions, of recovering persons have rebuilt their lives as the result of achieving and maintaining a sober life. In this regard, disease models are distinguished from other theories on addiction. On the issue of abstinence, the disease models are clear and direct. Other models dodge the issue a bit, do not address it directly, or contend that "it depends" on the individual client.

WEAKNESSES OF THE DISEASE MODELS

The weaknesses of the disease models have been identified throughout this chapter; they are not repeated here in detail. Simply put, some of the propositions of the disease models are not well supported by science. The notions that have been particularly discredited are that addiction is a "progressive disease" and that it involves a literal "loss of control." Clearly, the best-supported proposition is that alcoholism and other substance use disorders have varying degrees of genetic etiology. However, as argued earlier, the fact that a human trait, behavior, condition, syndrome, disorder, and so on is to some degree rooted in genes does not necessarily require us to think of it as disease. Furthermore, it is clear that environmental factors contribute greatly to all forms of substance use, abuse, and dependence.

The major limitation of the disease conception in general is that it gives too little emphasis to the impact of psychosocial variables and particularly the role of learning as etiological bases. Furthermore, the classical disease model has contributed little to skill-based relapse prevention strategies that rely on learning principles to enhance coping. Subsequent chapters in this volume explore some alternatives to the disease models. None of them is without significant limitations either, as we will see.

REVIEW QUESTIONS

1. Why are the disease models of alcoholism/addiction controversial in many quarters?

2. How does Peele distinguish between types of disease models?

3. Along which dimensions and among which groups do different conceptualizations of the disease models emerge?

4. What is meant by addiction as a "primary disease"?

5. In what ways do research data restrict the applicability of the primary-disease concept?

6. According to Kendler, what is the relationship between genes and the environment in influencing complex human traits?

7. What is meant by the terms "genes," "genotype," and "phenotype"?

8. Why should we be cautious about the assignment of numerical values to the contributions of "nature" and "nuture"?

9. How are MZ and DZ twin pairs different?

10. How is a twin study designed?

11. What are three assumptions on which twin studies rest?

12. According to the twin study research, what are the respective roles of genetics and environment in the etiology of alcoholism and other drug dependencies?

13. Do genetics characteristics influence nicotine metabolism?

14. What is the ADH pathway? What are the major limitations of the alcohol metabolism studies?

15. Why might the P3 wave findings be evidence of a true biological marker for alcoholism?

16. What is COGA?

14. What questions are raised by the prospect of genetic screening for alcohol and drug dependence? In the future, will such a test be widely used in the general population?

15. What should the addiction practitioner know about the genetics of addiction?

16. What is the structure and function of the neuron?

17. What is the significance of the mesolimbic dopamine pathway? How do various drugs interact with this system?

18. What is meant by "loss of control"? Why does Fingarette maintain that it is illogical?

19. Does laboratory research support the loss-of-control concept?

20. How do Johnson's and Milam and Ketcham's descriptions of the progression of alcoholism differ?

21. In what ways do research findings dispute the concept of alcoholism as a "progressive disease"?

22. What is "maturing out"? Is there evidence for this construct?

23. What is meant by addiction as a "chronic disease"?

24. Do research data support the use of controlled drinking as a treatment for alcoholism?

25. How is denial different from lying? What are the problems with calling it a "symptom" of a disease?

26. What are the strengths of the disease models?

27. What are the weaknesses of the disease models?

CHAPTER 3

Public Health
and Prevention Approaches

WHAT IS PUBLIC HEALTH?

The World Health Organization (1998) provides two definitions of public health. The one-sentence definition simply states that public health is "the science and art of promoting health, preventing disease, and prolonging life through the organized efforts of society" (p. 3). The elaborated definition distinguishes between traditional and more contemporary conceptions of public health:

> Public health is a social and political concept aimed at improving health, pro-longing life and improving the quality of life among whole populations through health promotion, disease prevention and other forms of health intervention. A distinction has been made in the health promotion literature between public health and a new public health for the purposes of emphasizing significantly different approaches to the description and analysis of the determinants of health, and the methods of solving public health problems. This new public health is distinguished by its basis in a comprehensive understanding of the ways in which lifestyles and living conditions determine health status, and a recognition of the need to mobilize resources and make sound investments in policies, programmes and services which create, maintain and protect health by supporting healthy lifestyles and creating supportive environments for health. Such a distinction between the 'old' and the "new" may not be necessary in the future as the mainstream concept of public health develops and expands. (World Health Organization, 1998, p. 3)

Public health, then, is often contrasted with medicine. Public health is concerned with promoting and protecting the health of populations, whereas medicine is primarily focused on the care of individual patients.

A Brief History of Public Health in America

The earliest attempts to address public health problems in America can be traced to the colonies of the 17th century (Duffy, 1992). Infectious diseases brought by western European settlers were the chief health problems of that period. Smallpox, malaria, diphtheria, yellow fever, diarrheas and dysenteries, scarlet fever, cholera, typhoid, and other diseases were endemic in the colonial period and contributed to enormous suffering. For instance, in Cotton Mather's diary, the famous New England minister noted that his wife, three children, and a maid died during a single measles outbreak in the winter of 1713–1714 (Duffy, 1992, p. 11). Colonists treated disabling conditions such as malaria and some forms of dysentery with resignation, but the more deadly diseases, such as smallpox, were feared because they appeared without apparent explanation and killed at random.

At that time, and until the 1880s, infectious disease was not well understood. The prevailing medical theories employed a poorly defined concept known as "miasma," which was thought to be an invisible, toxic matter coming from the earth or from rotting tissue or human waste, or other sources, that contaminated the atmosphere and led to widespread illness and death (Stone, Armstrong, Macrina, & Pankau, 1996). Thus, the early approaches to improve the public health were usually confined to the cities and took the form of municipal sanitary regulations that sought to reduce overcrowding in city buildings, controlling the dumping of garbage, improving the disposal of human waste, managing livestock better, and so on. These regulations were typically reactive in nature; that is, they were enacted in response to a local outbreak of disease. Their enforcement was often inconsistent and subsequently ignored after an illness waned (Duffy, 1992).

As the U.S. urban population grew in the 1800s, the health conditions in the cities deteriorated, particularly in impoverished sections of urban areas. Duffy (1992) noted that affluent families typically moved out of older parts of U.S. cities at this time, and they became filled with the poor. The great influx of Irish and immigrants from other countries in the 1840s and 1850s made this situation worse. Often entire poor families would live in small one- or two-room apartments. In most slum housing, the only water source was an outside well or standpipe, if the city had a water system at all. Frequently, multiple families would share a single toilet facility. Disease spread rapidly under these living conditions.

Public health advocates, often members of civic groups and sometimes well-educated, progressive physicians, led reform efforts in a number of cities during the 1800s (Duffy, 1992). Collectively, these reforms came to be known as the "sanitary movement," the forerunner for the modern public health movement that latter became institutionalized in the early part of the 20th century. Despite being based on the erroneous miasmatic disease concept, the sanitary reforms were mostly successful in reducing the incidence of infectious disease. In contrast, medicine played little part (Duffy, 1992). These developments clearly showed that the private medical treatment of individual sufferers was not an adequate community response. To prevent disease, there was a need to (1) focus on the environment, (2) alter the living conditions of citizens, and (3) educate citizens about how to protect themselves and their community. The origins of the tensions between medicine and public health then can be traced to the sanitary movement.

By the turn of the century, scientists had identified a number of the pathogenic organisms that caused common infectious diseases, including the germs causing tuberculosis, typhoid, and diphtheria (Stone et al., 1996). This new "germ theory" gradually supplanted miasmatic theory and revolutionized both public health and medicine. Better management and inspection of food and water supplies, preventive vaccines, the quarantine of the sick, and health education campaigns were remarkably successful in reducing the morbidity and mortality of common infectious diseases. Thus, public health began to rely more on science and research as a means to improve health conditions. However, even as more attention was being given to scientific methods, the experience with tuberculosis and infantile diarrheas in particular forced public health officials to recognize that environmental factors and living conditions, often associated with poverty, remained important causal factors in the development of disease (Duffy, 1992). Thus, the "new public health" official could not retreat into a narrow science based on germ theory. Political advocacy and activities directed to improving living conditions remained an important public health function (which continues today).

The 20th century saw a number of important developments in public health. One was the institutionalization of public health work. The federal government established a number of agencies with missions to focus on specific public health problems (e.g., the Substance Abuse and Mental Health Services Administration). Most of these agencies are under the umbrella of the U.S. Department of Health and Human Services. State, county, and municipal public health departments were created as well.

Another development was the professionalization of the public health field. Civic groups and some physicians spearheaded most of the reforms during the sanitary movement of the 1800s. The 20th century saw the advent of formal public health training provided typically by schools of public health. Initially, much of this training was geared toward the physician. Today, many students receive training in public health without a background in medicine.

The scope of public health also expanded greatly in the last century. Though much effort remains directed at infectious disease, many other health concerns are the focus of public health practice today. Chief among these problems are tobacco, alcohol, and other drug use. Some of the other major public health issues today include: HIV/AIDS, obesity, chronic disease, injuries and violence, and bioterrorism.

Furthermore, it is important to recognize that significant advances were made in public health during the 20th century (Centers for Disease Control and Prevention [CDC], 1999). Since 1900, the average lifespan of Americans increased by more than 30 years, and 25 years of this increase can be attributed to public health efforts (Bunker, Frazier, & Mosteller, 1994). Without ranking them in order of importance, the CDC (1999) has identified 10 great public health achievements of the 20th century (see Table 3.1).

Philosophical Foundations of Public Health

For some time, the public health enterprise in the United States has been involved in debate about the best approach to rely on to promote health and prevent disease in the population. The debate can be traced to the different social philosophies undergirding these approaches (Nijhuis & van der Maesen, 1994). The dominant approach of the 20th century was medical science. However, the view that public health practice is but one of many subdivisions of the field of medicine has had severe critics (e.g., McKinlay & Marceau, 2000). Proponents of a more progressive model have argued that to further strengthen the health of the population, a para-

---

TABLE 3.1. 10 Great Public Health Achievements in the United States, 1900–1999

 1. Vaccination
 2. Motor vehicle safety
 3. Safer workplaces
 4. Control of infectious disease
 5. Decline in deaths from coronary heart disease and stroke
 6. Safer and healthier foods
 7. Healthier mothers and babies
 8. Family planning
 9. Flouridation of drinking water
10. Recognition of tobacco use as a health hazard

Note. From Centers for Disease Control and Prevention (1999).

Social Philosophy	Conception of Health	Determinants	Public Health Activities
Individualism →	Absence of disease →	Physiological and lifestyle influences	→ Conventional medical care; early screening/detection; disease prevention; focus on treating patients
Collectivism →	Holistic/ecological view of health →	Physiological, lifestyle, social, and environmental influences	→ Advocacy for change in public health policies; increasing health care access; community-level intervention; health promotion initiatives; focus on population health

FIGURE 3.1. Competing visions of public health in the United States.

digm shift is needed in which medicine is subsumed under the more comprehensive structure of the public health system (Nijhuis & van der Maesen, 1994).

Figure 3.1 depicts the competing visions of the public health enterprise. McKinlay and Marceau (2000) contend that the conventional public health model is driven by a social philosophy of individualism, a dominant perspective in the United States today that emphasizes the traits, motives, and actions of distinct individuals as the primary determinants of one's health status. In this traditional approach, medical science is viewed as the means to best promote and preserve the health of the population. An alternative model arises from a collectivist social philosophy that is more holistic and ecological and points to multilevel intervention activities. In short, the holistic/ecological conception recognizes that health is a dynamic state influenced by determinants both within and outside the individual.

The conventional strategies employed in the United States for preventing and treating tobacco, alcohol, and other drug abuse has mostly followed the individualistic approach noted in Figure 3.1. That is, intervention strategies focus on risk factors usually "within the skin" of the individual, and have largely ignored multilevel strategies that seek to address community and environmental risk factors. Much of this chapter will be devoted to reviewing public health and prevention approaches that rely on innovative, multilevel interventions.

The Triad of Causation in Public Health

The public health experience with tuberculosis in the early part of the 20th century made clear that the disease was not caused merely by the presence of a germ, in this case—tubercle bacillus (Duffy, 1992). Gradually, public health officials came to recognize that more than one factor contributes to the occurrence of disease. For instance, it is now known that many persons exposed to tubercle bacillus do not develop tuberculosis, and that poverty, overcrowding, malnutrition, and alcoholism are important causal factors in its occurrence (Friedman, 1987). Thus, germ theory is an inadequate basis for understanding the development of disease and other health problems.

In public health, the triad model of causation, involving *host*, *agent*, and *environment*, is often used to explain the development of disease and other health problems. The model provides a better understanding of the interactive nature of the multiple factors that produce disease and other health problems, such as alcohol dependence, for example. Though the agent (i.e., alcohol), must be present for dependence to occur, its presence alone does not produce alcoholism in an individual (the host). Hence, the agent, in this case alcohol, is best considered a necessary factor, but not a sufficient factor, for a health problem, in this case alcohol dependence (or alcoholism), to occur. As depicted in Figure 3.2, the triad model proposes that the multiple characteristics of the host (in this case the alcoholic), determine susceptibility or resistance to the agent (alcohol). In general, host characteristics include such factors as genetic vulnerability, age, attitudes

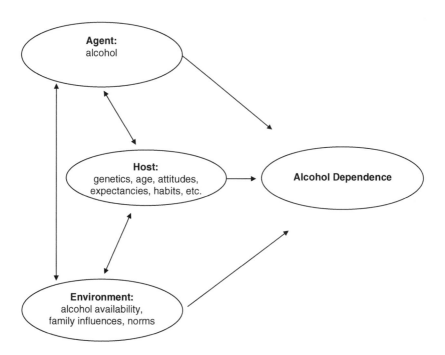

FIGURE 3.2. Agent–host–environment interaction model of alcohol dependence.

and expectancies, and habits (lifestyle variables), but with disorders that tend to be chronic, such as alcohol dependence, the range of determinants can be very broad and complex (Friedman, 1987). In addition, health problems, such as alcohol dependence, will be instigated or suppressed by the environment. Again, a wide range of environmental variables may be involved in the development of the disorder, including availability of the drug, community and peer drinking norms, family influences, and so on. Furthermore, subsets of agent, host, and environmental factors may interact to retard or promote disease and other health problems in specific populations. For example, Asian Americans appear to have lower rates of alcoholism than other ethnic and racial groups in the United States (NIAAA, 1997).

HEALTHY PEOPLE 2010: THE NATIONAL HEALTH PRIORITIES ON TOBACCO, ALCOHOL, AND DRUG USE

Healthy People 2010 is a public health initiative put in place to establish to set of health objectives for the Nation (U.S. Department of Health & Human Services [USDHHS], 2000). The initiative also monitors the progress made in achieving these objectives over the first decade of the new millennium. The two broad goals of Healthy People 2010 are (1) to increase the quality and years of healthy life of Americans and (2) to eliminate health disparities in different segments of the U.S. population. Healthy People 2010 is useful to many different types of organizations, agencies, and community groups in helping them create a vision and agenda for their work. Moreover, the initiative helps groups align their specific mission with national health priorities.

Among the 467 health objectives identified in Healthy People 2010, 45 of them address tobacco, alcohol, and other drug problems. Nine focus areas organize these 45 health objectives (see Table 3.2).

PUBLIC HEALTH SURVEILLANCE OF SUBSTANCE ABUSE

Public health surveillance is the ongoing assessment of the health of a community or population based on the collection, analysis, interpretation, and use of health data (Stone et al., 1996). Surveillance work provides the factual information needed for public health decision making, program promotion, and public advocacy. The data generated from surveillance activities provides an empirical basis for establishing priorities and planning programs that might not be well understood by the public or may even be controversial because they often address sensitive topics (e.g., regulation of

TABLE 3.2. Healthy People 2010: National Objectives for Tobacco, Alcohol, and Other Drug Use

<u>Tobacco use in population groups</u>

1. Reduce tobacco use by adults.
2. Reduce tobacco use by adolescents.
3. Reduce the initiation of tobacco use among children and adolescents.
4. Increase the average age of first use of tobacco products by adolescents and young adults.

<u>Cessation and treatment of nicotine dependency</u>

1. Increase smoking cessation attempts by adult smokers.
2. Increase smoking cessation during pregnancy.
3. Increase tobacco use cessation attempts by adolescent smokers.
4. Increase insurance coverage of evidence-based treatment for nicotine dependency

<u>Exposure to secondhand smoke</u>

1. Reduce the proportion of children who are regularly exposed to tobacco smoke at home.
2. Reduce the proportion of nonsmokers exposed to environmental tobacco smoke.
3. Increase smoke-free and tobacco-free environments in schools, including all school facilities, property, vehicles, and school events.
4. Increase the proportion of worksites with formal smoking policies that prohibit smoking or limit it to separately ventilated areas.
5. Establish laws on smoke-free indoor air that prohibit smoking or limit it to separately ventilated areas in public places and worksites.

<u>Social and environmental changes for smoking</u>

1. Reduce the illegal sales rate to minors through enforcement of laws prohibiting the sale of tobacco products to minors.
2. Eliminate tobacco advertising and promotions that influence adolescents and young adults.
3. Increase adolescents' disapproval of smoking.
4. Increase the number of tribes, territories, and states and the District of Columbia with comprehensive, evidence-based tobacco control programs.
5. Eliminate laws that preempt stronger tobacco control laws.
6. Reduce the toxicity of tobacco products by establishing a regulatory structure to monitor toxicity.
7. Increase the average federal and state tax on tobacco products.

<u>Adverse consequences of alcohol and other drug use</u>

1. Reduce deaths and injuries caused by alcohol- and drug-related motor vehicle crashes.
2. Reduce cirrhosis deaths.
3. Reduce drug-induced deaths.
4. Reduce drug-related hospital emergency department visits.
5. Reduce alcohol-related hospital emergency department visits.
6. Reduce the proportion of adolescents who report that they rode, during the previous 30 days, with a driver who had been drinking alcohol.

(continued)

TABLE 3.2. *(continued)*

Adverse consequences of alcohol and other drug use *(cont.)*

7. Reduce intentional injuries resulting from alcohol- and illicit drug-related violence.
8. Reduce the cost of lost productivity in the workplace due to alcohol and drug use.

Alcohol and other drug use

1. Increase the age and proportion of adolescents who remain alcohol and drug free.
2. Reduce past-month use of illicit substances.
3. Reduce the proportion of persons engaging in binge drinking of alcoholic beverages.
4. Reduce average annual alcohol consumption.
5. Reduce the proportion of adults who exceed guidelines for low-risk drinking.
6. Reduce steroid use among adolescents.
7. Reduce the proportion of adolescents who use inhalants.

Risks of alcohol and other drug use

1. Increase the proportion of adolescents who disapprove of substance abuse.
2. Increase the proportion of adolescents who perceive great risk associated with substance abuse.

Treatment of alcohol and other drug abuse

1. Reduce the treatment gap for illicit drugs in the general population.
2. Increase the proportion of inmates receiving substance abuse treatment in correctional institutions.
3. Increase the number of admissions to substance abuse treatment for injection drug use.
4. Reduce the treatment gap for alcohol problems.

State and local efforts to reduce alcohol and other drug abuse

1. Increase the proportion of persons who are referred for follow-up care for alcohol problems, drug problems, or suicide attempts after diagnosis or treatment for one of these conditions in a hospital emergency department.
2. Increase the number of communities using partnerships or coalition models to conduct comprehensive substance abuse prevention efforts.
3. Extend administrative license revocation laws, or programs of equal effectiveness, for persons who drive under the influence of intoxicants.
4. Extend legal requirements for maximum blood alcohol concentration levels of 0.08 percent for motor vehicle drivers ages 21 years and older.

Note. From U.S. Department of Health and Human Services (2000).

cigarette smoking in public areas and reducing HIV transmission). Further-more, as Duffy (1992) has noted, throughout U.S. history the public's attention span to health issues has been short (p. 313). There is a continual need to maintain awareness of their importance among the public. The sustained, ongoing nature of surveillance programs serves the important societal function of reminding the public about potential health threats and new emergencies.

Discussed next are three national surveillance systems of substance use operated by public health agencies of the U.S. federal government. Each relies on a different data collection method to collect data from nationally representative samples of Americans. The Youth Risk Behavior Surveillance Survey (YRBSS) is a school-based survey of high school students. The National Survey on Drug Use and Health (NSDUH) relies on a household survey, and the Drug Abuse Warning Network (DAWN) includes a survey of substance abuse-related visits to hospital emergency departments.

Youth Risk Behavior Surveillance Survey

The CDC (2004a) operates the YRBSS. The YRBSS collects self-report survey data on a biennial basis from a nationally representative sample of U.S. high school students (grades 9–12). The surveillance system monitors priority health risk behaviors that have been documented to contribute substantially to the social problems, disabilities, and death of American youth and adults. The multiple behaviors that are assessed include tobacco, alcohol and other drug use, sexual behaviors, violence, safety behaviors, eating behavior, and exercise behavior. These behaviors also are associated with educational outcomes and dropping out of school.

The YRBSS was designed with multiple purposes in mind. The system is used to (1) determine the prevalence of health risk behaviors among high students; (2) examine change in these behaviors over time; (3) study the co-occurrence of health-risk behaviors; (4) compare national, state, and local prevalence rates as well as those among subpopulations of adolescents (e.g., sex, age, and racial/ethnic groups); and (5) monitor progress toward achieving national health objectives (USDHHS, 2000). Table 3.3 shows the 30-day prevalence rates of each of five drugs found in 2003 to illustrate the type of data collected by the YRBSS.

In addition to documenting the relatively high prevalence of substance use among American high school students, the surveillance data in Table 3.3 reveals several noteworthy patterns. First, with the exception of inhalants, drug use prevalence rates increase with grade level. Second, alcohol clearly is the most commonly used drug, followed by cigarettes and marijuana, then cocaine and inhalants. Notice that the 9th-grade prevalence of

TABLE 3.3. Percentages of High School Students Using Each of Five Drugs in Past 30 Days: United States, Youth Risk Behavior Survey, 2003

Grade	Cigarettes	Alcohol	Marijuana	Cocaine	Inhalants
Ninth	17.4	36.2	18.5	3.6	5.4
Tenth	21.8	43.5	22.0	3.7	3.5
Eleventh	23.6	47.0	24.1	4.1	3.1
Twelfth	26.2	55.9	25.8	4.7	2.7

Note. Data from Centers for Disease Control and Prevention (2004b).

alcohol use (36.2%) is substantially higher than the similar 12th-grade rates for the other four drugs. Third, inhalant use decreases with grade level. Findings such as these can be useful for establishing prevention priorities and designing programs of intervention.

National Survey on Drug Use and Health

Another example of a national surveillance system is the NSDUH (Office of Applied Studies, 2004a). Formerly known as the National Household Survey on Drug Abuse, this surveillance survey is managed by the Substance Abuse and Mental Health Services Administration (SAMHSA). Conducted since 1971, the NSDUH is the primary source of data on the incidence and prevalence of tobacco, alcohol and other drug use in the civilian, non-institutionalized population 12 years of age and older in the United States. Data are collected in all 50 states and the District of Columbia.

Each year, about 67,500 face-to-face interviews are conducted in a representative sample of U.S. households (Office of Applied Studies, 2004a). Introductory letters precede the interviewer visits to the selected NSDUH households. Within these sampling units (can be a household or another type of living unit), survey participants are randomly selected using an automated program of a handheld computer. Prior to conducting these interviews, the interviewers explain the purpose of the study, how the data will be used, and the confidentiality protections provided under federal law. The names of the respondents are not collected and their addresses are stored separately from their survey responses.

The selected participant is asked to identify a private area in the home away from other household members for the purpose of conducting the 1-hour interview (Office of Applied Studies, 2004a). The interview relies on both computer-assisted personal interviewing (CAPI) and audio computer-assisted self-interviewing (ACASI). The interviewer begins the interview in

CAPI mode by reading the questions from the screen and entering the participant's responses into the database. For sensitive questions, the interviewer shifts to ACASI with the participant reading the questions silently on the screen and/or listening to them through available headphones. In ACASI mode, the participant enters their responses directly into the computer database. A $30 cash payment is given to each participant that completes a NSDUH survey.

One example of findings reported from the NSDUH appears in Figure 3.3. In 2003, a majority of those NSDUH respondents reporting any use of heroin in the past year (57.4%) also met DSM-IV-TR criteria for heroin abuse or heroin dependence (Office of Applied Studies, 2004a). Other drugs were associated with substantially lower rates of abuse and dependency. For instance, among those reporting past year use of cocaine, one-quarter (25.6%) were classified with either abuse or dependence on that drug, followed by sedatives (19.0%), marijuana (16.6 %), stimulants (13.7%), pain relievers (12.2%), and alcohol (11.5%). The co-occurrence of other drug use in the past year with DSM-IV-TR abuse/dependence criteria was less than 10% (tranquilizers, hallucinogens, and inhalants).

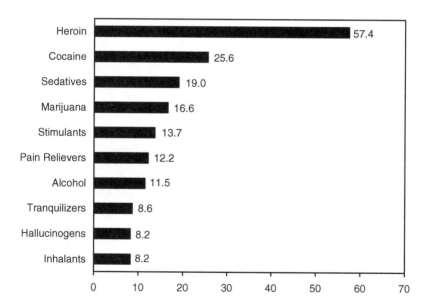

FIGURE 3.3. Percentage of past-year users with DSM-IV-TR abuse or dependence diagnosis, 2003. From Office of Applied Studies (2004a).

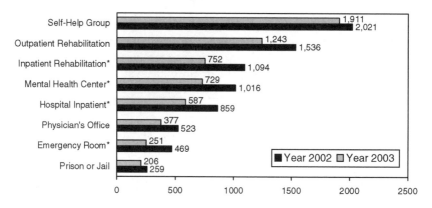

FIGURE 3.4. Numbers (in thousands) receiving treatment at a specific location in United States, 2002 and 2003. From Office of Applied Studies (2004a). Asterisks indicate that difference was statistically significant.

The data in Figure 3.4 also were collected by the NSDUH (Office of Applied Studies, 2004a). As can be seen, there were decreases in all types of treatment seeking between 2002 and 2003 in the United States. The decreases during this time period were statistically significant (i.e., unlikely due to sampling error) for the following locations: inpatient rehabilitation (–342,000), mental health center (–287,000), hospital inpatient (–272,000), and emergency room (–218,000). Recent changes in the NSDUH preclude examination of longer trends in treatment seeking (Office of Applied Studies, 2004a).

Drug Abuse Warning Network

A third example of a public health surveillance system of substance use is DAWN (Office of Applied Studies, 2004b). This system monitors trends in drug-related emergency department (ED) visits and deaths (data on deaths not reported here). DAWN also is sponsored by SAMHSA, which is required to collect these data under Section 505 of the Public Health Service Act (42 U.S.C. §290aa-4). The system provides estimates of drug-related ED visits for the coterminous United States by collecting data from a representative sample of hospitals.

Table 3.4 presents data generated by DAWN for the last 6 months of 2003. During that period, cocaine was the most mentioned drug category. It was involved in 20.0% of all drug-related ED visits. Alcohol-in-combination mentions were a close second and could be linked to 18.9% of all drug-related ED visits. Third was marijuana, followed by heroin, with substantially smaller percentages of mentions after these drug categories.

TABLE 3.4. Emergency Department Mentions for 15 Drug Categories: Coterminous United States, July–December, 2003

Rank	Drug category	Number of mentions	Percentage of total episodes
1.	Cocaine	125,921	20.0
2.	Alcohol in combination	118,724	18.9
3.	Marijuana	79,663	12.7
4.	Heroin	47,604	7.6
5.	Methamphetamine	25,039	4.0
6.	Alcohol alone (persons < age 21)	22,619	3.6
7.	Amphetamines	18,129	2.9
8.	PCP	4,581	1.0
9.	MDMA (Ecstasy)	2,221	< 1.0
10.	Inhalants	1,681	< 1.0
11.	GHB	990	< 1.0
12.	Miscellaneous hallucinogens	684	< 1.0
13.	LSD	656	< 1.0
14.	Ketamine	73	< 1.0
15.	Combinations not tabulated above	1,346	< 1.0

Note. From Office of Applied Studies (2004b).

AGE OF ONSET AND THE GATEWAY HYPOTHESIS

The Significance of Age of Onset

From a public health perspective, the optimal way to reduce the human costs associated with substance use is to prevent or delay the onset of tobacco, alcohol, and other drug use. Though a number of unanswered questions remain about the best way to characterize its developmental sequence, in the last 30 years much has been learned about the initiation of substance use and the risk factors associated with its onset. For instance, research has established that the onset of cigarette smoking can be predicted by early conduct problems in school, poor academic performance, weak school bonds, peer smoking and perceived peer norms, lower socioeconomic status, poor refusal skills, and other variables (Bryant, Schulenberg, Bachman, O'Malley, & Johnston, 2000; Conrad, Flay, & Hill, 1992; Olds, Thombs, & Ray-Tomasek, 2005). In turn, adolescents who currently smoke have been found to be to 3 times more likely than teen nonsmokers to drink alcohol, 8 times more likely to smoke marijuana, and 22 times more likely to use cocaine (CDC, 1994). Furthermore, teenage smoking has been linked to higher rates of other risk behaviors, including fighting and engaging in unprotected sex (CDC, 1994).

Research also has documented that the early onset of use (late childhood/early adolescence) of a particular drug increases the risk of experiencing problems with that same substance at a later point in life. For example, findings from the NSDUH (see Table 3.5) show that those Americans who initiated alcohol use before the age of 15 were almost four times more likely to have met criteria for alcohol abuse or alcohol dependence in the past year than those who started drinking at or after the age of 18, and about six times more likely to meet these same criteria than those starting to drink at or after the age of 21 (Office of Applied Studies, 2004c). Using data from a separate national probability sample, Grant and Dawson (1997) found that the odds of alcohol abuse in adulthood decreased 8% with each increasing year of age at drinking onset, whereas the odds of alcohol dependence decreased 14% with each increasing year of age at drinking onset. From a public health perspective, these findings suggest that a goal of prevention strategies should be to delay or postpone the onset of alcohol use until at least the age of 18, when the risk for alcohol abuse or dependence has fallen to a relatively low level (as shown in Table 3.5).

The Gateway Hypothesis

Though early onset is clearly a risk factor for subsequent alcohol and drug abuse problems, there are more complex models that seek to explain the progression into use of so-called hard drugs, such as cocaine and heroin (see Klein & Riso, 1993). The most prominent (and probably controversial) model is the "gateway hypothesis" (MacCoun, 1998). The hypothesis proposes that there is a predictable sequence to the process by which people

TABLE 3.5. Rates of Alcohol Abuse or Dependence in the Past Year among American Adults by Age of Drinking Onset: National Survey on Drug Use and Health, 2003

Age at first use of alcohol	Percentage experiencing alcohol abuse or dependence
Before age 12	16.0
12–14	15.5
15–17	9.0
18–20	4.2
At or after age 21	2.6

Note. Data from Office of Applied Studies (2004c). Respondents were 21 years of age or older at the time of the survey.

become involved in drug use (Kandel & Faust, 1975; Kandel, Yamaguchi, & Chen, 1992). The sequence involves four stages in which the use of beer or wine is followed by hard liquor or cigarettes, which in turn is followed by marijuana and then other illicit drugs (see Figure 3.5). An important point to keep in mind is that although the large majority of persons who reach stages 3 and 4 have previously used gateway substances, most people at stages 1 and 2 never advance to stages 3 or 4.

A compelling piece of evidence supporting this developmental sequence is that though not every drug user follows this specific sequence, only about 1% began their substance use with marijuana or another illicit drug. Thus, for young people, the legal drugs (i.e., alcohol and cigarettes) seem to function as a "gateway" to marijuana and possibly other illicit drug use. Furthermore, Kandel et al. (1992) have found that the progression to a subsequent stage is strongly predicted by both age of onset and frequency of use in the previous stage.

Without doubt, the most controversial aspect of the gateway hypothesis is whether the sequence and association of drug use identified in Figure 3.5 should be considered a *causal* model (Kandel, 2003; MacCoun, 1998). In public policy debates about the legal control of cannabis, proponents of laws prohibiting marijuana use and distribution frequently assert that the gateway sequence involves causation; that is, marijuana use is a cause of hard drug use (methamphetamine, heroin, cocaine, etc.). Thus, those in favor of restrictive cannabis laws may argue that even though the use of marijuana by itself may sometimes not be highly addictive or dangerous, it often leads young people to other more serious drug use that is very harmful to the individual, his/her family, and society.

Opponents of strong legal controls on marijuana typically argue that the stage sequence in Figure 3.5 does not establish causality but, rather, represents a series of spurious correlations. In this view, it is contended that there is no plausible biological mechanism by which drug use at one stage would cause drug use at a subsequent stage. Therefore, the observed correlation between marijuana and hard drug use is the result of some third factor, such as an underlying proneness to deviance, that puts individuals at risk for use of both cannabis and hard drugs as well as a range of other unconventional behavior (Jessor, Donovan, & Costa, 1991). Furthermore, opponents of marijuana prohibitions maintain that the gateway hypothesis

Stage 1	Stage 2	Stage 3	Stage 4
Beer or wine→	Hard liquor or cigarettes →	Marijuana	→ Other illicit drugs

FIGURE 3.5. The gateway hypothesis: A developmental sequence of drug involvement.

is simplistic and directs attention away from the actual root causes of hard drug use which are believed to be such factors as: limited economic opportunity and poverty, poor education, weak family bonds and inadequate parental supervision, neighborhood disorganization, and so on.

Two twin studies conducted to test the gateway hypothesis have arrived at somewhat different conclusions about the role of marijuana use as a possible cause of other drug abuse and dependence. In one study, Lynskey et al. (2003) assessed 311 monozygotic (MZ) and dizygotic (DZ) same-sex twin pairs discordant for early marijuana use (before age 17). The participants ranged in age from 24 to 36 (median = 30 years). The design of their investigation was based on the assumption that same-sex twins share the same environmental and family experiences, and that the MZ pairs share the same genetic risk factors. Therefore, if the relationship between early marijuana use and other drug use later in life can be explained by shared environmental factors, then in those twin pairs who were discordant for early marijuana use, the co-twin who did not initiate early marijuana use should be at the same risk for developing later drug problems as co-twin who did start using marijuana early. In addition, if shared genetic variables explained the relationship between early marijuana use and other drug use in later life, then the MZ twin pairs discordant for early marijuana should still have the same risk for developing later drug problems (Lynskey et al., 2003). Alternatively, if the relationship between early marijuana use and other drug use in later life is causal, or accounted for nonshared environmental factors, it would be expected that higher rates of later drug problems would be observed in the twins who had initiated marijuana early in life.

Lynskey et al. (2003) found that the relationship between early marijuana use and other drug use later in life could not be adequately explained by either shared environmental factors or genetic factors, providing support for the gateway hypothesis. (The investigators controlled for a host of other known risk factors, such as parental conflict/separation, sexual abuse during childhood, conduct disorder, social anxiety, etc.) Compared to the twins who had not used marijuana by the age of 17, those who had done so were 2.1 to 5.2 times more likely to have experienced other drug use, alcohol dependence, and drug abuse/dependence. The investigators speculated that the gateway mechanism operates within a social context of peers to reduce the perceived barriers against other drug use and to increase access to them. They also cautioned that their findings do not provide definitive evidence that early marijuana use plays a causal role in producing other drug use. Rather, they suggested that their study lends strong support to the view that individuals who start smoking marijuana early in life are at greatly elevated risk for other subsequent drug abuse and drug dependence (Lynskey et al., 2003).

In a separate twin study, Agrawal, Neale, Prescott, and Kendler (2004) evaluated an expanded set of relational models (compared to those examined by Lynskey et al., 2003). Using data from a sample of 1,191 male and 934 female same-sex twin pairs, the investigators tested 13 genetically informed models that offered distinct explanations about the nature of the association between marijuana use and other illicit drug use. Agrawal et al. (2004) found that a correlated liabilities model provided the best fit to the data for marijuana use and its association with both other illicit drug use and abuse/dependence. Distinct from the gateway hypothesis which maintains that marijuana use directly increases the subsequent risk of other drug use and abuse/dependence, the correlated liabilities model proposes that "cannabis use and other illicit drug use are influenced by genetic and environmental factors that are correlated across the drugs" (Agrawal et al., 2004, p. 219). That is, they found evidence that the co-occurrence of marijuana use and other illicit drug use arises from correlated genetic and environmental influences that exist for both classes of drugs—not a causal mechanism involving marijuana. This finding is supported by previous research that examined these relationships in a sample of men (Tsuang et al., 1998).

However, Agrawal et al. (2004) acknowledge that their study yielded some evidence to support a modified gateway model for *high-risk* marijuana users. In this model, individuals are at risk for other illicit drug use only after they reach a high threshold of risk for marijuana use. This finding appears to be consistent with the earlier epidemiological work of Kandel et al. (1992). Furthermore, the Agrawal et al. (2004) study did not account for the impact of age of onset of marijuana use as did Lynskey et al. (2003). Thus, the existing evidence establishes that there is an observable sequence and relatively strong association between marijuana use and other illicit drug use, which may involve a marijuana risk gradient. However, at this time, it is probably premature to conclude that the co-occurrence arises from a causal mechanism.

TYPES OF PREVENTION PROGRAMS AND STRATEGIES

Today, the categorization of substance abuse prevention programs is most often based on the target population they are designed to assist (National Institute on Drug Abuse [NIDA], 2003). In an attempt to clarify confusion about different types of prevention, the following classification scheme has been proposed by the Institute of Medicine (1994): (1) *universal prevention*—programs designed for the general population, such as all students in a school; (2) *selective prevention*—programs targeting groups at risk or subsets of the general population, such as students performing poorly in school or children of drug abusers; and (3) *indicated prevention*—programs designed for people already using drugs, such as high-risk youth and their families. Effective prevention programs within each of these three categories address the protective factors and risk factors associated with substance use (NIDA, 2003).

At different stages of development, youth will be exposed to different sets of protective factors and risk factors, and these influences may be altered by the presence of preventive interventions. For instance, it has been found that children and adolescents who have been exposed to positive youth development programs are less likely to use tobacco, alcohol, and other drugs (Catalano, Bergland, Ryan, Lonczak, & Hawkins, 1998a; Flay & Allred, 2003). Moreover, it is important that negative behaviors in early childhood, such as aggression, be changed because they can lead to social and academic difficulties that further heighten risk for later drug abuse.

One important aim of all preventive interventions is to alter the balance between protective factors and risk factors such that the former outweigh the latter in the life experience of children and adolescents (NIDA, 2003). Table 3.6 provides examples of common protective factors and risk factors that affect young people in five developmental spheres.

Evidence-Based Prevention Programs

Over the past two decades, the federal government has invested a considerable amount of money into the research and development of programs to prevent substance use and abuse (Botvin, 2004). These efforts have been fruitful and today a number of effective prevention approaches, both school and community based, have been identified through rigorous testing and evaluation. As a result, several federal government agencies maintain

TABLE 3.6. Protective Factors and Risk Factors for Youth Substance Use

Protective factors	Developmental sphere	Risk factors
Positive self-concept	Individual	Negative self-concept
Parental monitoring	Family	Inadequate parental monitoring and supervision
Primary friendships with positive youth	Peers	Primary friendships with troubled youth
Academic success with strong school bonds	School	Academic difficulties with weak school bonds
Strong neighborhood attachment	Community	Weak neighborhood attachment

registries or lists of recommended prevention programs for communities and schools. For example, SAMSHA, (2004) maintains the National Registry of Effective Programs and Practices to identify "model programs" in substance abuse and mental health. Through an ongoing, formal review process, SAMSHA (2004) classifies evidence-based substance abuse prevention programs into one of three categories: "promising," "effective," or "model." In a report titled *Exemplary, and Promising Safe, Disciplined, and Drug-Free Schools Programs*, the U.S. Department of Education (2001) published the results of a formal review of school-based prevention programs. In this report, an expert panel classified school programs as either "promising" or "exemplary." Third, in their report *Preventing Drug Use Among Children and Adolescents: A Research-Based Guide for Parents, Educators, and Community Leaders*, NIDA (2003) provided selected examples of research-based drug prevention programs.

Several of these recommended programs are discussed here to provide some perspective on the range of prevention strategies that have empirical support. The identification of these three programs should not be considered an endorsement of them. Readers interested in learning about the full range of prevention options should consult the three federal government reports identified earlier.

LifeSkills® Training

Today, LifeSkills® Training (LST) is one of the most widely used, evidence-based prevention programs (National Health Promotion Associates, 2004). LST is a universal, school-based program designed for both elementary and middle school students. The program has been successfully tested in white, suburban student populations as well as in ethnic and minority populations and inner-city schools (National Health Promotion Associates, 2004).

The LST program does not spend a great deal of time reviewing information about the pharmacological actions of drugs or on the medical and legal consequences of drug use. Instead, the program addresses protective and risk factors by attempting to build skills in three areas: drug resistance skills, personal self-management skills, and general social skills. For example, through coaching and practice, students learn to deal with social pressures to use drugs, they learn how to reevaluate personal challenges in an optimistic manner, and they learn ways to overcome shyness.

LST can be taught once a week over an extended period of time or it can be offered in an intensive miniseries format where it is taught every day or two to three times a week (National Health Promotion Associates, 2004). The elementary school LST curriculum is normally taught in 24 class sessions (30–45 minutes long) over a 3-year period in either grades 3–5 or grades 4–6. Ideally, the elementary curriculum is followed by booster sessions in middle school. The LST curriculum designed for middle school is normally taught in 30 class sessions (45 minutes long) over a 3-year period in either grades 6–8 or grades 7–9.

In the first test of LST, Botvin, Eng, and Williams (1980) examined short-term cigarette smoking outcomes in 281 8th- to 10th-grade students in suburban New York. The program appeared to produce a 75% decrease in the number of new cigarette smokers after an initial posttest and a 67% decrease in new smoking at 3-month follow-up (Botvin et al., 1980). During the 1980s and early 1990s, Botvin and colleagues continued to be successful in testing LST with longer-term follow-ups for reducing tobacco use (e.g., Botvin & Eng, 1982; Botvin, Renick, & Baker, 1983), for reducing alcohol and other drug use (Botvin, Baker, Botvin, Filazzolla, & Millman, 1984; Botvin, Baker, Dusenburg, Tortu, & Botvin, 1990), and in minority populations (Botvin et al., 1992).

LST began to draw serious attention in 1995 when Botvin and colleagues published their work in the prestigious *Journal of the American Medical Association*. Botvin et al. (1995) reported the long-term outcomes of a randomized trial involving 56 public schools that were assigned to LST or a control condition. School, telephone, and mail surveys were used to collect follow-up data for 6 years after baseline. The investigators detected significant reductions in both drug and polydrug use for the groups that received LST with strongest effects observed among those who received the program implemented with greatest fidelity. The Botvin et al. (1995) investigation was one of the first studies to provide compelling evidence that a properly implemented, school-based prevention program could produce meaningful and sustained reductions in student tobacco, alcohol, and marijuana use.

More recent evaluations of LST have offered further verification that the program is effective for other populations and drug problems. For instance, Botvin, Griffin, Paul, and Macaulay (2003) conducted another randomized trial of LST in elementary school students (grades 3–6). In 20 schools, rates of knowledge, attitudes, normative expectations, and substance use and related variables were assessed among students who were assigned to either LST (9 schools; n = 426) or to a control group (11 schools; n = 664). Individual-level analyses revealed that after controlling for gender, race, and family structure, students in LST reported less cigarette smoking in the past year, higher antidrinking attitudes, increased substance use knowledge and skills-related knowledge, lower normative expectations for smoking and alcohol use, and higher self-esteem at a posttest assessment (Botvin et al., 2003). Furthermore, at the posttest assessment, school-level analyses showed that the annual prevalence rate was 61% lower for smoking and 25% lower for alcohol use in schools that received the LST than in control schools. These findings suggest that LST reduces substance use at the elementary school level.

Botvin, Griffin, Diaz, and Ifill-Williams (2001) examined the efficacy of LST in a predominantly minority student population (29 New York City schools; n = 3,621), and Griffin, Botvin, Nichols, and Doyle (2003) evaluated LST in a subsample of this group that had been identified as being at high risk for substance use initiation. In both the total sample (Botvin et al., 2001) and the high-risk sample (Griffin et al., 2003), students who received LST reported less cigarette smoking, alcohol consumption, drunkenness, inhalant use, and polydrug use compared with controls. LST also had a direct positive effect on several cognitive, attitudinal, and personality variables that have been theoretically linked to adolescent substance use (Botvin et al., 2001). These findings support the use of LST in schools that serve disadvantaged, urban, minority adolescents and in assisting high-risk, adolescent populations (Botvin et al., 2001).

Guiding Good Choices®
(Formerly Known as Preparing for Drug-Free Years®)

Another example of a universal prevention program is Guiding Good Choices® (Catalano, Kosterman, Haggerty, Hawkins, & Spoth, 1998b; Channing Bete Company, 2005). This program was designed for parents of preadolescents. As implied by the name of the program, the aim of the Guiding Good Choices curriculum is to reduce the risk for alcohol and other drug problems during adolescence by empowering parents of 8- to 14-year-olds. Specifically, Guiding Good Choices teaches parents how to enhance important protective factors and reduce risk factors during the later elementary and middle school years. An important feature of the program is that it was designed for adult learners with varying learning styles and levels of education.

The conceptual foundation of Guiding Good Choices is the social development model (Catalano & Hawkins, 1996). A unifying construct of this framework is "bonding," which is viewed as consisting of both attachment and commitment. In the context of a family, a strong parent–child bond is expected to lead to the child's acceptance of the beliefs and standards of the parent. When a bond generates beliefs that are prosocial and healthy, it serves as a protective factor. Of course, children can bond with antisocial parents, peers, or other harmful persons as well. The social development model and its Guiding Good Choices application stress the importance of bonding to prosocial family, school, and peers as a protection against the development of conduct problems, school misbehavior, and drug abuse (Catalano et al., 1998b).

The Guiding Good Choices program was originally developed in 1987 for use in the Seattle Social Development Project, a longitudinal research study funded by the NIDA (Catalano et al., 1998b). According to Catalano and colleagues, more than 120,000 families have been trained in the program. The Guiding Good Choices program is a 3-day parent-training course, comprised of five 2-hour sessions. For use in the workplace, the program has been offered as a series of 10 1-hour sessions. In most cases, two trained leaders from the community conduct the workshops. The content of Guiding Good Choices focuses on three core beliefs:

1. parents can play an important role in the reduction of risk factors for other drug and alcohol use by their children;
2. parents can take an active role in the enhancement of protection for their children by offering them opportunities for involvement within the family, teaching them skills to be successful, recognizing and rewarding their involvement, and communicating clear family norms on alcohol and other drug use;
3. regular family meetings provide a mechanism for family involvement and serve as a tool to transfer content and skills learned in the workshop into the home environment." (Catalano et al., 1998b, pp. 135–136)

The initial evaluations of Guiding Good Choices were focused mostly on dissemination issues, for example, answering such questions as whether parents would participate in the program and use recommended family management practices. In attempting to reach parents, these are important issues to consider in designing a prevention program. Dissemination obstacles can range from logistical problems, such as lack of transportation or child care, to the manner in which the program is marketed to parents (Catalano et al., 1998b).

In Oregon, Heuser (1990) evaluated the statewide dissemination of Guiding Good Choices in 32 counties and within four state agencies. Television, radio, and newspaper announcements; posters and brochures; and announcements at public agencies, schools, and churches were used to recruit parents. It was found that the largest proportion of participants learned of the Guiding Good Choices workshops through their child's school (45%) or from a friend or family member (34%). Overall, attendance dropped about 33% during the course of the workshops. Again, participant ratings of the workshops were quite favorable, and between 49% and 61% of the parents reported that they had organized and held a family meeting in the past week, as instructed in each session (Heuser, 1990).

In the Seattle metropolitan area, Hawkins, Catalano, and Kent (1991) had broadcast a 1-hour television special on the local NBC affiliate (at 9:00 P.M. on a Tuesday evening) that vividly documented the risk factors and consequences of adolescent drug abuse and presented strategies that parents could use to prevent these problems. About 98,000 households were estimated to have viewed the program. In addition, public service announcements were broadcast to alert parents to the availability of 87 local Guiding Good Choices workshops.

Hawkins et al. (1991) found that about 2,500 participants attended the voluntary Guiding Good Choices workshops in the Seattle area. About 90% of the parents were identified as "European American," and a majority had children in the targeted age (grades 4–7). Most of the participants had seen the television special (53%) and had learned about the workshops either through this special (29%) and/or through their child's school (72%). At the final session, about 69% of the original attendees remained in the program. Overall, the participants provided very favorable program ratings, and at posttest, there was evidence of increases in knowledge about good family management and utilization of program parenting strategies (Hawkins et al., 1991).

Guiding Good Choices has been tested among families with sixth- and seventh-graders in rural Iowa (Catalano et al., 1998b). Through nine different schools, parents were invited to participate. The families were nearly all white and mostly working class. At the initial assessment, data were collected from 209 families. At the final assessment, 175 of these families (84%) provided posttest data. The relatively high participation rate was probably motivated by the use of financial incentives (approximately $10 per hour per family member for completing assessments). However, the incentives were not given for program participation itself. About 88% of participating mothers and 69% of participating fathers attended at least three of the five sessions (mean attendance rate for mothers = 3.9 sessions; fathers = 3.1 sessions). In addition to responding to questionnaires, participating families also were videotaped in two structured interaction tasks. One task involved responding to general questions about their family life, such as chores, roles, and parental monitoring. The other task was focused on family problems and attempts at problem solving.

Families were randomly assigned to either the Guiding Good Choices intervention condition or a wait-list control condition (to receive the Guiding Good Choices program after the trial). Families were administered posttest assessments 2 to 9 weeks following completion of the program. Trained community members conducted the workshops. The investigators collected data on the fidelity of the delivery of the workshops. Across workshops, it was found that 74% to 82% of the complete Guiding Good Choices curriculum was delivered by the community members (Catalano et al., 1998b).

The analysis of parent outcomes revealed that there was significant improvement in parenting behavior, child management, and the affective quality of parent–child relations, for both mothers and fathers in the intervention group (Catalano et al., 1998b). Specifically, mothers who had participated in Guiding Good Choices were significantly more likely to report that they (1) provided rewards to their child for prosocial behavior, (2) communicated rules about substance use, (3) appropriately punished their child for misbehavior, (4) restricted alcohol use by their child, (5) expected their child to refuse a beer if offered by a friend, (6) expressed less conflict toward their spouse, and (7) attempted to involve themselves more with their child. Fathers in the Guiding Good Choices program were significantly more likely to report that they (1) communicated rules about substance use and (2) attempted to involve themselves more with their child.

The effects of the Guiding Good Choices program on adolescent substance use have been positive as well. In a study reporting the adolescent outcomes of the Iowa trial, Spoth, Redmond, and Shin (2001) found that in families in which the parents had received the Guiding Good Choices program, 3½ years later their 10th-grade children were 19% less likely to report ever being drunk, 37% less likely to report ever smoking marijuana, and 41% less likely to have used alcohol in the past month—compared to 10th graders in a no-treatment control condition. These long-term outcomes are particularly impressive given that Guiding Good Choices is a brief, five-session intervention for parents. Also, it is possible that the differences between adolescents in the intervention and control groups could have continued to increase over time (Spoth et al., 2001).

The research on the Guiding Good Choices program suggests that one viable universal prevention strategy is parent education and training delivered via community-based workshops. It appears that with appropriate promotion and marketing, parents can be successfully recruited to participate, and that the content of a program such as Guiding Good Choices is found to be acceptable to most parents. Furthermore, the program appears to strengthen parental family management practices that are critical for enhancing protective factors and reducing risk factors for adolescent substance use.

Project Towards No Drug Abuse

Project Towards No Drug Abuse (Project TND) is an example of an intervention that can be classified as both a selective and an indicated prevention program (Sussman, Dent, & Stacy, 2002). The program is designed for the heterogeneous population of high school youth, ages 14–19, who may or may not have prior experience with substance use and violence. In three experimental trials, Project TND has been tested in both traditional and alternative high schools in southern California. At 1-year (Sussman et al., 2002) and 2-year (Sussman, Sun, McCuller, & Dent, 2003b) follow-up assessments, reductions in cigarette smoking, alcohol use, marijuana use, hard drug use, and victimization have been detected in these trials. (The investigators defined a "hard" drug as any one of the following: cocaine/ crack, hallucinogens, stimulants, inhalants, depressants, PCP, steroids, heroin, etc.)

The conceptual framework of Project TND is the Motivation–Skills–Decision-Making Model (Sussman, 1996). This model proposes that teenage problem behavior such as drug use arises from deficits in three classes of variables. The motivational deficits that are viewed to instigate teen drug use are (1) believing that drug use is not wrong, (2) misunderstanding the effects of drugs, and (3) possessing a desire to use them. Skill deficits, which decrease the likelihood of bonding with lower-risk peer groups, include poorly developed social conversation skills and weak self-control. Third, problems with rational decision making comprise a distinct set of deficits.

The current Project TND curriculum consists of a set of 12 40-minute interactive sessions for the high school classroom (Sussman et al., 2002). The goals of these sessions are to teach active listening skills, challenge stereotypes that drug use is the norm among teens, debunk various myths about drug use, learn about the consequences of substance dependence, teach ways to deal with stress and the importance of health as a means of achieving life goals, learn skills for bolstering self-control and assertiveness, learn how to avoid unproductive ways of thinking, encourage the adoption of more conservative views on drug use, and make a personal commitment to about drug use. Rather than using a lecture format in class, the teaching of these topics relies heavily on prescribed interactive activities, including role plays, mock talk shows, and games (Sussman, Rohrbach, Patel, & Holiday, 2003a).

The first randomized trial of Project TND involved 21 continuation (or alternative) high schools assigned to one of three conditions: a nine-session classroom curriculum combined with a school-led extracurricular-activities component, the nine-session curriculum by itself, and a "standard care" control (Sussman, Dent, Stacy, & Craig, 1998). In California, continuation high schools serve students who are unable to remain in the traditional high school setting because of conduct problems related to poor attendance, academic underachievement, drug use, and so on. At 1-year follow-up (Sussman et al., 1998), it was found that compared to those in the control schools, the students in both of the intervention conditions had 25% lower rate of hard drug use and a 21% lower rate of weapon carrying. Among males in the intervention conditions, there was a 23% reduction in being a victim of violence. Furthermore, among students who were using alcohol at baseline, there was a 7% decrease in alcohol use. Project TND did not appear to have an impact on either cigarette use or marijuana use (Sussman et al., 1998). The school-led extracurricular-activities component did not appear to offer any protective benefit to students above and beyond that provided by the classroom curricula at the 1-year follow-up.

A long-term evaluation also was conducted of the nine-session Project TND trial (Sun, Skara, Sun, Dent, & Sussman, in press). At 5-year follow-up, no intervention effects were detected for 30-day use of cigarettes, alcohol, or marijuana. However, there was approximately a 50% decrease in the 30-day rate of hard drug use among the students who received the classroom-only intervention and about an 80% reduction in the 30-day rate of hard drug use among those students who had received the classroom-plus-extracurricular-activities component. The investigators speculate that hard drug use may be more amenable to intervention because compared to tobacco, alcohol, and marijuana, use of these substances is viewed as more immediately dangerous (Sun et al., in press).

A second Project TND trial tested the program in three regular high schools in California (Dent, Sussman, & Stacy, 2001). Within each school, classrooms were assigned to either the nine-session TND curriculum or a no-treatment control condition. The results paralleled those found in the first trial. At 1-year follow-up, hard drug use was reduced by 25% and alcohol use was reduced by 12% in the baseline users. Among males, weapon carrying was reduced by 19% and being a victim of violence was reduced by 17%. Cigarette and marijuana use did not appear to be reduced by the TND curriculum.

In the third Project TND trial, the curriculum was expanded to 12 sessions (Sussman et al., 2002; Sussman et al., 2003b). The new sessions were added to better address tobacco and marijuana use as well as violence prevention. A total of 18 alternative high schools were assigned to one of three conditions: the 12-session TND classroom curriculum, a self-instructed TND curriculum, or control. The findings of this trial revealed that the teacher-led TND curriculum reduced substance use and violence at both a 1-year (Sussman et al., 2002) and a 2-year (Sussman et al., 2003b) follow-up assessment (the self-instruction version did not reduce substance use or violence relative to the control condition). At 1-year follow-up, a 27% reduction in cigarette use was observed followed by other reductions of 26% for hard drug use, 22% for marijuana use, and 9% for alcohol use among baseline users (Sussman et al., 2002). Furthermore, a 6% decrease in being a victim of violence was observed among males and a 37% decrease in weapon carrying was detected in baseline non-weapon-carrying students. At 2-year follow-up, the reductions in substance use associated with having been exposed to the teacher-led program appeared to increase further: cigarette use, 50%; hard drug use, 80%; alcohol use, 13%. Marijuana use was reduced by 88% in the subsample of male students who never used the drug at baseline (Sussman et al., 2003b). Though Project TND needs further testing in other populations, these findings indicate that school-based curricula can be developed and used to prevent substance use and violence in high school students. In addition, the results suggest that classroom interactivity is a critical feature of effective substance abuse curricula (Sussman et al., 2003a).

Research to Practice: The Challenges of Dissemination and Implementation

Unfortunately, the transfer of research findings to practice is a relatively slow process. To assess the extent of this problem in the United States, Ennett et al. (2003) studied the prevention practices of middle school program providers in 1999. The 1,795 providers were selected from a national sample of public and private middle schools. The investigators administered surveys to these personnel after determining that they were the person most knowledgeable about the substance abuse program in their middle school. The assessment compared the substance use prevention practices in place in the schools against standards previous research has determined necessary for effective curriculum content and delivery.

The findings of this study highlighted the limited extent to which prevention research findings had been disseminated or transferred to the nation's schools (Ennett et al., 2003). For instance, in 1999, only 35% of the middle school providers reported that they had implemented an evidence-based prevention program at their school ("evidence-based programs" were identified by using criteria established by organizations such as SAMHSA [2004]). A majority of the providers were found to teach effective content (62%), but only a small proportion used effective delivery (17%), and even a smaller percentage relied on both effective content and delivery (14%). The providers most likely to have implemented both effective content and delivery were those who had adopted evidence-based programs, such as LST. In addition, the use of effective content and delivery methods was found to be positively related to (1) being recently trained in substance use prevention, (2) being comfortable with using interactive teaching methods in the classroom, (3) possessing a graduate degree, and (4) being female. Use of effective content and methods was not related to specific set of school capabilities, number of years the provider had been teaching substance use prevention, provider age, school status (public vs. private), school enrollment, geographic location of the school, and other variables (Ennett et al., 2003). Clearly, a great deal of works needs to be done to strengthen the prevention capacity of schools.

The Diffusion of Innovation

One way to understand the speed at which communities and schools adopt evidence-based drug prevention programming is to apply the diffusion of innovation model. According to Rogers (1995b), "an innovation is an idea, practice, or object that is perceived as new by an individual or other unit of adoption" (p. 11). The study of the diffusion of innovation has revealed that new ideas and practices are often adopted slowly, even when they appear to have advantages over traditional views and practices. As indicated previously, this is frequently the case with evidence-based prevention programming in many communities and schools.

The speed at which an innovation is adopted is thought to be influenced by five general factors: (1) the perceived attributes of the innovation; (2) the type of innovation decision; (3) the communication channels; (4) the nature of the social system, including the views of opinion leaders and community norms; and (5) promotion efforts by change agents. The specific perceived attributes that foster diffusion are the innovation's *relative advantages* over the customary practice, its *compatibility* with existing values, past experiences and needs of potential adopters, its *complexity* to use, its *trialability* or the degree to which the innovation can be experimented with on a limited basis, and its *observability* or the degree to which the effects of the innovation are visible to others (Rogers, 1995b). Adoption decisions that depend on an individual making a decision generally speed up diffusion of innovation, whereas adoption decisions that requires a large number of stakeholders in a community, school, or organization to decide slows down diffusion. Furthermore, when diffusion depends on interpersonal communication channels, it will generally occur more quickly than when it depends on mass media. In social systems in which the views of opinion leaders and the norms of the community support change, innovation is more likely to occur. Finally, the intensity of change agents' efforts to promote the adoption of an innovation may make it more likely to occur. Figure 3.6 depicts these factors as they apply to the decision to adopt a new drug prevention program in a community.

The Politics of Diffusion: DARE and the School Superintendent

Schools throughout the United States have been confronted with the decision whether to replace Drug Abuse Resistance Education (DARE), a popular but ineffective prevention program (Ennett et al., 1994; Lynam et al., 1999). By the mid-1990s, DARE's continuing popularity, despite its lack of empirical support, had already drawn the attention of a number of investigators and social critics interested in the diffusion of evidence-based drug prevention programs (e.g., Clayton, Leukefeld, Harrington, & Cattarello,

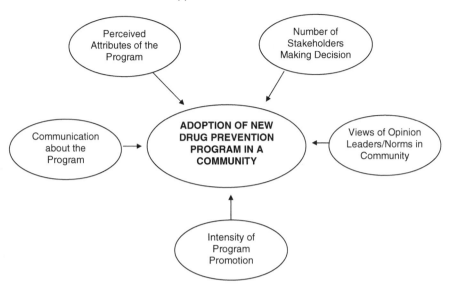

FIGURE 3.6. Factors determining adoption of new drug prevention programs.

1996; Elliot, 1995). Thus, in more recent years, the pressure to replace DARE with an evidence-based program kept increasing as the reviews conducted by the SAMHSA (2004), the U.S. Department of Education (2001), and NIDA (2003) failed to identify it as a model program, or even a promising one.

In most communities, the public school superintendent is an important opinion leader on school-based drug prevention practices. As the senior school district official, superintendents are expected to provide leadership on issues affecting students' academic performance, health, and safety. These officials also are significant change agents who can wield considerable influence on a school district's approach to drug abuse prevention, if they choose to do so.

Thus, in a study I conducted with a colleague, we examined the specific role of the public school superintendent in the decision to keep or replace DARE (Thombs & Ray-Tomasek, 2001). The specific aim of the study was to explain superintendents' intentions toward future reliance on the DARE program. In June 2000, we mailed an anonymous survey to all 611 superintendents in the state of Ohio (response rate was 71%). At that time, we found that DARE was used by 85%–87% of the state's public school districts. A large majority of the superintendents (88%) reported that they intended to continue using the program in the future. Most of the superintendents held either incorrect knowledge about DARE's effectiveness in deterring substance use (29%) or acknowledged that they were uniformed about DARE outcome research (34%).

Results from a multivariate analysis indicated that the intention to use DARE in the future was positively associated with the superintendent's beliefs about community support for the program and negatively associated with perceptions of their ability to replace drug prevention curricula in their district. Perhaps most troubling was the finding that accurate knowledge of the research on DARE outcomes had no relationship to intentions toward DARE, suggesting that these school officials do not use research findings as a guide for making decisions about prevention programming. Overall, the findings suggested that superintendents' positive intentions toward continued use of DARE were formed to avert conflict with adults in the school district and community (Thombs & Ray-Tomasek, 2001). This study provides some insight into the challenges of adopting evidence-based programs.

COMMUNITY COALITION BUILDING

During the past 20 years, coalition building has become a common grassroots response to public health problems in communities throughout the United States (Kreuter, Lezin, & Young, 2000; Wolff, 2001a). There are many reasons for the rise of the community coalition. Recent interest comes from the increasing recognition that problems such as substance abuse do not result only from characteristics within the individual but are instigated and maintained by conditions in the community as well (Kreuter et al., 2000; Wolff, 2001a). Interest in coalitions also comes from (1) the shift of responsibility for health and social problems from the federal government to state and local levels; (2) the societal expectation that these problems will be adequately addressed with fewer resources; (3) the widespread belief that health and human service systems are too bureaucratic to adequately address community needs; and (4) the hope that volunteer work in coalitions will restore civic engagement in the United States (Wolff, 2001a).

Though not well documented, public health officials and other community practitioners typically report that the process of coalition building is not well understood, and that the many coalition success stories are probably matched by a comparable number of failures (Wolff, 2001b). However, according to Wolff (2001a), it also is possible to identify a number of functional features of effective community coalitions (see Table 3.7).

The research base on community coalitions is limited at this time. The systematic studies that have been conducted raise questions about their potential to have a positive impact on public health problems, such as sub-

TABLE 3.7. Seven Functional Features of Effective Community Coalitions

1. *Holistic and comprehensive.* Breadth allows a community to address those issues that it believes are a priority.

2. *Flexible and responsive.* Adaptability allows a coalition to respond to emerging needs and sudden threats.

3. *Build a sense of community.* The coalition serves as a recognized forum for problem solving in a community.

4. *Build and enhance citizen engagement in community life.* The coalition promotes civic engagement and connectedness.

5. *Provide a vehicle for community empowerment.* The coalition creates the capacity to impact a problem.

6. *Allow diversity to be valued and celebrated as a foundation for the wholeness of the community.* The coalition can assist with finding common ground on issues that generate conflict.

7. *Serve as an incubator for innovative solutions to large problems facing not only their community, but also the nation as a whole.* The coalition can challenge government and other established institutions to think differently about a problem.

Note. Data from Wolff (2001a).

stance abuse (e.g., Green & Kreuter, 2002; Hallfors, Cho, Livert, & Kadushin, 2002). One problem may be the insistence of funding agencies that community initiatives adopt "best practices," as identified by past research conducted in different locations and/or with different populations. Unfortunately, these so-called best practices may not be well suited for a specific community or culture. Conversely, community initiatives can make the mistake of ignoring research altogether in favor of its own unproven, "homegrown" intervention (Green & Kreuter, 2002, p. 305). These problems reveal the complexities of public health interventions that rely on community collaboration.

In one comprehensive review of the research literature, Kreuter et al. (2000) found that only 6 of 68 published studies reported that a coalition or consortium produced a positive health status or health system change. Based on the descriptions found in these 68 studies, the investigators concluded that there were three overlapping, possible explanations for the lack of positive coalition outcomes: "(1) Collaborative mechanisms are inefficient and/or insufficient mechanisms for carrying out planning and implementation tasks. (2) Expectations of health status/health systems change outcomes are unrealistic. (3) Health status/health systems change may occur but may go undetected because it is difficult to demonstrate a cause-and-effect relationship" (Kreuter et al., 2000, p. 52). These conclusions should not be considered the definitive and final word on community coalition building. However, they should be sobering to those who advocate for coalitions as a means of changing community conditions that promote substance abuse.

RESULTS FROM COMMUNITY INTERVENTION TRIALS

Increasing Cessation among Adult Smokers

The COMMIT Trial

Although the prevalence of cigarette smoking among Americans steadily dropped in the 1980s (CDC, 1987), to reduce morbidity and mortality associated with tobacco use there was a need to identify ways to assist adult smokers to quit. Thus, in 1986, the National Cancer Institute funded the Community Intervention Trial for Smoking Cessation, known more simply as the COMMIT Trial (COMMIT Research Group, 1995a, 1995b). The large randomized trial involved 10 matched pairs of communities in the United States and one pair in Canada (within each pair, one community was randomly assigned to the intervention). The research design of the trial relied on rigorous, state-of-the-art methods to test the following hypothesis: "a defined intervention, delivered through multiple community sectors and organizations over a 4-year period and using limited external resources, would result in higher quit rates among heavy cigarette smokers in the intervention communities than in the comparison communities" (COMMIT Research Group, 1995a, p. 184). The trial was based on a collaborative conceptual framework that sought to bring together diverse organizations, institutions, and individuals for the purpose of conducting smoking cessation activities in the community. This framework was based on the premise that a comprehensive community-based strategy would decrease the likelihood that adult smokers could avoid exposure to cessation messages and opportunities for quitting smoking.

The COMMIT Trial was carried out in communities with populations ranging from 49,421 to 251,208 residents (COMMIT Research Group, 1995a). Prior to implementation, a community board, comprised of key community representatives, was formed in each community. These boards had responsibility for overseeing the implementation of COMMIT in their communities. The intervention activities were implemented via four channels, including (1) public education delivered by media and at community events, (2) health care providers, (3) workplaces and other organizations, and (4) smoking cessation resources. The intervention protocol required that 58 activities had to be implemented in each of the intervention communities. Systematic monitoring indicated that across the 11 intervention communities, the mean attainment rates for implementing intervention activities was 90%–93%. Optional intervention activities also were encouraged to allow for variability in community needs.

In each community, about 550 light-to-moderate smokers (1–24 cigarettes per day) and 550 heavy smokers (25 or more cigarettes per day) were
randomly selected at baseline and tracked over the 4-year trial (COMMIT
Research Group, 1995a). All these smokers were 25 to 64 years of age. The
data collected from the two cohorts of 10,328 light-to-moderate smokers
and 10,019 heavy smokers were analyzed separately in the study.

At the end of the COMMIT trial, there was no difference between the
intervention and comparison communities on a measure of current smoking status in either the light-to-moderate smoking cohort or the heavy
smoking cohort. The observed "quit smoking" rate appeared to be mod-
estly increased by the intervention (1.8%) in the light-to-moderate smoking
cohort, but there was no observed increase on this same measure in the
heavy smoking cohort. Consistent with these findings, it was found that in
the light-to-moderate smoking cohort, the 4-year intervention appeared to
slightly reduce the "daily number of cigarettes smoked" (mean reduction of
2.7 cigarettes per day in the intervention condition). There was no significant change in daily number of cigarettes smoked in the heavy smoking
cohort. Overall, the COMMIT intervention appeared to have a small, positive impact on cigarette smoking in light-to-moderate smokers but no significant effect on heavy smokers (COMMIT Research Group, 1995a).

Profiling the "Hard-Core" Smoker

Research conducted after the COMMIT Trial sheds some light on the failure of the community-based intervention to reduce cigarette use in heavy
smokers. Emery, Gilpia, Ake, Farkas, and Pierce (2000) defined "hard-
core" smokers as those reporting that they (1) smoke at least 15 cigarettes
per day, (2) have no recent quit attempts, and (3) have no intention to quit
smoking at anytime. In a random sample of California households, these
investigators found that an estimated 1.3% of the state's population, 26
years of age or older, met criteria for being classified as a hard-core smoker
(Emery et al., 2000). This group of smokers made up 5.2% of the smoking
population (26 years of age or older). Hard-core smokers were typically
retired, white men living alone, with 12 years or less of education, and
annual income below $50,000. In addition, these smokers were distin-
guished from other smokers by being less likely to believe that (1) negative
health consequences were associated with their smoking, (2) tobacco is an
addictive drug, and (3) secondhand smoke harms other people. Compared
to other smokers, the hard-core smokers also were more likely to have
begun experimenting with smoking at a younger age and to report that they
were younger when they became regular smokers (Emery et al., 2000). This
relatively unique profile suggests that it may be unrealistic to expect some
individuals to ever quit smoking.

Neighbors for a Smoke-Free North Side

Another example of a community intervention seeking to increase smoking cessation among adult smokers was the Neighbors for a Smoke Free North Side Project (Fisher et al., 1998). The intervention sites were located in three predominately low-income neighborhoods in St. Louis. Three similar neighborhoods in Kansas City were selected as the comparison group. The intervention stressed neighborhood-based governance and resident involvement in the design of strategies to reduce smoking. Using neighborhood volunteers and paid staff members, wellness councils were established to carry out the program for a 24-month period. The program relied on smoking cessation classes, billboard advertisements, door-to-door promotion campaigns, and a "gospel fest." In 1990 and 1992, results from random-digit dial telephone surveys indicated that smoking prevalence in St. Louis declined 7% compared to only 1% in Kansas City—a difference that was statistically significant.

The investigators speculated that the Smoke Free North Side intervention was more successful than COMMIT because the former program was developed in the targeted St. Louis neighborhoods and thus may have had greater "community ownership" (Fisher et al., 1998). In contrast, COMMIT was centrally developed at the national level and then delivered to communities with only a limited number of tailoring options.

Decreasing Youth Access to Tobacco

Other community interventions have sought to restrict youth access to tobacco products. For instance, Rigotti et al. (1997) compared three communities in Massachusetts that increased enforcement of youth tobacco laws with three matched comparison communities. In the intervention communities, health departments started quarterly compliance checks with underage tobacco purchase attempts. At baseline, 68% of vendors sold to minors. The difference between the intervention and control communities was not statistically significant at baseline. At a 2-year follow-up, only 18% of the vendors in the intervention communities, compared with 55% in the comparison communities, sold tobacco to minors. Yet, three annual surveys of more than 17,600 respondents revealed only a small decrease in underage adolescents' perceived ability to purchase tobacco and no decline in tobacco use itself.

The Tobacco Policy Options for Prevention Project (TPOP) was 32-month intervention that attempted to restrict tobacco among youth through a community mobilization effort (Forster et al., 1998). This initiative centered its energy on changing local ordinances, altering retailer and other adult practices regarding the provision of tobacco to youth, and increasing the enforcement of laws that prohibit sales to underage youth. A total of 14 Minnesota communities were randomly assigned to intervention and control conditions. In June 1993 and June 1996, youth under the control of investigators attempted to purchase tobacco at all tobacco outlets in the communities.

During the trial (1993–1996), school surveys of more than 6,000 students indicated that adolescent smoking had increased in both sets of cities, but less in the intervention communities (Forster et al., 1998). It appeared that the intervention had little effect on perceptions of tobacco availability through social sources such as peers or parents, but it reduced perceived availability through commercial sources. Furthermore, in the intervention communities, purchase attempts declined significantly during the trial. In all communities in the trial, there was a large decrease in youth purchase attempts that resulted in sales, and it was not significantly greater in the intervention cities. The overall reduction in tobacco purchase success in both the intervention and the control communities was attributed by the investigators to changes in state laws that restricted youth access to tobacco, and to the increased awareness created by news reports of these changes in law that took place during the course of the trial (Forster et al., 1998).

A similar intervention program designed to bolster tobacco enforcement took place in Erie County, New York (Cummings et al., 1998). Six pairs of communities were matched on number of tobacco outlets, population size, and other demographic variables. Directed by police, underage purchase compliance checks were conducted in 366 tobacco outlets at baseline and 319 outlets at follow-up. In the intervention communities, all retailers were sent a letter about tobacco laws and sales to minors that also warned that compliance checks were planned for the area. Distribution of the letter was followed by a dramatic increase in purchase compliance in both enforcement and nonenforcement communities. Interestingly, compliance rates between the two groups of communities did not vary however. It seems that most vendors in both areas learned about the enforcement program and perceived enforcement as more vigilant in the entire region.

Gemson et al. (1998) conducted a similar trial in central Harlem (New York City). In a randomized trial of 15 tobacco vendors, retail outlets selling tobacco were randomly assigned to three conditions: enforcement, education, and control. In October 1993 and April 1994, surveys of underage tobacco purchase compliance were conducted in the community. During both surveys, violators from the outlets in the enforcement condition only were fined (in accordance with the state law). At 6-month follow-up, underage sales had declined 56% among enforcement outlets, 34% among education outlets, and 16% among control stores (Gemson et al., 1998).

Decreasing Youth Access to Alcohol

Another community intervention was designed to decrease the availability of alcohol to youth. At the University of Minnesota, Wagenaar et al. (2000a) have developed and tested a community intervention known as Communities Mobilizing for Change on Alcohol. This community-organizing project aimed to reduce the number of outlets selling alcohol to underage youth and restrict the availability of alcohol to youth through noncommercial sources, such as peers and parents. A total of 15 communities were randomly assigned to intervention and comparison conditions. A leadership strategy team worked to strengthen numerous policies, procedures, and practices in the intervention communities. Community action was pursued through public and private organizations including: city councils, school and enforcement agencies, alcohol merchants, business associations, and the media.

Several assessments were made to evaluate the project. Approximately 4,500 12th graders were surveyed in 1992 and 1995. In addition, a telephone survey of 3,095 18- to 20-year-olds was conducted in 1992 and repeated in 1995. Also, during the same years, alcohol purchase compliance checks, using study confederates who appeared underage, were conducted at more than 25 off-sale outlets.

Relative to the communities in the comparison condition, those in the intervention condition showed a 17% greater rate of checking age identification of youthful-looking purchasers and a 24% lower rate of sales to potential underage purchasers at bars and restaurants. Furthermore, in the intervention communities, there was a 25% decrease in the proportion of older teens providing alcohol to younger teens, and a 7% decrease in underage respondents who reported drinking in the previous 30-day period. There also was a statistically significant decrease in DUI (driving under the influence) arrests among 18- to 20-year-olds (Wagenaar, Murray, & Toomey, 2000b).

Community-Based Prevention for Youth

The Midwestern Prevention Project

Several community interventions have been tested for their ability to delay the onset of substance use among adolescents with no history of use and to decrease use in adolescents who have previous experience with one or more drugs. The Midwestern Prevention Project (MPP) attempted to deter cigarette, alcohol, and marijuana use among 10- to 14-year-olds in two U.S. cities: Kansas City, Missouri, and Indianapolis, Indiana. A quasi-experimental design in Kansas City (Pentz et al., 1989) and a randomized experimental design in Indianapolis (Chou et al., 1998) evaluated the program. From

September 1984 to January 1986, the Kansas City students received a 10-session training program that included skills for resisting substance use, homework exercises relying on interviews of others, and role plays with parents and family. Most students interviewed parents and family members about family rules on substance use, effective techniques for avoiding use, and how to deal with media and community influences. Among other activities, teen participants also made statements of public commitments to avoid tobacco, alcohol, and other drug use, practiced role playing of resistance skills, and discussed homework results.

Among the 42 schools in the MPP trial, 4 were randomly assigned to the intervention condition and 4 to the control condition (Pentz et al., 1989). The remaining 34 schools were assigned based on their willingness to participate—20 were willing, 14 were not. School willingness may have been associated with perceptions that substance abuse was or was not a high-priority concern in the school. The 20 willing schools received the intervention, increasing the total number of intervention schools to 24 (18 schools served as controls).

At 1-year follow-up, students in the intervention condition reported lower rates for all three drugs compared to those in the control condition: 17% versus 24% for cigarette use, 11% versus 16% for alcohol use, 7% versus 16% for marijuana use. Although cigarette, alcohol, and marijuana use had increased in both groups of schools, two years after the program, the increases for these three substances were significantly lower in the intervention group. This finding provides evidence that the MPP effects were sustained, at least for 2 years following the intervention (Pentz et al., 1989).

Chou et al. (1998) implemented and evaluated the MPP in Indianapolis by tracking 1,904 students in intervention schools and 1,508 students in control schools. The schools were randomly assigned to these conditions, and after baseline, student follow-up assessments were conducted at 6 months, 1½ years, 2½ years, and 3½ years. After statistically adjusting for ethnicity, gender, socioeconomic status, father's occupation, and school type and grade, the researchers discovered that among those adolescents who had a baseline history of tobacco, alcohol, or other drug use, alcohol use had been decreased at the 6-month and 1½-year follow-ups and for tobacco use at 6-month follow-up only. Results for marijuana use were not consistent over time.

Project Northland

Located in Minnesota, Project Northland was designed to reduce alcohol use among preteens and younger adolescents (Perry et al., 1996). The intervention was community based but had a significant school component. A 3-year behavioral curriculum was provided to sixth, seventh, and eight graders that emphasized peer leadership, parental involvement, and community task force activities. The program taught students to resist negative peer influence and sought to instill conservative norms about the use of alcohol. In addition, students learned about methods to bring about community social, political, and institutional change in alcohol-related programs and policies. Students interviewed parents, local government officials, law enforcement personnel, retail alcohol merchants, schoolteachers, and administrators to learn about their views and activities relative to teenage drinking. Students also conducted "town meetings" and developed recommendations for community action to deter adolescent drinking.

Project Northland also organized community task forces to press for passage of local ordinances to prevent sales of alcohol to minors and intoxicated patrons of drinking establishments (Perry et al., 1996). The task forces consisted of government officials, law enforcement personnel, school representatives, health professionals, youth workers, parents, concerned citizens, and teenagers. In addition, students who pledged to be alcohol and drug free were eligible for discounts at local businesses.

At baseline, 2,351 students were surveyed in Project Northland (Perry et al., 1996). The investigators were able to obtain 2-year follow-up rates greater than 80% in both the intervention and control groups. At baseline, a higher percentage of students in the intervention group were alcohol users. However, at follow-up, the proportions of students that had used alcohol in the past week and past month were lower in the intervention group than in the control group. The intervention effects of Project Northland appeared to be greatest (and statistically significant) among students with no history of alcohol use at baseline. The intervention did not reduce cigarette smoking or marijuana use in the participating youth (Perry et al., 1996).

Reducing Impaired Driving and Alcohol-Related Injuries and Deaths in the General Population

Community Prevention Trial Program

Two community interventions have attempted to reduce alcohol-related injuries and deaths in the general population. The Community Prevention Trial Program was a 5-year project designed to decrease the number of alcohol-related injuries and death in three experimental communities (Holder 1997; Holder et al., 2000). The model for this intervention relied on five reinforcing components to change individual behavior by changing the environmental, social, and structural contexts of drinking in the community. The first component of the intervention model was community mobilization. Local residents were organized to press for public policy change. These efforts increased general awareness and concern about alcohol-related trauma. In each community, the media, mobilization and intervention activities had specific objectives tailored to their needs. The second component of the intervention model was responsible beverage service. This component attempted to reduce sales to intoxicated patrons in drinking establishments and to strengthen local enforcement of alcohol-control laws by collaborating with restaurants, bars, and hotel associations; beverage wholesalers; and the Alcohol Beverage Control Commission. The third component of the intervention was a drinking and driving component to improve traffic safety. This component sought to increase the number of DWI (drinking while intoxicated) arrests in the community through officer training, use of passive alcohol sensors (at DWI checkpoints), and media-publicized sobriety checkpoints. The fourth intervention component was a media advocacy initiative. These efforts attempted to focus news attention on underage drinking, enforcement of underage sales laws, and training of personnel to prevent alcohol sales to minors. The fifth intervention component sought to reduce alcohol outlet density through local zoning regulations.

The Community Prevention Trial Program relied on a quasi-experimental design to evaluate the effects of each intervention component in intervention and comparison communities as well as the overall project effects on alcohol-related injuries (Holder et al., 2000). During the trial, local regulation of alcohol outlets and public sites for drinking were altered in all three experimental communities. Furthermore, compliance checks at 150 outlets revealed a significant decrease in successful alcohol purchases by youth.

Holder et al. (2000) found that the DWI intervention component produced increased news coverage about drinking and driving, heightened police enforcement, and increased their use of roadside breath-testing equipment. Data collected via telephone surveys indicated a significant increase in the perceived likelihood of DWI arrest and a decrease in the self-reported frequency of driving and drinking. Data collected at roadside surveys corroborated the reduction in driving after drinking found in the telephone survey. Most important, alcohol-related crashes, as measured by single-vehicle night crashes, fell by 10–11% in the intervention communities, and alcohol-related trauma visits to emergency departments declined by 43% in the intervention communities.

Massachusetts Saving Lives Program

The Massachusetts Saving Lives Program was a comprehensive community intervention designed to reduce drinking and driving and alcohol-involved traffic deaths (Hingson, McGover, Howland, & Hereen, 1996). The intervention began in 1988 and ended in 1993. A competitive proposal process was used to select six program communities for the trial. The six intervention communities were compared with five matched communities that also submitted applications but were not funded. The remaining communities of Massachusetts served as a comparison group as well. Outcome data were collected for the period 5 years before and after the intervention.

From the mayor's office in each intervention community, a full-time coordinator organized a task force of private citizens and organizations and public officials. Each year, the intervention communities received approximately $1 per inhabitant in program funds. One-half of these funds supported the program coordinator. The balance provided for increased law enforcement, other program activities, and educational materials. The intervention also encouraged citizens to volunteer their time to program activity. In each intervention community, active task force participation ranged from 20 to 100 individuals, and about 50 organizations participated in each of these cities (Hingson et al., 1996).

In the Massachusetts Saving Lives Program, the intervention communities were responsible for developing most of the program activities. Communities adopted such objectives as reduce alcohol-impaired driving, speeding, "running" red lights, failing to yield to pedestrians in crosswalks, and failing to use seat belts. To address the problems of drinking and driving and speeding, intervention communities implemented media campaigns, sobriety checkpoints on roadways, speed-watch telephone hotlines, alcohol-free prom nights, beer keg registration, police surveillance of alcohol outlets, and a number of other activities. To address the problems of pedestrian safety and seat belt use, intervention communities conducted media campaigns and police checkpoints, posted crosswalk signs warning motorists of fines for failure to yield, increased the number of crosswalk guards at schools, and other activities (Hingson et al., 1996). The effects of the Massachusetts Saving Lives Program were positive. For example, among drivers under the age 20, the proportion reporting driving after drinking in random-digit-dialing telephone surveys decreased from 19% in the first year of the trial to 9% in subsequent years. In the comparison cities, there was little change on this measure. A 7% increase in seat belt use was observed in the intervention cities, a significantly greater increase than found in the comparison cities. Fatal motor vehicle crashes declined from 178 during the 5 preintervention years to 120 during the 5 intervention years, representing a 25% greater reduction than existed in the remainder of the state. Moreover, fatal crashes involving alcohol decreased by 42%, and the number of fatally injured drivers with positive blood alcohol levels was reduced by 47% compared to the rest of the state. The evaluation found that all six of the intervention cities had greater decreases in fatal and alcohol-related fatal crashes than did the comparison cities or the rest of the state (Hingson et al., 1996).

Lessons Learned about Community Interventions

Four conclusions can be drawn from this review of comprehensive community interventions. First, most of the trials reviewed here produced reductions in substance abuse and related problems (e.g., drinking and driving) and/or increased protective actions in the community (e.g., refusing alcohol sales to minors). These findings indicate that community interventions can be designed to effectively address substance abuse problems. Second, though community interventions have the potential to produce far-reaching effects, including an impact on high-risk, "hard-to-reach" groups, the *size* of the effects generated from these interventions is often relatively small. For instance, the MPP reduced adolescent alcohol use by an estimated 5% (Pentz et al., 1989). Thus, it becomes a matter of judgment as to whether the costs of an intervention are justified when the effect size is not large. Third, the design of the interventions reviewed here suggests that positive outcomes depend on combining community mobilization and local policy change with public education and awareness activities (Hingson & Howland, 2002). Sole reliance on substance abuse education and awareness activities does not seem to be adequate community prevention strategy. Fourth, interventions that can somehow foster and promote community collaboration, input, and ownership seem to be more likely to succeed than those interventions that are imported from outside the community.

THE PARTICIPATORY RESEARCH APPROACH

In the field of public health, there has long been a tension between researchers, who believe it necessary to investigate research questions, and practitioners and citizens, who favor action, community development, and possibly social change. These tensions have led to appeals to better serve the needs of community members by treating them more as research "users" than merely as research "subjects." On this point, Brownson, Baker, and Kreuter (2001) commented: "It is recognized increasingly that effective research in communities should be conducted *with* and *in* communities rather *on* communities" (p. vii). Thus, researchers have been challenged to be more attentive to the application of research findings, their dissemination, and the formulation of best-practice guidelines for practitioners. It is in this context that the concept of "participatory research" has become a dominant theme in public health practice in recent years (Green & Mercer, 2001).

Participatory research is not a specific research method but, rather, a mind-set and an approach that attempts to engage all potential users of the research in the community (and possibly elsewhere, e.g., state health department) in the generation of the research questions and the implementation of the research itself (Green et al., 1995). The core beliefs of the participatory research approach are that public health research can be (1) sensitive to unique circumstances in a specific locale, (2) under local control, (3) trusted to communities and involve collective decision making, and (4) conducted without compromising the quality of the evaluation (Brownson et al., 2001; Mercer, MacDonald, & Green, 2004). A range of participatory research exists, such that any specific community's participation in public health research will vary by project (Green & Mercer, 2001). Maximum community participation would involve collaborating with stakeholders to identify research questions, select research methods, and assist in data analysis and interpretation and the application of findings. Minimum community participation is limited to formative work at the beginning of a research project and to interpretation and application at the end of an investigation. Proponents argue that integrating stakeholder values into the design of participatory research projects does not compromise the scientific integrity of the study and its evaluation.

Though U.S. government funding for participatory research has been limited thus far, the approach has shown promise (Frankish et al., 1997; Langton, 1995; Mercer et al., 2004; Minkler & Wallerstein, 2003). This optimism is based on the democratic and inclusive values that are implicit in the approach. Nevertheless, at this point, significant questions remain about (1) the extent to which communities are interested in, and capable of, participating in public health research and (2) the potential of this research process to produce knowledge that has generalizibility and usefulness beyond the specific community or communities in which it was applied (Green et al., 1995).

THE COMMUNITY MOBILIZATION APPROACH

Wagenaar, Gehan, Jones-Webb, Toomey, and Forster (1999) have outlined a *process* for mobilizing communities to take action to change local institutional polices on substance abuse issues. The seven stages identified in Table 3.8 are not sequential sets of activities. During a mobilization effort, there typically is ongoing work in other stages, but perhaps at a lower level of intensity, when the focus turns to a new stage. Action and vigor characterize community organizing. Wagenaar et al. (1999) describe the functions of the organizers at each stage as "advising, teaching, modeling, persuading, selling, agitating, facilitating, coaching, confidence-building, guiding, mobilizing, inspiring, educating, and leading" (p. 317).

Both the community mobilization model and the participatory research model recognize the need for collaborative work and community

TABLE 3.8. A Community Organizing Process for Changing Local Institutional Policy

1. *Comprehensive assessment of community interests, needs, and resources.* What is the range of perceptions on various tobacco, alcohol, and other drug problems? Who wields power on these issues in the community? Who are likely supporters and opponents of local policy changes? What arguments should be anticipated from opponents of a policy change? Where do the self-interests of various stakeholders collide with potential policy changes?

2. *Establishing a core group of support.* Who supports local policy change? Who is connected to a network of potential supporters? How do we find supporters from diverse public and private sectors of the community?

3. *Development of an action plan.* Which local policy or policies do we work to change? How do we develop a consensus on identifying a policy for change? Do we focus on one policy at a time or on multiple policies? Are we willing to develop an action plan that may be perceived to be controversial in some circles in the community?

4. *Expanding the base of support for the action plan.* What activities should the core group implement to build broad support for the action plan? (write letters, mass mailings, making phone calls, one-to-one negotiating, public speaking, working with news media, etc.)

5. *Implementation of the action plan.* What specific strategies do we need to secure changes in local policy? When do we propose policy change to various public and private groups?

6. *Maintaining the effort and institutionalizing it.* How do we continue this work without grant support? Where can we find other sources of funding?

7. *Evaluating and disseminating the results of the community mobilization effort.* What are the outcomes of our work? Who are the stakeholders that need to have knowledge of these outcomes?

Note. Data from Wagenaar, Gehan, Jones-Webb, Toomey, and Forster (1999).

input. However, the community mobilization model is the more strategic and targeted approach; the investigator determines the specific aims of the research and these goals may not be the highest health priorities in the community. In contrast, the participatory research model is more egalitarian and allows communities to set the priorities and decide the direction of the research to best meet their needs. Although this latter emphasis may present communities with special opportunities, and thus at first appear to be an obvious advantage of the participatory research model, it should be kept in mind that substance abuse problems may become secondary or even low priorities in comprehensive initiatives seeking to enhance public and community health. For example, Green (1992), a proponent of participatory research, has suggested that alcohol abuse would seldom if ever be identified by a community as its number-one health problem. The community mobilization model might be more appropriate for public health problems that require the community to be *coaxed* to address.

CURRENT U.S. DRUG CONTROL POLICY
AND THE PROSPECTS OF A PUBLIC HEALTH APPROACH

Historically, the federal government of the United States has spent most of its drug control dollars on interdiction and law enforcement with substantially smaller amounts of funds directed to prevention and treatment (Haaga & Reuter, 1995; U.S. Office of National Drug Control Policy, 2004). The public health approaches to substance use and abuse described in this chapter generally challenge this traditional approach to drug control policy. How would U.S. drug control policy change if it were based on a public health framework? According to Des Jarlais (2000), there would be five significant changes in how the United States would go about addressing problems in tobacco, alcohol, and other drug use.

First, instead of relying on historical precedents, cultural biases, and emotion, *scientific knowledge* would be used as the foundation for developing drug control policy. This knowledge base would be multidisciplinary, depending on such diverse disciplines as neuroscience, behavioral science, and epidemiology. Furthermore, Des Jarlais (2000) notes that this would require the recognition that psychoactive drug use (broadly defined) is nearly a universal human experience rather than the deviant conduct of a small segment of the population. Second, heavy emphasis would be placed on the *prevention* of substance use, particularly the primary prevention of cigarette smoking. Decisions to adopt prevention programs would rest on evidence-based criteria. Third, there would be a shift in public policy so that *treatment* would become the primary method for addressing problems of illicit drug abuse. Arrest and incarceration would be deemphasized as a means for dealing with active illicit drug users. Fourth, *harm-reduction strategies* (see Chapter 10) would be adopted by communities to help active users protect themselves from modifiable risks and to possibly motivate them to move toward abstinence. Fifth, the development of a drug-control policy would explicitly *consider the potential benefits* of some forms of psychoactive drug use in some situations. This change in policy development may reduce the likelihood of adopting unrealistic policies and initiatives that if implemented, could have unintended consequences (Des Jarlais, 2000).

Obviously, the near-term prospects of the United States turning to public health approaches for dealing with substance use and abuse problems are not good, particularly those approaches that seek to address illegal drug use. Higher levels of enthusiasm exist for public health approaches that are directed to preventing tobacco, alcohol, and other drug use in youth. However, for the foreseeable future, illegal drug use will almost certainly continue to be defined as a law enforcement problem in this country.

Why is it not likely that law enforcement-driven policies will be supplanted by those based on public health concepts? Among the impediments is a fear of pleasure (Des Jarlais, 2000). Throughout U.S. history, the widespread ambivalence about the experience of pleasure has been the fuel for drug regulation and prohibition. Another obstacle to a public health approach is simply the fear of change. Many citizens underestimate the hazards of some current forms of legal drug use, such as cigarette smoking, and possibly overestimate the dangers of some types of drug use that are currently illegal, such as marijuana use as an adjunct to cancer chemotherapy. Misplaced moral judgments also serve as hindrances to adopting a public health model (Des Jarlais, 2000). The tendency to condemn the drug user is well ingrained in U.S. culture. Finally, the widespread adoption of public health approaches could threaten the economic status quo of U.S. industries (e.g., tobacco companies) that benefit from either the manufacture of legal drugs or the incarceration of illicit drug users (Des Jarlais, 2000).

REVIEW QUESTIONS

1. What is the focus of public health and how is it different from medicine?

2. What were public health problems of colonial America?

3. What was the sanitary movement?

4. What were the important developments in public health field in the 20th century?

5. What were the great achievement public health achievements of the 20th century?

6. What are the competing visions of public health in the United States?

7. How can the triad model of causation be applied to substance abuse and dependence?

8. What is Healthy People 2010 and what are the national health priorities on tobacco, alcohol, and other drug use?

9. What is the purpose of public health surveillance of substance use?

10. What are examples of national surveillance systems on substance use and abuse?

11. From a prevention perspective, why is age of onset an important issue?

12. What is the gateway sequence?

13. Does existing scientific evidence support the view that marijuana use is a gateway to other illegal drug use?

14. What are the three types of prevention programs?

15. Have prevention programs been shown to reduce substance use in youth?

16. What are the different features and target populations of LifeSkills Training, Guiding Good Choices, and Project Towards No Drug Abuse?

17. How rapidly do schools adopt evidence-based prevention programs?

18. What factors influence the diffusion of prevention programs and what influence might school superintendents have on decisions about adopting new programs?

19. Does the research literature support the use of community coalitions to address substance abuse problems in the community?

20. What has been learned about increasing cessation among adult smokers in the community?

21. What approaches have been used to decrease youth access to tobacco and alcohol?

22. What were the major outcomes of the Midwestern Prevention Project and Project Northland?

23. What were the major outcomes of the Community Prevention Trial Program and the Massachusetts Saving Lives Program?

24. Overall, what lessons have been learned from community interventions seeking to reduce substance use and abuse?

25. What is the participatory research approach and how is it different from the community mobilization approach?

26. What are the prospects in the United States for a drug-control policy based on public health concepts?

Toward an Understanding of Comorbidity

Historically, the classification of mental disorders by the psychiatric profession was driven by a desire to identify discrete, independent illnesses (Faraone, Tsuang, & Tsuang, 1999). Although comorbidity was recognized, early versions of the American Psychiatric Association's *Diagnostic and Statistical Manual of Mental Disorders* (DSM) encouraged diagnostic hierarchies that focused attention on a "primary" disorder while assigning less clinical significance to the "secondary" disorder, and frequently substance abuse or dependence was considered the secondary disorder. However, as a result of epidemiological research (reviewed later) as well as clinical experience, the emphasis on hierarchical approaches to diagnosis and treatment gradually waned (Mueser, Noordsy, Drake, & Fox, 2003).

Today the co-occurrence of substance use disorders with other psychiatric conditions is recognized as a pervasive feature of the mental health problems experienced in the general population and in clinical samples. In part, the comorbidity of substance abuse, and severe mental illness specifically, can be traced to the deinstitutionalization movement that began in the United States in the 1960s and continued through the 1980s (American Hospital Association, 1995). Prior to the 1960s, persons with severe mentally illness (typically schizophrenia) were confined indefinitely in state psychiatric facilities. Now they are treated in community-based programs and thus are often left unprotected from the dangers of street life, including alcohol and illicit drugs. As Drake and Wallach (1999) have observed, "Like homelessness itself, a comorbid substance use disorder is an unintended consequence of a deinstitutionalization policy that paid more attention to closing hospitals than to providing affordable housing that is also safe from the predators of urban street culture" (p. 589). Thus, the co-occurrence of substance abuse and *severe* mental illness has become an obvious public health problem in the United States (Dickey & Azeni, 1996).

This chapter first reviews the epidemiology of comorbid disorders to establish the broadest picture of the problem in the United States. Comorbidity should be recognized as a heterogeneous problem in the general population—it clearly takes many forms. Consistent with conventional clinical practice, in this chapter the term "dual diagnosis" is reserved for the subset of co-occurrences that involve substance use disorder and a severe mental illness, such as schizophrenia or bipolar disorder (Drake & Mueser, 2000). After the epidemiology section, the chapter reviews explanatory models of comorbidity and integrated treatment.

THE EPIDEMIOLOGY OF COMORBIDITY
IN THE UNITED STATES

The National Epidemiologic Survey on Alcohol and Related Conditions (NESARC) is the largest ($n = 43,093$) and most comprehensive surveillance study ever conducted on alcohol and drug use and their associated comorbidities (Grant et al., 2004c). Conducted by the National Institute on Alcohol Abuse and Alcoholism (NIAAA) in 2001–2002, the NESARC is a nationally representative face-to-face survey of American adults, ages 18 and older. The 2001–2002 survey was the first wave of an ongoing longitudinal study (second wave conducted in 2004–2005). Interviews were conducted in households randomly selected from a U.S. Census Bureau sampling frame. The sampling frame also included group living quarters such as college residence halls, boarding houses, and shelters.

The NESARC relied on a structured diagnostic interview that assessed alcohol and drug use, mood, anxiety, and personality disorders and treatment seeking for these same disorders. DSM-IV (American Psychiatric Association, 1994) criteria were used to design the survey instrument. Efforts were made to distinguish between psychiatric symptoms that represent independent mental disorders and those that were the consequence of drug intoxication and withdrawal. The NESARC assessed the following drugs: sedatives, tranquilizers, heroin, opiates other than heroin and methadone, stimulants, hallucinogens, cannabis, cocaine and crack, inhalants/solvents, and other drugs. Schizophrenia and bipolar disorder were not assessed by the interview (though mania and hypomania were included). The overall survey response rate was 81%.

Findings from the NESARC document the pervasiveness of mental health and substance abuse problems in the United States. In 2001–2002, the survey yielded estimates indicating that about 15% of the U.S. population met DSM-IV criteria for one or more personality disorders, followed by any anxiety disorder, 11%; any mood disorder, 9%; alcohol depend-ence, 4%; and any drug dependence, 1% (Grant et al., 2004b; Grant et al., 2004c). Table 4.1 shows the prevalence of mood, anxiety, and personality disorders among adult Americans who also met criteria for alcohol depend-ence and other drug dependence.

Among individuals with alcohol dependence in the general U.S. popu-lation, it appears that about 40% met criteria for a personality disorder, 28% had a mood disorder, and 23% had an anxiety disorder. The most common specific diagnosis among alcohol-dependent individuals was major depression (20.5%). These comorbid conditions appeared at consid-erably higher rates in drug-dependent individuals. For instance, 70% of drug-dependent persons met criteria for a personality disorder, with 55% having had a mood disorder and 43% an anxiety disorder. Among those with a drug dependency, major depression (40%) and antisocial personality disorder (39%) were the most common specific diagnoses. These findings clearly document that the co-occurrence of mood, anxiety, and personality

TABLE 4.1. Prevalence of Mood, Anxiety, and Personality Disorders among Alcohol and Drug Dependent Adults in the U.S. Population: Findings from the NESARC, 2001–2002

Coexisting condition	Alcohol dependent (%)	Drug dependent(%)
Any mood disorder	27.5	55.0
Major depression	20.5	40.0
Dysthymia	4.6	16.7
Mania	7.6	18.0
Hypomania	5.0	4.8
Any anxiety disorder	23.4	43.0
Panic disorder with agoraphobia	1.8	5.3
Panic disorder without agoraphobia	4.7	10.3
Social phobia	6.2	12.9
Specific phobia	13.8	22.3
Generalized anxiety disorder	5.7	17.2
Any personality disorder	39.5	69.5
Avoidant	7.7	18.2
Dependent	2.5	10.1
Obsessive–compulsive	15.2	28.7
Paranoid	15.8	33.2
Schizoid	8.2	21.0
Histrionic	10.2	20.6
Antisocial	18.3	39.5

Note. n = 43,093. Data from Grant et al. (2004b) and Grant et al. (2004c).

disorders with both alcohol dependence and drug dependence are pervasive in the U.S. population (Grant et al., 2004b; Grant et al., 2004c).

The NESARC 2001–2002 data also establish that the associations between substance dependence and mood, anxiety, and personality disorders are of substantial magnitude and unlikely to be due to sampling error (Grant, Hasin, Chou, Stinson, & Dawson, 2004a; Grant et al., 2004b; Grant et al., 2004c). The odds ratios (ORs) appearing in Table 4.2 represent the odds of having a coexisting condition among individuals with nicotine, alcohol, or any other drug dependence relative to the odds of having the same coexisting condition in those individuals not dependent on that specific substance. An OR equal to 1.0 indicates no difference between the two groups in the odds of having a coexisting condition. When the accompanying 95% confidence interval (CI) does *not* encompass the OR of 1.0, then we can be confident that the observed co-occurrence between the specific type of substance dependence and a mental health problem is not likely due to chance (i.e, statistically significant).

As can be seen in Table 4.2, the ORs range from 2.2 to 26.0, representing relatively strong associations that are all statistically significant. For instance, nicotine-dependent individuals were 3.3 times more likely than non-nicotine-dependent individuals to have had major depression in the past 12 months; alcohol-dependent persons were 3.1 times more likely than non-alcohol-dependent persons to have had generalized anxiety disorder in the past 12 months; and drug-dependent individuals were 13.9 times more likely than non-drug-dependent individuals to have had mania in the past 12 months (each mental health condition unrelated to drug intoxication or withdrawal).

Many of the largest ORs in Table 4.2 represent associations involving personality disorders. For example, compared to nondependent individuals, drug-dependent persons were 18.5 times more likely to have met criteria for antisocial personality disorder and 26.0 times more likely to have been diagnosed with dependent personality disorder. Also of significant interest were the associations involving nicotine dependence and alcohol/drug dependence in men and women. For example, among women, cigarette smokers were 16.4 times more likely to have a drug dependency (other than nicotine) than non-cigarette smokers.

Comorbidity Among Persons Who Seek Treatment

The 2001–2002 NESARC found that relatively small percentages of persons with substance use, mood, and anxiety disorders sought out treatment for these conditions (Grant et al., 2004b). In the previous 12-month period, only 5.8% of those diagnosed with alcohol abuse or alcohol dependence sought treatment, compared to 13.1% meeting criteria for any drug abuse

TABLE 4.2. Comorbidity in the U.S. Adult Population: Odds Ratios from the NESARC, 2001–2002

Coexisting condition	Odds ratios (95% CI)		
	Nicotine dependence	Alcohol dependence	Any drug dependence
Any mood disorder	3.3 (3.0–3.6)	4.1 (3.5–4.8)	12.5 (8.8-17.7)
Major depression	3.3 (3.0–3.7)	3.7 (3.1–4.4)	9.0 (6.5–12.7)
Dysthymia	3.3 (2.8–4.0)	2.8 (2.0–3.8)	11.3 (7.5–17.2)
Mania	3.9 (3.2–4.7)	5.7 (4.4–7.4)	13.9 (8.9–21.7)
Hypomania	3.5 (2.7–4.5)	5.2 (3.9–6.8)	4.4 (2.2–8.7)
Any anxiety disorder	2.7 (2.4–3.0)	2.6 (2.2–3.0)	6.2 (4.4–8.7)
Panic disorder with agoraphobia	4.6 (3.4–6.2)	3.6 (2.0–6.5)	10.5 (5.6–19.7)
Panic disorder without agoraphobia	3.9 (3.2–4.8)	3.4 (2.5–4.7)	7.6 (4.7–12.2)
Social phobia	2.6 (2.2–3.1)	2.5 (1.8–3.3)	5.4 (3.5–8.3)
Specific phobia	2.6 (2.3–2.9)	2.2 (1.8–2.6)	3.8 (2.5–5.8)
Generalized anxiety disorder	3.4 (2.8–4.2)	3.1 (2.3–4.1)	10.4 (6.5–16.7)
Any personality disorder	3.3 (3.0–3.6)	4.0 (3.6–4.6)	13.5 (9.9–18.2)
Avoidant	3.3 (2.7–3.9)	3.8 (3.0–4.9)	9.6 (5.9–15.6)
Dependent	5.5 (3.9–7.7)	6.1 (3.6–10.1)	26.0 (13.3–50.6)
Obsessive–compulsive	2.3 (2.0–2.6)	2.2 (1.8–2.6)	4.8 (3.3–6.9)
Paranoid	3.8 (3.4–4.4)	4.6 (3.8–5.5)	11.3 (7.8–16.2)
Schizoid	3.3 (2.8–3.8)	2.9 (2.3–3.9)	8.6 (5.7–13.0)
Histrionic	4.5 (3.7–5.5)	7.5 (6.0–9.4)	14.8 (9.5–23.0)
Antisocial	5.7 (4.8–6.6)	7.1 (6.0–8.4)	18.5 (13.6–25.1)
Substance dependence by sex			
Alcohol dependence—men	5.7 (4.8–6.7)	N/A	N/A
Alcohol dependence—women	7.5 (6.0–9.5)	N/A	N/A
Any drug dependence—men	14.8 (9.6–23.1)	N/A	N/A
Any drug dependence—women	16.4 (10.0–26.8)	N/A	N/A

Note. n = 43,093. Data from Grant, Hasin, Chou, Stinson, and Dawson (2004a); Grant et al. (2004b); and Grant et al. (2004c). ORs represent the odds of having a coexisting condition among individuals with nicotine, alcohol, or any other drug dependence relative to the odds of having the same coexisting condition in those individuals not having the specific type of substance dependence.

or drug dependence diagnosis. Among those with mood disorders, 26.0% sought treatment for these conditions. Among those with anxiety disorders, 12.1% sought treatment.

An important set of findings from the 2001–2002 NESARC reveals that many persons who seek treatment for a mood or anxiety disorder also have some type of substance use disorder (Grant et al., 2004b). Table 4.3 shows that 15.4% (panic disorder without agoraphobia) to 31.0% (hypomania) of persons seeking treatment for specific mood anxiety disorders had coexisting substance use problems. These findings are of considerable clinical significance because if a substance use disorder is not recognized in the treatment of mood and anxiety disorder, the prognosis for both disorders may be poor.

TABLE 4.3. Prevalence of Substance Use Disorder among Respondents Seeking Treatment for Mood and Anxiety Disorders in Past 12 Months: Findings from the NESARC, 2001–2002

Treatment sought for following condition:	Percentage with any substance disorder
Any mood disorder	20.8
Major depression	20.3
Dysthymia	18.5
Mania	22.5
Hypomania	31.0
Any anxiety disorder	16.5
Panic disorder with agoraphobia	21.9
Panic disorder without agoraphobia	15.4
Social phobia	21.3
Specific phobia	16.0
Generalized anxiety disorder	15.9

Note. n = 43,093. Data from Grant et al. (2004b).

The findings from the 2001–2002 NESARC indicate that the co-occurrence of alcohol/drug problems with mental health problems represent a common psychiatric syndrome in the U.S. population. Thus, comorbidity should be an expectation rather than viewed as the exception (Substance Abuse and Mental Health Services Administration, 2002). Persons with substance dependence disorders (nicotine, alcohol, and other drugs) are much more likely to have a coexisting mood, anxiety, or personality disorder than persons without substance dependence diagnoses. These mental health problems appear to be independent of alcohol/drug intoxication and withdrawal. Furthermore, many persons who seek treatment for mood and anxiety disorders have a substance use disorder as well, which highlights the needs for careful, systematic client assessment and integrated treatment of both disorders. As noted by the Substance Abuse and Mental Health Services Administration (2002) in a report to the U.S. Congress: "Improving the Nation's public health demands prompt attention to the problem of co-occurring disorders" (see Executive Summary).

Levels of Comorbidity across Patterns of Substance Dependence

In a separate national probability sample, Kandel, Huang, and Davies (2001) examined the extent to which persons with one or more drug dependencies had coexisting major depression or any anxiety disorder (i.e., a mood disorder of some type). The investigators found that a *single* dependence on nicotine, alcohol, or illicit drugs had similar degrees of association with the mood disorders. However, dual dependence on both a licit (nicotine or alcohol) and an illicit drug was associated with nearly a doubling of the odds of a coexisting mood disorder. The odds of having a coexisting mood disorder did not appear to be elevated by a dual dependence on nicotine and alcohol, however. Kandel and colleagues concluded that persons seeking treatment for dependencies that involve both a licit and an illicit drug will likely be those most in need of mental health services. In other words, a dual dependence of this type may be a marker for other psychiatric problems.

Lifetime Comorbidity in Cannabis-Dependent Persons

The use of cannabis (marijuana) is a significant public health issue. Among the illegal substances, cannabis is the most widely used drug in the United States, with an estimated 14.6 million past-month users in 2003 (Office of Applied Studies, 2004a). The drug also is the source of a great deal of controversy and public debate because many users and groups that advocate for reform of marijuana laws contend that the drug causes little harm (see www.norml.org).

In this context, it is useful to consider the rates of *lifetime* comorbidity among cannabis dependent persons. The findings summarized in Table 4.4 were obtained by diagnostic interviews conducted in a national probability sample of Americans, ages 15–54 (Agosti, Nunes, & Levin, 2002). They indicate that with the exception of mania, cannabis dependent persons are much more likely to have had a DSM-III diagnosis in their lifetime than non-cannabis-dependent persons. For instance, individuals dependent on cannabis at the time of a diagnostic interview were found to be almost 18 times more likely to also have met criteria for alcohol dependence in their lifetime, compared with individuals not dependent on cannabis. Furthermore, among the cannabis-dependent subsample, fully 70% also had been alcohol dependent at some point in life. Overall, Agosti et al. (2002) found that 90% of the cannabis-dependent persons had some mental disorder in their lifetime, compared to 55% of those persons who were not dependent on cannabis.

Although the correlations reported in Table 4.4 should not be interpreted as evidence that cannabis causes mental disorder or that cannabis is used to self-medicate psychological disturbance, it does appear that dependence on the drug is often one feature of a broader psychiatric profile. Clearly, persons dependent on marijuana have elevated lifetime risks for a variety of mental disorders. These findings underscore the need to identify coexisting conditions among cannabis-dependent persons who present themselves for treatment or other forms of professional assistance.

TABLE 4.4. Lifetime Comorbidity among Cannabis–Dependent Persons in the U.S. Population, Ages 15–54: Results from the NCS, 2001–2002

Lifetime diagnosis	Among cannabis dependent population	
	%	Odds ratio (95% CI)
Alcohol dependence	70.0	17.8 (13.4–23.6)
Antisocial personality disorder	21.4	11.2 (7.9–15.8)
Conduct disorder	44.4	6.0 (4.6–7.9)
Nonaffective psychosis	2.0	3.5 (1.3–9.0)
Social phobia	29.0	3.3 (2.4–4.5)
Posttraumatic stress disorder	18.5	3.0 (2.1–4.2)
Hypomania	4.4	2.9 (1.5–5.4)
Generalized anxiety disorder	12.1	2.7 (1.8–4.0)
Major depression	32.7	2.4 (1.8–3.2)
Dysthymic disorder	13.3	2.3 (1.5–3.3)
Panic disorder	6.9	2.3 (1.5–3.3)
Agoraphobia	11.3	1.8 (1.2–2.7)
Simple phobia	18.1	1.8 (1.3–2.5)
Mania	6.9	0.9 (0.1–6.2)

Note. $n = 5,877$. Data from Agosti, Nunes, and Levin (2002). ORs represent the odds of having a lifetime diagnosis among cannabis-dependent persons relative to the odds of having the same lifetime diagnosis among persons not cannabis dependent.

Comorbidity among Adolescents

At this time, relatively little is know about the prevalence of comorbid substance abuse and psychiatric disorder in the general population of adolescents. In a review of the existing literature, Armstrong and Costello (2002) found just 15 studies that investigated this issue. A synthesis of these studies led these investigators to estimate that about 60% of teenagers with substance use, abuse, or dependence probably had a coexisting psychiatric condition. Most commonly associated with substance use, abuse, and dependence were conduct disorder and oppositional defiant disorder, followed by depression. The association between substance use disorder and attention-deficit/hyperactivity disorder was not found to be strong. Evidence was found to support the view that psychopathology in childhood (particularly conduct disorder) is predictive of early-onset substance use and abuse in adolescence. These epidemiological findings are consistent with results from a twin study that sought to elucidate the relationship between conduct disorder and alcohol dependence by teasing out the specific influence of "behavioral undercontrol" (i.e., the personality traits of impulsivity, thrill seeking, rebelliousness, nonconformity, and aggressiveness). In that study, Slutske et al. (2002) found that genetic variables influencing the expression of behavioral undercontrol may account for about 40% of the variation in risk for conduct disorder and alcohol dependence.

EXPLANATORY MODELS

The epidemiological data reviewed thus far indicates that substance use disorders co-occur with other psychiatric disorders at rates far exceeding that explained by chance or coincidence. Unfortunately, these data do little to elucidate the nature of these comorbid conditions. Much work has been devoted to establishing the onset order of the co-occurring disorders (e.g., Does alcohol dependence typically predate the onset of major depression?). Though important, questions about order of onset fail to address the most fundamental issues at a nosological level. When comorbidity is observed, does it truly represent the presence of two distinct disorders or instead an uninformed appraisal which does not recognize a third *independent disorder* that encompasses the broader symptomatology of the comorbid condition? In the co-occurrence of substance use and other psychiatric problems, these issues of classification are among the most pressing questions for both clinical practitioners and researchers.

Table 4.5 identifies 10 models that attempt to clarify the association between substance use and other psychological problems (Neale & Kendler, 1995). The question each model attempts to address also appears in the table. Chance, sampling bias, and population stratification are models that assert that comorbid conditions are nothing more than artifacts (i.e., the co-occurrence is not significant or meaningful). Clearly, the epidemiological data reviewed here indicate that this is not the case. However, these models are useful for helping us to clarify our understanding of the nature of comorbidity, and thus have been included in Table 4.5.

The model labeled "alternative forms" maintains that the co-occurrence of substance use and other psychological problems arises from a single risk factor with a single threshold of severity (Agrawal et al., 2004). Others have referred to this as a "common factor model" (Mueser, Drake, & Wallach, 1998; Mueser, et al., 2003; NIAAA, 1994). Regardless, the model proposes that a risk factor increases the risk for both substance use and psychiatric disorder. The common risk factors most discussed in the research literature are genetic vulnerability, antisocial personality disorder, disordered mesolimbic activity in the brain, and poverty (Mueser et al., 2003). One landmark study in molecular genetics study has found that a variation in the muscarinic acetylcholine receptor M2 is a risk factor for the associated clinical characteristics of alcohol dependence and major depression (Wang et al., 2004). This finding gives rise to speculation that in the future, other shared and specific genetic risk factors may be found to underlie a variety of comorbid conditions.

Random multiformity and extreme multiformity are models that assume that one disorder can take heterogeneous or atypical forms (Klein & Riso, 1993). In such situations, symptoms will appear that are typically

TABLE 4.5. Models of Comorbidity

Name	Question posed by the model
Chance	Is the co-occurrence of the disorders due simply to chance?
Sampling bias	Do we overestimate the prevalence of comorbid condition in the general population because our observations are derived from a clinical population that has been referred for treatment?
Population stratification	Do we overestimate the prevalence of comorbid condition in the general population because we fail to account for subgroup differences, such as socioeconomic status or other stratification variables?
Alternate forms	Is there one underlying risk factor that gives rise to both disorders?
Random multiformity	Does the comorbid condition represent an atypical form of one of the disorders with symptoms that overlap with those of the second disorder?
Extreme multiformity	Does the atypical form arise only after risk factors for either or both of the disorders reach extreme levels?
Three independent disorders	Does the comorbid condition represent a third disorder that is distinct from the other two disorders?
Correlated liabilities	Do the two disorders have a high probability of co-occurring because they arise from a set of shared risk factors?
Causation	Is one disorder a risk factor for the subsequent onset of the other disorder?
Reciprocal causation	Regardless of which disorder appears first, do the two disorders exacerbate one another with the passage of time?

associated with other disorders. Thus, multiformity does not represent true comorbidity but, instead, "indicates that the boundaries of a disorder have been drawn in the wrong place" (Klein & Riso, 1993, p. 44). Extreme multiformity is a variant model that assumes the atypical form will appear only when the severity of the risk factors for either or both of the disorders are at elevated thresholds. For instance, the co-occurrence of cannabis dependence and social phobia (an anxiety disorder) might not be likely to occur unless the frequency of marijuana smoking reaches some high threshold or there exists an extensive family history of anxiety disorder. These models challenge conventional diagnostic criteria, such as those found in DSM-IV-TR (American Psychiatric Association, 2000).

The model known as "three independent disorders" assumes that the comorbid condition is actually a distinct disorder itself. Neale and Kendler (1995) describe this model as "somewhat implausible" (p. 941). It is the only model that asserts that the co-occurrence arises from a process that is completely separate from those that instigate the development of the other two disorders.

The correlated liabilities model proposes that comorbid conditions arise because prevalent forms of co-occurrence tend to share common sets of risk factors (Neale & Kendler, 1995). Though any two disorders will have common and unique risk factors, the overlapping of them will contribute to a rate of co-occurrence that is higher than that expected by chance. For example, the co-occurrence of substance dependence and depression in adolescence may arise from a variety of forms of neglect and abuse experienced during childhood.

The straightforward causation model asserts that one disorder operates as a risk factor for the subsequent onset of a second disorder. For instance, alcohol dependence causes major depression. Causation models assert that one disorder predates the other in time of onset. Two types of causation models have been proposed to specific the order of onset of substance use and other psychiatric disorders (Mueser et al., 2003). The secondary substance abuse model proposes that psychopathology precedes and causes substance abuse. In contrast, the secondary psychiatric disorder model maintains that substance abuse precedes and causes psychopathology.

Finally, the reciprocal causation model proposes that over time, substance use and psychopathology will exacerbate one another. Arising from clinical observations, this model is less concerned with the order of onset of the disorders and is more focused on integrated treatment options (Mueser et al., 2003). In addition, the reciprocal causation model tends to emphasize the role of multiple risk factors in the immediate social environment of the dual-diagnosis patient, including negative peer influences, employment problems, and limited recreational opportunities.

Problem Behavior Theory: A Social-Psychological Framework for Explaining Comorbidity

One alternative framework for understanding the co-occurrence of substance abuse and other mental health problems is problem behavior theory (Jessor & Jessor, 1977; Jessor et al., 1991). The result of longitudinal research on the development of adolescents and young adults, this social psychological model maintains that human behavior is the result of person–environment interaction. The theory consists of three interdependent systems of variables: the behavior system, which encompasses a conventional behavior syndrome or a problem behavior syndrome (substance abuse, low academic achievement, aggression, etc.); the personality system, which particularly includes such variables as achievement motivation, affiliation/ alienation, self-esteem, and mental health; and the perceived environmental

system, which includes "perceived controls and instigations from significant others in the life space, particularly parents and friends" (Jessor et al.,
1991, p. 29).

In problem behavior theory, the variables from each system represent
either instigations or controls that, in combination, generate "proneness"
or the probability of resultant problem behavior. Although proneness can
exist in one, two, or all three of the systems, overall psychosocial proneness
is the central concept of the theory and is used to predict and explain variation in problem behavior. Psychological proneness can be considered the
"outcome of the balance of instigation toward and controls against engaging in problem behavior" (Jessor et al., 1991, p. 19). In essence, the psychological concepts of "instigations" and "controls" can be thought of as anal-
ogous to the epidemiological notions of "risk" and "protective" factors.

A major proposition of problem behavior theory is that problem
behaviors are highly interrelated (Jessor & Jessor, 1977). That is, *multiple*
problem behaviors (often more than two) tend to co-occur within individuals. The data collected by Jessor and colleagues suggest that it is relatively
unusual for individuals to have just one problem behavior. Instead, they
tend to co-occur in prone individuals. For instance, Jessor and colleagues
have noted that individuals who smoke cigarettes are much more likely to
engage in a range of risk behavior, including sexual risk taking, drinking
and driving, and other deviant behavior.

The tendency of multiple problem behaviors to cluster within individuals is described as "problem behavior syndrome." The syndrome concept
implies that a common factor (psychosocial proneness) underlie the development of different types of problem behaviors. The structural equation
models created by Jessor et al. (1991) provide strong evidence to support
the syndrome concept of both problem behavior and conventional (nonproblem) behavior. More than one-half of the variance in both problem
behavior involvement and conventional behavior involvement can be
explained by the psychosocial measures assessed in their longitudinal investigation (Jessor et al., 1991). An important point is that "problem behavior" does not necessarily imply antisocial behavior. Rather, the term is
reserved for a broad range of behaviors that undermine conventional (or
normal) human psychosocial development.

Problem behavior theory does not encompass psychiatric/medical conceptions of mental illness but, instead, relies on traditional measures used
in the field on social psychology. Nevertheless, the theory rests on a strong
empirical foundation. Thus, the propositions of problem behavior theory
have great significance for helping to understand the co-occurrence of substance use disorder and mental health problems. In particular, the rather
narrow psychiatric perspective focusing on two coexisting DSM disorders may not be an adequate or rich enough model for capturing the

many psychosocial problems and life challenges of so-called dual-diagnosis patients (Drake, Wallach, Alverson, & Mueser, 2002). Our understanding of coexisting substance abuse and mental disorder may be enhanced by further interdisciplinary inquiry.

The Possible Role of Discounting Delayed Consequences

The findings from an emerging body of research in the area of behavioral economics suggest that persons with substance use disorders tend to *discount* both the value of delayed reinforcement and the severity of reinforcement losses encountered at a later time, compared to persons without these disorders (Bickel & Marsch, 2001; Higgins, Heil, & Lussier, 2004). In other words, substance abusers appears to prefer immediate reinforcement, even if it is of smaller magnitude, over delayed reinforcement of greater magnitude, and they prefer that punishment be delayed, even if it means that its magnitude will increase. An intriguing possibility is that increased rates of discounting may be associated with comorbidity. Substance abusers with co-occurring antisocial personality disorder (Petry, 2002) and gambling problems (Petry & Casarella, 1999) have been found to discount delayed consequences more than substance abusers without these comorbid conditions. Thus, it is possible that in the population of mentally ill persons, comorbidity may be most likely to occur in those that are less sensitive to the longer-term contingencies associated with alcohol and drug use. More research is needed in this area.

Substance Abuse/Dependence and Severe Mental Illness

The term "dual diagnosis" is often used to refer to the subset of possible comorbidities that involve a substance use disorder and a severe mental illness—usually schizophrenia or bipolar disorder. Persons with dual diagnoses pose special challenges to communities and the treatment systems that offer them assistance (Carey, 1995). Some dual-diagnosis clients find it difficult to comply with treatment. Others may frequently drop out of treatment or become involved in the "revolving door" of brief inpatient treatment admissions to resolve crises associated with bouts of substance abuse. Care of dual-diagnosis patients also stretches the fiscal resources of the treatment system. One study found that dual-diagnosis patients had treatment costs that were almost 60% higher than those for psychiatric patients without a substance use disorder (Dickey & Azeni, 1996). In addition, it has been estimated that at least 20% of the homeless population are persons with dual diagnoses (Drake, Osher, & Wallach, 1991).

In a review of the literature on substance use disorders and severe mental illness (schizophrenia or bipolar disorder), Mueser et al. (1998) suggested that these associations may be explained by more than one model. They proposed that the features of these comorbid conditions may be of two types: an antisocial personality disorder (ASPD) model and a supersensitivity model. The ASPD model conceptualizes the co-occurrence of substance use disorder and severe mental illness as a problem of developmental psychopathology. That is, ASPD—and its childhood precursor, conduct disorder—is viewed to be the common factor that increases risk for the subsequent development of both substance use disorder and serious mental illness in young adulthood. In contrast, the supersensitivity model posits that persons with a coexisting substance use disorder and severe mental illness are extremely vulnerable to stress. Psychotherapeutic medications usually decrease this vulnerability. However, alcohol and street drug use, even in relatively small quantities, may greatly exacerbate the psychiatric symptomatology. In essence, persons with dual diagnoses are "supersensitive" to the negative consequences of alcohol and drug use, even at low doses or infrequent use. Table 4.6 identifies the features of these two proposed models.

Clozapine Use Associated with Reductions in Alcohol Use

Clozapine is an antipsychotic medication used to treat schizophrenia. In a 3-year study of 151 patients diagnosed with schizophrenia or schizoaffective disorder and coexisting substance abuse treated in a dual-disorder program, 36 were given clozapine for standard clinical indications (Drake,

TABLE 4.6. Two Models Explaining the Co-Occurrence of Substance Use Disorder and Severe Mental Illness

Feature	ASPD model	Supersensitivity model
Age of onset of substance use disorder	Earlier	Later
Quantity of substance use	Higher	Lower
Physical dependence on a drug	More likely	Less likely
Family history of substance abuse	More likely	Less likely
Age of onset of severe mental illness	Earlier	Later
Premorbid social functioning	Marginal	Good
Social functioning	Poor	Good
Psychiatric symptoms	More severe	Less severe
Aggression	More likely	Less likely
Prognosis	Guarded	Good

Note. Adapted from Mueser, Drake, and Wallace (1998). Copyright 1998 by Elsevier. Adapted by permission.

Xie, McHugo, & Green, 2000). The clozapine patients who abused alcohol averaged 12.5 drinking days while taking the medication and 54.1 drinking days during 6-month intervals that the medication was withheld. The clozapine patients also improved more than patients in the study who did not receive the medication. At the end of 3 years, 79% of the clozapine patients had been in remission from alcohol use disorder for at least 6 months, compared to only 33.7% in the nonclozapine group. Though there is a need for larger, controlled trials to test clozapine further, this study suggests that use of the medication is associated with reductions in alcohol abuse among persons with schizophrenia. Clozapine effectiveness in this population suggests that the development of better explanatory models of comorbidity may depend on advances in the neuroscience of severe mental illness.

INTEGRATED TREATMENT FOR DUAL DIAGNOSIS

Not long ago, discussions about treating persons with co-occurring substance use disorder and severe mental illness tended to focus on the most appropriate sequence of independently delivered treatment regimens (see NIAAA, 1994, pp. 51–53). Persons experiencing these problems were either treated at the same time in separate substance abuse and mental health treatment programs (i.e., parallel treatments) or they were treated in one program first, discharged, and then treated in the second program (i.e., sequential treatment). The advantages and disadvantages of these two approaches were weighed and evaluated in the context of traditional treatment delivery systems. Over the last 15 years or so, innovations have led to the development of the integrated treatment model (Drake & Mueser, 2001). Though still evolving, the core feature of this model is the coordinated, concurrent treatment of two or more disorders in programs designed specifically for those patients with comorbid substance abuse and severe mental illness (Mercer, Mueser, & Drake, 1998).

During the 1990s, the dissatisfaction with the traditional treatment modalities gave rise to a set of guiding principles for the provision of integrated treatment (Drake, Mercer-McFadden, Mueser, McHugo, & Bond, 1998). For substance-abusing patients who also suffer from severe mental illness, such as schizophrenia, treatment should be provided by one integrated program that is designed to address both disorders. It is not adequate to sequentially treat one disorder and then the other at a later time. One feature then of integrated treatment is the employment of clinical staff members who are trained to treat both substance abuse and severe mental disorder. Another feature of integrated treatment is that many of the traditional practices used in addiction treatment programs need to be modified to properly assist those with severe mental illness. For instance, in integrated treatment, the emphasis is placed on establishing a relationship with patients and helping them to cope, whereas in traditional addiction treatment, confrontation often was used to break down denial. Furthermore, to engage patients, integrated treatment endorses a harm-reduction approach that may not insist on immediate abstinence from alcohol and illicit drugs. Consistent with this approach, there is recognition that treatment will probably be long term—at least for most patients. Thus, counseling is stage based and motivational—not confrontational. In addition, to adequately attend to crises, integrated treatment needs to be provided in facilities that can offer around-the-clock access to treatment staff. In such an environment, 12-Step programs must be available, but participation should be voluntary. Finally, in integrated treatment programs, the patient's severe mental illness is recognized as a biological disorder that usually needs treated with psychotherapeutic medication. Medication is not thought to compromise the treatment goals set for the substance use disorder. Table 4.7 summarizes these principles.

TABLE 4.7. Guiding Principles of the Integrated Treatment Model

1. Treatment is provided by one integrated program designed to address both substance use disorder and severe mental illness.

2. The substance use disorder and the severe mental illness are treated by one team of dually trained clinicians.

3. The treatment for substance use disorder deviates from traditional "detox" and "rehab" practices and is tailored to the needs of those with severe mental illness.

4. Emphasis is placed on reducing anxiety—not breaking through denial about substance abuse.

5. Attempts are made to build trust and engage the patient in treatment—confrontation is avoided.

6. Priority is placed on reducing the harm associated with substance abuse—insistence on immediate abstinence may be counterproductive.

7. Recognition that treatment will probably be long term—rapid detoxification and short-term treatment followed by discharge is not realistic.

8. Counseling is stage based and motivational—not confrontational and time limited.

9. Around-the-clock access to treatment staff—not limited to daytime office hours.

10. Participation in 12-Step programs is available and encouraged—but not mandatory.

11. Use of psychotherapeutic medications is based on the patient's psychiatric and medical needs—the goals of substance abuse treatment are not seen as comprising reliance on these medications.

Effectiveness of Integrated Treatment

In two reviews of studies on integrated treatment, Drake et al. (1998) and Brunette, Mueser, and Drake (2004) concluded that the methodological limitations of the research conducted to date preclude any firm conclusions to be reached about the effectiveness of the approach. Brunette et al. (2004) added that the integrated treatment model should be tested in a large, randomized clinical trial. With these caveats in mind, the available evidence suggests that simply adding dual-diagnosis groups to traditional services is not effective. Also, integrated treatment when delivered via *intensive* inpatient, residential, or day treatment does not appear effective. The dropout rate in these programs is high, presumably because of the insistence on abstinence. Low-intensity programs may be more effective. The authors found some reason to be optimistic about the prospects of newer comprehensive, integrated treatment approaches that rely on long-term, stage-based, motivational counseling. The somewhat better outcomes may be attributed to assertive outreach and possibly not insisting on immediate abstinence from alcohol and other illicit drugs.

Results from other studies bolster the view that long-term, comprehensive treatment is important for "engaging" dual-diagnosis patients (i.e, keeping them in treatment). For instance, one comparison of long-term and short-term residential programs found that at follow-up, dual-diagnosis patients in the former type of program were more likely to stay in treatment, more likely to maintain abstinence, and less likely to experience homelessness (Brunette, Drake, Woods, & Hartnett, 2001). There were no statistically significant differences between the two groups on measures of psychiatric hospitalization, incarceration, or number of moves. The investigators concluded that dual-diagnosis patients need safe, stable, sober living environments to learn skills for maintaining abstinence, and that the acquisition of these skills is less likely to occur in intensive, short-term programs that may be too challenging. Another study of long-term outcomes of integrated treatment followed 126 dual-diagnosis patients for up to 3 years (Judd, Thomas, Schwartz, Outcalt, & Hough, 2003). The study found that integrated treatment produced statistically significant improvements in quality of life, substance use, and psychiatric symptoms. Moreover, these improvements were associated with decreases in health care and criminal justice costs (Judd et al., 2003).

Unfortunately, there are significant policy and organizational impediments associated with the adoption, implementation, and maintenance of dual-diagnosis treatment programs (Mercer et al., 1998). Although many states have implemented services for dual-diagnosis clients, high-quality treatment programs are the exception, not the rule (Drake et al.,

2001; Drake & Wallach, 1999; Torrey et al., 2002). Public investment in these programs may depend on research that can demonstrate cost-effectiveness.

SUMMARY

Comorbidity remains one of the most poorly understood areas in the substance abuse and treatment services fields. Although surveillance studies have begun to document the patterns of association between substance use disorders and mental disorders and have established that these associations are not due to chance, much remains to be understood about the etiology of comorbid conditions. Interdisciplinary research efforts may yield new insights because the questions about comorbidity range from problems in molecular genetics to those in the social environment and the public policy arena. Among the most pressing needs is further research on integrated approaches to treating persons with dual diagnoses (i.e., substance abuse and severe mental illness). The integrated treatment model holds promise for helping this population of clients, but at this time the evidence supporting its use is not compelling.

REVIEW QUESTIONS

1. How is the deinstitutionalization movement implicated in the problem of dual diagnosis?

2. What is the NESARC?

3. In the NESARC, how prevalent are mood, anxiety, and personality disorders among alcohol and drug dependent persons?

4. Compared to nondependent persons, how likely are nicotine-, alcohol-, and drug-dependent persons to have a mental disorder? (based on odds ratios from the NESARC)

5. When people seek treatment for a mood disorder, how often do they have a coexisting substance use disorder? (based on the NESARC)

6. According to research conducted by Kandel and colleagues, what is the significance of being dependent on both a licit and illicit substance?

7. To what extent is cannabis dependence associated with lifetime risk of alcohol dependence and mental disorder?

8. Which mental disorders are most closely associated with substance abuse in adolescence?

9. According to Neale and Kendler, what are the 10 possible models of comorbidity?

10. In problem behavior theory, why is it predicted that multiple problem behaviors cluster in individuals?

11. What are the ASPD and supersensitivity models for explaining dual diagnosis?

12. What are the features of integrated treatment for dual diagnosis?

13. How effective is integrated treatment?

Psychoanalytic Formulations

Sigmund Freud (1885–1939) made the first systematic attempt to explain the origins of mental disorders. His theory is known as "psychoanalysis." His ideas have had a lasting impact on our culture. For example, he originated the notion of defense mechanisms (denial, rationalization, etc.). He brought attention to the significance of anxiety in the human experience. He was the first to give an extensive description of unconscious mind. He pointed to the importance of early childhood experience, and he was the first to insist that human sexual behavior is an appropriate subject for scientific scrutiny.

Freud derived psychoanalytic concepts from his clinical practice. His patients were predominantly white female residents of Vienna, Austria, from the 1890s to the 1930s. Psychoanalytic models continue to influence clinical practitioners in the mental health field today, particularly in some psychiatric circles (Gabbard, 1999). These concepts also have historical significance and provide perspective on the evolution of addictions treatment.

PSYCHOANALYSIS: A TYPE OF PSYCHOTHERAPY

The terms "psychoanalysis" and "psychotherapy" are not synonymous, though they are sometimes mistakenly thought to be. "Psychotherapy" is a more general term describing professional services aimed at helping individuals or groups overcome emotional, behavioral, or relationship problems. There are more than 240 methods of counseling and psychotherapy (George & Cristiani, 1995). Psychoanalysis is one of these approaches.

Traditional psychoanalysis involves an "analyst" and an "analysand" (i.e., the client). Typically, the analysand lies comfortably on a couch while the analyst sits behind him/her, out of view. Often, the analyst takes notes while the analysand describes whatever comes into his/her mind. Interestingly, Freud discouraged analysts from taking notes; he cautioned that doing so would distract their attention (Gay, 1988).

Interpretation

Psychoanalysis relies heavily on the analyst's interpretation of the analysand's concerns. To this end, the analyst encourages the analysand to say absolutely everything that comes to mind. By contrast, the analyst remains as silent as possible, hoping that this silence will stimulate uninhibited verbal activity on the part of the analysand. Gay (1988) describes the process in this way:

> In the strange enterprise that is psychoanalysis, half the battle and half alliance, the analysand will cooperate as much as his neurosis lets him. The analyst for his part is, one hopes, not hampered by his own neurosis; in any event, he is required to deploy a highly specialized sort of tact, some of it acquired in his training analysis, the rest drawn from his experience with analytic patients. It calls for restraint, for silence at most of the analysand's productions and comments on a few. Much of the time patients will experience their analyst's interpretations as precious gifts that he doles out with far too stingy a hand. (p. 298)

Free Association

According to Freud, the fundamental principle of psychoanalysis is that "free association" should be encouraged. The analysand should be free to reveal the most sensitive things that come to mind, so that the analyst can interpret them. For this reason, the analyst positions him/herself behind the analysand. The analyst's reactions to shocking disclosures could cause the analysand to be distracted and inhibit the free flow of associations.

Dream Interpretation

Another feature of psychoanalysis is dream interpretation. Its purpose is to uncover unconscious material, which the analysand typically represses. The task of the analyst is to study the symbols presented in the dreams and to interpret their disguised meanings. Psychoanalysts believe that dreams have two types of content: "manifest" and "latent." The manifest content is the dream as it appears to the dreamer, while latent content is what is disguised to the dreamer. The latent content consists of the analysand's actual motives that are seeking expression but that are very painful or personally unacceptable (Coleman, Butcher, & Carson, 1980).

Resistance

In *The Interpretation of Dreams*, Freud (1900/1953) defined resistance as simply "whatever interrupts the progress of analytic work" (p. 555). According to Gay (1988), Freud warned: "Resistance accompanies the treatment at every step; every single association, every act of the patient's must reckon with this resistance, represents a compromise between the forces aiming at cure and those opposing it" (p. 299).

For the psychoanalyst, resistance arises because the analysand becomes threatened by the uncovering of unconscious material. At such times, the analysand may attempt to change the subject, dismiss its importance, become silent, forget dreams, hold back essential information, be consistently late for appointments, become hostile, or employ other defensive mechanisms. Gay (1988) describes resistance as a "peculiarly irrational" but universal human tendency. The contradictory nature of resistance is underscored by the pointlessness of voluntarily seeking help (and paying for it) and then fighting against it.

Resistance can be viewed as a significant problem in counseling individuals with alcohol and other drug problems. Addiction practitioners who value the concept will see it in their clients and adopt helping strategies in accordance with it. Though traditional psychoanalytic thinking maintains that resistance arises from personality dynamics, Taleff (1997) and others have recognized that it has sources outside the person as well, such as counselor practices, inadequate treatment models, family and group dynamics, and the structure of treatment programs. To a great extent, the challenge in helping persons with substance abuse problems is properly assessing and attending to these issues (Taleff, 1997).

Transference

In the process of psychoanalysis, the relationship between analyst and analysand becomes emotionally charged. In this situation, the analysand frequently applies to the analyst particular feelings, thoughts, attributes, and motives that he/she had in a past relationship with a parent or other significant person (a teacher, coach, clergyman, etc.). As a result, the analysand may respond to the analyst as he/she did to that particular person in the past. If the past relationship was characterized by hostility or indifference, the analysand may feel the same way about the analyst. The tasks of the analyst, then, are to help the analysand (1) "work through" these feelings, (2) recognize that the analyst is not the parent or significant other figure, and (3) stop living within the confines of past relationships.

PERSONALITY STRUCTURE

In the psychoanalytic perspective, human behavior is thought to result from the interaction of three major subsystems within the personality: the "id," "ego," and "superego." Although each of these structures possesses unique functions and operating principles, they interact so closely with one another that it is often impossible to separate their distinct effects on behavior. In most cases, behavior is the result of the dynamic interaction among the id, ego, and superego. Each subsystem does not typically function in the absence of the other two (Hall & Lindzey, 1978).

The id is the original source of the personality and consists largely of instinctual drives. Psychoanalytic theorists have a specific understanding of the term "instinct." It is defined as an "inborn psychological representation of an inner somatic source of excitation" (Hall & Lindzey, 1978, p. 39). The psychological representation is more commonly referred to as a "wish," "internal urge," or "craving." The bodily excitations that give rise to wishes or urges are called "needs." Thus, the sensation of hunger represents the physiological need of the body for nutrients. Psychologically, this need is expressed as a wish or craving for food. In addiction, drugs become sources of bodily excitation, which in turn give rise to cravings for that chemical. The chemical craving serves to motivate the addict to seek out the drug of choice. Psychoanalysts note that addicts' instinctual drives make them hypersensitive to environmental stimuli (offers from friends to "get high," the smell of a burning match, advertisements for alcohol, etc.). These stimuli elicit cravings and make them vulnerable to "slips" and relapses.

The id is present from birth. It is the basic life force from which the ego and superego begin to differentiate themselves. It supplies the psychic energy necessary for the operation of the ego and superego. "Psychic energy" is defined as mental activity, such as thinking and remembering. Freud believed that the id is a bridge that connects the energy of the body to that of the personality. Interestingly, Freud noted that this psychic energy is not bound by logic and reality. It allows us to do such impossible things as to be in two places at once, or to move backward in time.

Some of the instinctual drives of the id are constructive (e.g., sex). However, others are destructive (e.g., aggression, destruction, and death). Because the id cannot tolerate increases in psychic energy (they are experienced as uncomfortable states of tension), it is identified as the component of personality that is completely selfish. The id is only concerned with immediate gratification (i.e., discharge of tension). It has no consideration for reality demands or moral concerns.

The id is said to operate via the "pleasure principle." That is, high tension levels (e.g., sexual urges or drug cravings) prompt the id to act to reduce the tension immediately and return the individual to a comfortably constant level of low energy. Thus, the id's aim is to avoid pain (e.g., the discomfort of abstinence) and to increase pleasure (e.g., drug-induced euphoria). The operation of the pleasure principle makes frustration and deprivation difficult to tolerate. Obviously, both frustration and deprivation are common in early recovery, and they make the addict susceptible to relapse.

The ego emerges from the id in order to satisfy the needs of the individual that require transactions with the external world (i.e., reality). Survival requires the individual to seek food, water, shelter, sex, and other basic needs. The ego assists in this effort by distinguishing between subjective needs of the mind (an id function) and the resources available in the external world.

Ultimately, the ego must answer to the demands of the id. However, it does so in such a way as to ensure the survival and health of the individual, which requires the use of reason, planning, delay of immediate gratification, and other rational resources in dealing with the external world. In "normal" individuals, the ego is able, to some degree, to control the primitive impulses of the id. As a result, the ego is said to operate via the "reality principle." The aim of the ego is to suspend the pleasure principle temporarily, until a time at which an appropriate place and object can be found for the release of tension. In this way, the ego is the component of personality that mediates between the demands of the id and the realities of the external world.

The third subsystem of the personality is the superego, which is the moral component of the personality. It emerges from the learning of moral values and social taboos. The superego is essentially that which is referred to as the "conscience"; it is concerned with "right" and "wrong." The superego develops during childhood and adolescence, as a result of reward and punishment. It has three main functions. One is to suppress impulses of the id, particularly sexual and aggressive urges. The second function is to press the ego to abandon realistic goals in exchange for moralistic ones. The third is to impel the individual to strive for perfection.

Though the three subsystems of personality operate as a whole, each represents distinct influences on human behavior (see Figure 5.1). The id is the biological force that influences human behavior. The ego represents the psychological origins of behavior, whereas the superego reflects the impact of social and moral forces. Both the id and superego can be thought of as the irrational components of personality; the id strives for pleasure at all costs whereas the superego always works to prevent it.

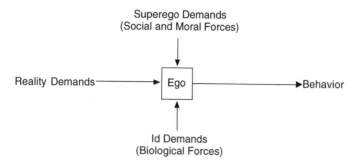

FIGURE 5.1. Influence of the id, ego, and superego and of reality demands on human behavior.

ANXIETY, DEFENSE MECHANISMS, AND THE UNCONSCIOUS

Anxiety plays a prominent role in psychoanalytic theory. The purpose of anxiety is to warn the individual that there is impending danger (i.e., pain). It is also a signal to the ego to take some preventive measure to reduce the threat.

Often the ego can cope with anxiety by rational measures. For example, a nervous student with an upcoming exam can spend extra time studying. A stressed-out employee can exercise, meditate, or turn to other constructive diversions. A parent can begin to save money now for a child's college education in 15 years. A recovering alcoholic who has cravings can call his/her Alcoholics Anonymous (AA) sponsor. Such actions require reason, the ability to plan, and the delay of immediate gratification for long-term gain.

However, the ego is often overcome by anxiety it cannot control. In such situations, rational measures fail and the ego resorts to irrational protective mechanisms, which are often referred to as "defense mechanisms." The defense mechanisms, such as denial and rationalization, alleviate the anxiety. However, they do so by distorting reality instead of dealing directly with the problem. This creates a discrepancy or gap between actual reality and the individual's perception of it. As a consequence, the ego's ability to cope with reality demands becomes increasingly diminished. Such is the case with alcoholics, who, upon being confronted with their problematic drinking, rely on denial and rationalization. These defenses, in turn, allow the abusive drinking to continue and to become increasingly dysfunctional.

Typical ego defense mechanisms among the chemically dependent include the following:

1. *Compensation*: making up for the deprivation of abstinence by overindulging in another pleasure. (Example: A recovering drug addict becomes compulsive about gambling, work, eating, etc.)
2. *Denial*: inability to perceive an unacceptable reality. (Example: An employee denies he is suffering from alcoholism when confronted about the bottle he keeps hidden in his desk.)
3. *Displacement*: directing pent-up feelings of hostility toward objects less dangerous than those that initially aroused the anger. (Example: An addict in treatment comes home from a group counseling session and screams at his wife. In group, he had received feedback from the faciliator indicating that he was not actively participating.)
4. *Fantasy*: gaining gratification from the loss of intoxicants by imagining the euphoria and fun of one's past drug abuse. (Example: While in rehabilitation, a group of addicts experience cravings as they reminisce about the "good ol' times.")
5. *Isolation*: withdrawing into a passive state in order to avoid further hurt. (Example: A depressed alcoholic in early recovery refuses to share her problems.)
6. *Projection*: assuming that others think badly of one even though they have never communicated this in any way. (Example: An addict unexpectedly blurts out to a counselor, "I know you think I'm worthless.")
7. *Rationalization*: attempting to justify one's mistakes or misdeeds by presenting rationales and explanations for the misconduct. (Example: An addict reports that he missed a 12-Step meeting because he had to take a very important telephone call from his attorney.)
8. *Regression*: retreating to an earlier developmental level involving less mature responses. (Example: In a therapeutic community, an adult resident "blows up" and makes a huge scene when she learns that iced tea is not available for lunch that day.)
9. *Undoing*: atoning for or making up for an unacceptable act. (Example: An alcoholic goes to a bar after work and gets "smashed." He doesn't get home until 4:00 A.M. His wife is furious. The next day he brings her flowers and cooks dinner.)

The defense mechanisms and other processes operate on an unconscious level. The unconscious, according to Freud, represents the largest part of the human mind. The individual is generally unaware of the content and process of this part of mind. The conscious mind, by contrast, is a function of the ego that has often been likened to the "tip of an iceberg" (see Figure 5.2).

The unconscious mind holds forbidden desires, painful memories, and unacceptable experiences that have been "repressed," or pushed out of con-

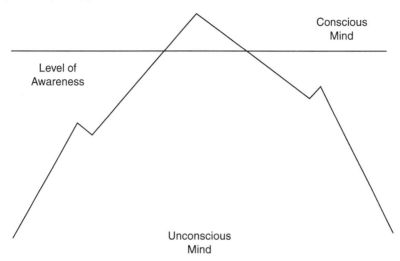

Conscious
Mind

Level of
Awareness

Unconscious
Mind

FIGURE 5.2. The "iceberg" view of the conscious versus the unconscious mind.

sciousness. Although individuals are unaware of unconscious material, it possesses energy and seeks expression. Thus, at times, unconscious material successfully penetrates the conscious mind. Typical examples of this are so-called Freudian slips (e.g., using the word "sex" when the word "stress" would have been appropriate). Unconscious material also surfaces during fantasies, dreams, and hypnosis. In each case, ego controls are lowered, allowing the unconscious to appear. Psychoanalysts believe that as long as unconscious material is repressed and not integrated into the ego (presumably through psychoanalysis), maladaptive behavior (e.g., addictions) will be maintained.

INSIGHTS INTO COMPULSIVE SUBSTANCE USE

Early psychoanalytic formulations insisted that substance dependence stems from unconscious death wishes and self-destructive tendencies of the id. It was believed that among alcoholics and drug addicts, the id is oriented toward death instincts rather than constructive (e.g., sexual) instincts. Thus, many early psychoanalysts viewed compulsive substance abuse as a form of "slow suicide" (Khantzian, 1980). The focus in treatment was on the tendencies of the id. This traditional school of thought, known as "drive reduction," holds that substance abuse is merely a manifest symptom of a repressed idea (or memory) that comes to consciousness. The repressed idea is unrecognizable; that is, it appears as substance abuse, because it is distorted by psychological defenses (Leeds & Morgenstern, 1996). In essence, substance abuse can be thought of as a compromise resulting from the conflict between a repressed idea and the defense against it (Leeds & Morgenstern, 1996).

A second school of thought, within the psychoanalytic tradition, is sometimes referred to as "ego psychology." Contemporary psychoanalytic treatment of chemical dependence seems to draw heavily on this conceptualization of addiction (Murphy & Khantzian, 1995). Here, substance abuse is seen as a symptom of a deficient ego. According to Murphy and Khantzian (1995), "it is the vulnerable and disregulated self which is the central problem in addiction" (p. 162). Individuals with addiction problems are seen as lacking the capacity to adequately care for themselves; they expose themselves unnecessarily to a variety of risks: health, safety, financial, legal, and so on. The consequences of risky or dangerous behavior can be ignored because a sense of well-being, security, and pleasure is provided by the drug intoxication (Murphy & Khantzian, 1995). In this psychoanalytic approach, the goal of treatment is to build ego strength by helping the person develop the capabilities to cope with the demands of the external world.

Despite the differences described previously, psychoanalytic formulations of addiction share a set of assumptions. According to Leeds and Morgenstern (1996), these are:

1) the act of drug use is a symptom of some type of underlying psychological disorder,
2) the psychological problems of the addict precede and cause the substance abuse—there is little recognition that psychological problems are the consequence of substance abuse,
3) addiction is seen as a uniform disorder—there is relatively little consideration given to disorder subtypes, different drugs of abuse, to the course or severity of the addiction problem, etc.,
4) the presence of addiction indicates severe psychopathology. (p.76)

Contemporary psychoanalysts tend to view chemical dependency as a symptom of a deficient ego. Essentially, they believe that substance abuse is only the obvious and outward manifestation of deeper personality problems. The goal of treatment in such cases is to build ego strength, so that the demands of the id can be better managed.

Two Necessary Conditions

According to Wurmser (1974), two general factors are always present in the development of compulsive substance use. The first is described as the "addictive search." This internal urge is a psychological hunger or craving for an entire group of activities; the urge precedes the onset of chemical dependency but accompanies it and follows it, even after abstinence has been established. The activities may include compulsive gambling, overeating, indiscriminate sexual activity, irresistible violence, compulsive shoplifting, endless television viewing, and/or running away. All these activities can be used to provide external relief from overpowering internal drives.

The second necessary factor is referred to as the "adventitious entrance" of chemicals (Wurmser, 1974). This is the random introduction (in terms of accessibility and seductiveness) of alcohol or drugs into a person's life. They are typically introduced by peers, or perhaps by drug dealers in the case of illicit drugs. Without access to and experimentation with these substances, addiction is obviously not possible.

Together, these two predisposing factors (i.e., the addictive search and the adventitious entrance) set the stage for the development of chemical dependency. Both must be present for the disorder to appear. According to Wurmser (1974), some people are driven by an addictive search, but they have not been exposed to the world of drug or alcohol abuse. In such cases, "there is no compulsive drug use without this trigger factor; but there is still an overriding emotional compulsiveness directed toward other activities and objects" (Wurmser, 1974, p. 829). This may also be the case for many chemically dependent persons in recovery. That is, they have removed themselves from the drinking/drugging scene and are abstinent, but they may continue old compulsions or develop new ones. They may be said to be continuing an addictive search even though they are abstinent.

These two predisposing factors may also explain why some people who gain access to the world of drug or alcohol abuse never become dependent on such substances. Despite the availability of various drugs, they may not possess the psychological hunger that is necessary to initiate or maintain compulsive drug or alcohol abuse. In other words, they may not need external relief from internal cravings or urges. Of course, an alternative "disease" explanation is simply that such individuals lack the *genetic* vulnerability to alcoholism and other drug addictions.

Abuse as Affect Defense

Contemporary psychoanalytic thinking maintains that substance abuse itself is a defense mechanism (Khantzian, 1980; Wurmser, 1980). Addicts abuse alcohol or drugs to protect themselves from overwhelming anxiety, depression, boredom, guilt, shame, and other negative emotions. Wurmser (1974) has stated that compulsive drug use is "an attempt at self-treatment" (p. 829). That is, it represents an attempt at self-medication, a way to relieve psychic pain.

For the most part, contemporary psychoanalysts do not view negative affective states (e.g., anxiety and depression) as consequences of substance abuse but, rather, as its causes. According to Khantzian (1980):

> I have become convinced, as has Wurmser, that becoming and remaining addicted to drugs is in most instances associated with severe and significant psychopathology. Necessarily, some of the deserved pathology evident in addicts is the result of drug use and its attendant interpersonal involvements. However, it is my opinion that drug-dependent individuals are predisposed to use and become dependent upon their substances mainly as a result of severe ego impairments and disturbances in the sense of self. . . . (p. 29)

Wurmser's (1978) analysis of this problem goes further. He believes that the greater the legal penalties and social stigma against a drug, the more likely its user is to have severe psychopathology. The lack of internal controls to resist engaging in conduct which society condemns is seen as pathology. Thus, Wurmser (1978) concludes that "a compulsive alcohol or nicotine abuser shows far less preexisting psychopathology than a compulsive (or even casual) user of heroin, LSD, or cocaine" (p. 9).

Wurmser (1978) refers to the link between severe psychopathology and addiction as the "hidden problem." He contends that drug control bureaucrats, law enforcement officials, many physicians (including psychiatrists), and drug users themselves are in denial about this relationship. According to Wurmser (1978), this collective unwillingness to acknowledge the emotional conflict underlying addiction has led to the development of misguided drug control policy and ineffective approaches to prevention and treatment. He believes legal controls do little to address the demand for drugs and that much treatment is superficial because it focuses on the use/nonuse of substances rather than on underlying personality and emotional issues.

Does Research Support the "Self-Medication" Hypothesis?

The psychoanalytic belief that individuals are predisposed to addiction by negative affective states is not supported by research findings. According to Cox's (1985) review of the personality correlates of substance abuse, there is little evidence that psychological distress (e.g., anxiety, depression, and low self-esteem) leads to addiction. Rather, studies of young people indicate that future substance abusers tend to show three character traits: independence, nonconformity, and impulsivity (Cox, 1985). It appears that negative affective states are usually the consequences of years of substance abuse, not the precursors, as claimed by psychoanalysts. Chapter 4 provides more contemporary perspectives on the nature of comorbid substance abuse and mood disorders.

Specific Drugs to Correct Different Affects

Psychoanalysts generally dispute the notion that an addict's drug of choice is determined by economic, environmental, or sociocultural factors. Instead, they maintain that addicts become dependent on the drug that will correct or counteract the specific negative emotional state from which they want relief. For example, Wurmser (1980) puts it this way:

> The choice of drugs shows some fairly typical correlations with otherwise unmanageable affects (moods): narcotics and hypnotics are deployed against rage, shame, and jealously, and particularly the anxiety related to these feelings; stimulants against depression and weakness; psychedelics against boredom and disillusionment; alcohol against guilt, loneliness, and related anxiety. (p. 72)

Khantzian, Halliday, and McAuliffe (1990) have recently outlined the differing types of emotional pain that they believe lead to dependence on opiates, sedative–hypnotics, or cocaine. They propose that opiate or narcotic addicts are typically the victims of traumatic abuse and violence. As a result, they eventually become perpetrators of violence themselves. Their history causes them to suffer with acute and chronic feelings of hostility and anger for which opiates provide relief. In contrast, these authors propose that individuals who are anxious and inhibited use sedative–hypnotics, including alcohol, to overcome deep-seated defenses and fears about interpersonal intimacy. Cocaine addicts are thought to select cocaine for its energizing qualities. These addicts are seeking relief from depression, boredom, or emptiness. Cocaine is found to be appealing because it bolsters feelings of self-esteem and assertiveness (Khantzian et al., 1990).

As noted previously, empirical data often appear to refute psychoanalytic concepts. This seems to be the case for "specific drugs to correct different affects." For example, alcoholism appears to co-occur frequently with antisocial personality disorder and depression (Holdcraft, Iacono, & McGue, 1998), which is somewhat inconsistent with the psychoanalytic profile of the alcoholic as guilt-ridden, lonely, and anxious. In teenagers, epidemiological data indicate that marijuana abuse is correlated with delinquency and depression (Greenblatt, 1998). These associations do not neatly fit in the psychoanalytic model either.

STAGES OF RECOVERY FROM ADDICTION

According to the psychoanalytic perspective, there are three stages to complete recovery, as shown in Table 5.1 (Zimberg, 1978). Stage I is characterized by the self-statement "I can't drink or drug." In this stage, external control (e.g., detoxification and Antabuse) is important. In essence, clients need protection from their own impulses. The second stage is characterized by the self-statement "I won't drink or drug." Here, the control becomes internalized. Many AA/NA members remain at this level indefinitely. The third stage is represented by "I don't have to drink or drug." Many recovering persons never complete this stage, nor do they necessarily relapse. According to the psychoanalytic perspective, insight-oriented therapy is appropriate at this stage (Zimberg, 1978). However, because a recovering client's perception of the need for change is usually diminished at this point (life is relatively normal or manageable), few recovering persons pursue insight-oriented therapy.

PSYCHOANALYTIC CONCEPTS IN CLINICAL PRACTICE TODAY

Psychoanalytic concepts are widely employed in the practice of substance abuse counseling. However, many practitioners are not aware that they are derived from psychoanalytic theory. For example, many make attempts to identify clients' defense mechanisms in an effort to help the clients recognize their perceptual distortions. Denial, rationalization, and fantasy are typical protection mechanisms employed by chemically dependent clients.

TABLE 5.1. A Contemporary Psychoanalytic View of Treatment Stages

Stages	Client status	Treatment
Stage I	"I can't drink or drug" (need for external controls)	Detoxification, directive psychotherapy, Antabuse, drug testing, AA/NA, family therapy
Stage II	"I won't drink or drug" (control becomes internalized)	Directive psychotherapy, supportive psychotherapy, AA/NA; Antabuse and drug testing may be discontinued
Stage III	"I don't have to drink or drug" (conflict over abstinence is resolved)	Psychoanalytic psychotherapy

Note. Adapted from Zimberg (1978). Copyright 1978 by Plenum Publishing Corporation. Adapted by permission.

Closely intertwined with them is the unconscious, an indisputable influence on at least some classes of human behavior.

However, many psychoanalysts today recognize that traditional analytic treatment methods are largely ineffective with substance-dependent clients (e.g., Brickman, 1988). This is not to say that psychoanalytic concepts have no place in clinical practice. As Leeds and Morgenstern (1996) have noted, there often has been confusion between the psychoanalytic *understanding* of addiction and the psychoanalytic *treatment* of the disorder. It should not be assumed that one necessarily leads to the other. In fact, the theory itself seems to predict that traditional psychoanalytic methods would not work well with substance abusers.

Contemporary psychoanalysts have pointed out that the persons with substance dependence suffer from poor ego controls. This makes them poor candidates for psychoanalysis, a process that requires significant ego strength. Wurmser (1974), himself a leading psychoanalyst, states that most compulsive drug users are relatively inaccessible by psychoanalysis. There are various reasons for this poor match. Many persons with substance dependence enter treatment with little initial motivation for personal change. Many others require assistance with the ordinary, mundane challenges of staying sober and "straight" a day at a time (e.g., remembering to take Antabuse and finding a ride to an AA meeting). Still others need strong guidance and structure to avoid relapse. These pressing reality-based concerns are not readily addressed in traditional psychoanalysis, with its emphasis on the intellect, the origins of problems, and protracted self-analysis.

In recent decades, several psychoanalytically oriented clinicians have recommended that traditional psychoanalytic practice be modified for the treatment of persons with substance dependence (Yalisove, 1989). The following modifications have been recommended:

1. The initial stage of treatment should be supportive and didactic in nature.
2. Management issues must be emphasized in early phases of treatment (i.e., hospitalization, dangerous behavior, and withdrawal symptoms).
3. Sessions should be held once or twice a week.
4. The "couch" should not be used.
5. Interpretation should be minimized.
6. Abstinence should be encouraged.
7. AA attendance should be emphasized.

A consideration of these "modifications" gives rise to this question: Is it still psychoanalysis? The extent of the modifications eliminates most (possibly all) of the distinctive features of traditional psychoanalysis. That which is left appears to be conventional psychotherapy.

REVIEW QUESTIONS

1. What are the origins of psychoanalysis?

2. How are psychotherapy and psychoanalysis distinguished from each other?

3. What are major features of the process of psychoanalytic therapy?

4. What are the chief characteristics of the id, ego, and superego? How do they interact?

5. What is a defense mechanism? How are defense mechanisms related to anxiety and the unconscious?

6. How do "drive reduction" and "ego psychology" hypotheses differ in explaining addiction?

7. What are the "addictive search" and the "adventitious entrance"?

8. What is meant by "abuse as affect defense"?

9. Is the self-medication hypothesis of psychoanalysis supported by empirical research?

10. What specific affects are different drugs thought to correct?

11. Why do addicts not recognize the risks associated with their compulsive use?

12. What are the three stages of contemporary psychoanalytic treatment?

13. What are the criticisms of psychoanalysis as a treatment of addiction?

14. Today, do psychoanalysts recommend traditional methods to treat substance abusers?

CHAPTER 6

Conditioning Models and Approaches to Contingency Management

The principal aims of "behaviorism" are to elucidate the conditions of human learning and to develop a technology for behavior change. Behaviorists believe that most or all human behavior is learned, including not only adaptive but also maladaptive behavior (e.g., addiction). One of the major premises, then, is that certain fundamental laws (known and unknown) govern the initiation, maintenance, and cessation of human behavior. Alcohol or drug use is considered a behavior subject to the same principles of learning as driving a car, typing a letter, or building a house.

Behavioral psychology, for the most part, restricts itself to the study of overt behavior—that is, behavior which is observable and measurable. There is a heavy emphasis on empirical evidence, as behaviorists are interested in building a true science of human behavior. For this reason, they are usually not interested in internal "mentalistic" constructs, such as mental illness, self-esteem, affective states, thoughts, values, personality structure (e.g., the ego), defense mechanisms, or the unconscious. These concepts cannot be directly observed or measured, and there is no way to prove or disprove their existence. It is thus believed that they are not appropriate subjects for scientific inquiry.

The most prominent behaviorist of the 20th century, B. F. Skinner, commented on how the use of mentalistic constructs has distorted (in his view) our society's understanding of addiction and other problem behaviors. He did not believe that it is useful to describe persons as immoral, irresponsible, or diseased. According to Skinner (1975),

When the control exercised by others is thus evaded or destroyed (by the individual), only the personal reinforcers are left. The individual turns to immediate gratification, possibly through sex or drugs. If he does not need to do much to find food, shelter, and safety, little behavior will be generated. His condition is then described by saying that he is suffering from a lack of values. As Maslow pointed out, valuelessness is variously described as anomie, amorality, anhedonia, rootlessness, emptiness, hopelessness, the lack of something to believe in and be devoted to. These terms all seem to refer to feelings or states of mind, but what are missing are effective reinforcers. Anomie and amorality refer to a lack of the continued reinforcers which induce people to observe rules. Anhedonia, rootlessness, emptiness, and hopelessness point to the absence of reinforcers of all kinds. . . . If people do not work, it is not because they are lazy or shiftless but because they are not paid enough or because either welfare or affluence has made economic reinforcers less effective. . . . If citizens are not law abiding, it is not because they are scofflaws or criminals but because law enforcement has grown lax. . . . If students do not study, it is not because they are not interested but because the standards have been lowered or because subjects taught are no longer relevant to a satisfactory life. (pp. 112–113)

Skinner (1975) noted that individuals do not choose to become addicted to drugs. Rather, he believed that they are conditioned to engage in frequent drug-taking behavior by a society that is afraid to implement a scientific technology of behavior. In his view, individuals abuse drugs (or alcohol) because they have not been reinforced for engaging in other kinds of constructive behavior.

CONDITIONED BEHAVIOR

Learned behavior is usually classified according to whether it is the result of "respondent conditioning" or "operant conditioning." This distinction is an important one. However, the two types of conditioning do not represent different kinds of learning but, instead, different types of behavior (McKim, 1986). Respondent behavior is under the control of a well-defined stimulus, whereas operant behavior appears voluntary and is not directly elicited by a stimulus situation. Most human behavior falls into the latter category.

Respondent Conditioning

Respondent conditioning is also known as "classical conditioning" or "Pavlovian conditioning." It was the first type of learning to be studied systematically and was first investigated by the great Russian physiologist Ivan Pavlov. Respondent behavior is reflexive in the sense that it is under the control of well-defined environmental stimuli. Examples of respondent behavior include the following:

1. Blinking in response to a bright light.
2. Pulling one's hand away from a hot stove.
3. Salivating at the sight or smell of food.
4. Perspiring as the result of walking into a hot room.
5. Jerking one's leg forward when struck on the knee with a physician's hammer.

When a dog salivates at the sight of food, the salivation is considered respondent behavior, under the control of the stimulus of food. Pavlov found that if he paired the sight of food with a neutral stimulus like a ringing bell, the bell alone would eventually elicit the salivation. Thus, the bell became a conditioned stimulus able to elicit salivation—a strange situation indeed. Figure 6.1 diagrams the respondent or Pavlovian conditioning model.

Interestingly, research conducted by Siegel (1982) has demonstrated that drug tolerance can become partially conditioned to the environment in which the drug is normally used via respondent conditioning procedures. If a drug is administered in the presence of usual cues (i.e., the paired stimulus situation depicted in Figure 6.1), the drug effect will become somewhat diminished over time. In behavioristic jargon, "the drug effect is reduced by these anticipatory conditioned compensatory responses" (Brick, 1990, p. 178). In other words, repeated drug use in the same environment will gradually produce diminishing effects. This is one process for building behavioral tolerance. Thus, while cellular adaptation (a biological process) is clearly involved in the development of drug tolerance, learning also plays an important role.

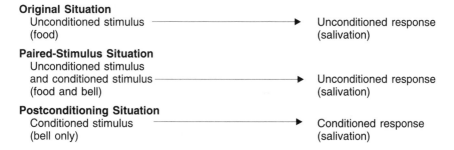

FIGURE 6.1. Model of respondent or Pavlovian conditioning.

Operant Conditioning

Operant behavior is different from respondent behavior in that operant behavior appears to be voluntary. In most cases, it does not seem to be directly elicited, or caused by, a specific stimulus in the environment. Furthermore, operant behavior is conditioned if it is followed by a reinforcer. In other words, operant behaviors are those that are maintained by events occurring *after* the behavior, not before it. If a behavior is followed by a reinforcer, the behavior will probably appear again. The subsequent change in rate of behavior is considered "learning."

A "reinforcer" is best defined as any event that increases the probability or rate of a behavior (Miller, 1980). Reinforcers can be any number of things. Some examples include alcohol, drugs, food, sex, verbal praise, money, a good grade, public recognition, and job promotion. Each person finds different things reinforcing. For example, actively drinking alcoholics find alcohol to be a potent reinforcer. Furthermore, the potency of a reinforcer is determined by an individual's state of deprivation. For instance, in all probability, a soldier who returns from 6 months of combat duty in a place where no alcohol was available is going to generate much more behavior to obtain a beer than a civilian who has ready access to alcohol.

The varying effectiveness of alcohol as a reinforcer is further illustrated by the ability of researchers to breed strains of alcohol-craving mice (McKim, 1986). Some strains show a strong fondness for alcohol; others demonstrate a dislike for the beverage. Alcohol-craving mice prefer alcohol to sugar water and will occasionally drink to drunkenness. For these mice, alcohol is a potent reinforcer. They will learn new behaviors and engage in high rates of a behavior to continue to get alcohol; in other words, they will work for it. Among the mice that do not care for alcohol, the drink cannot be used as a contingency to train them. For this group, alcohol has little reinforcement value.

An important distinction in operant conditioning involves the difference between "positive reinforcement" and "negative reinforcement." In both situations, the rate or probability of a behavior increases. Furthermore, negative reinforcement is not punishment. A negative reinforcement procedure begins with an aversive stimulus; the behavior generated to remove the stimulus results in relief from the noxious stimulus. Thus, in a negative reinforcement procedure, *relief* is the reinforcer. The use of an alarm clock is a good example of negative reinforcement. The alarm sounds until one awakens in order to shut it off. The reinforcer in this case is silence (i.e., relief from noise), and the behavior change is reaching to turn off the alarm.

With addictive behavior, the classic example of negative reinforcement is withdrawal sickness. In alcoholic withdrawal, the symptoms include tremors, irritability, restlessness, anxiety, insomnia, and cravings. These symptoms are known by the alcoholic to almost disappear immediately upon taking a drink. Thus, in chronic alcoholism where an abstinence syndrome is present, drinking is reinforced by relief from the symptoms of withdrawal. Notice that the reinforcer is not alcohol or withdrawal itself but, rather, *relief from withdrawal*. In cases of alcohol dependence in which there is no withdrawal sickness (among teens, young adults, heavy episodic drinkers, etc.), drinking behavior is contingent upon positive reinforcers, such as euphoria and enhanced sociability.

"Punishment" can be defined as any event that decreases the probability or rate of a behavior (Miller, 1980). Again, punishment and negative reinforcement have opposite effects: The former decreases behavior; the latter increases it. Punishers can also be any number of things or events. They can include a "dirty" look, ignoring a comment, or even physical abuse.

In regard to substance use and punishment, it is known that some people have particularly negative physical or psychological reactions to small amounts of alcohol or a drug. The examples of the person who becomes flushed, dizzy, and nauseated after one drink and the person who becomes extremely paranoid and panicky after a couple of puffs on a joint of marijuana illustrate this point. Such persons are essentially punished for substance use. The punisher (i.e., sickness or a panic attack) decreases the probability of future substance use. In cases such as these, there is little likelihood that substance dependencies will develop.

Generalization and Discrimination

Generalization and discrimination are two types of learning that are influenced by environmental stimuli as well as by reinforcement. "Generalization" can be defined as the "tendency to perform a response in a new setting because of the setting's similarity to the one in which the response was learned, with the likelihood of the response's occurring being proportional to the degree of similarity between settings" (Mehr, 1988, p. 153). For example, let us imagine that a cocaine addict, 4 years into recovery, goes on a business trip to a distant city. After arriving at the airport, he heads to the subway to catch a train for a downtown meeting. While riding on the subway train, he experiences intense cravings for cocaine. The last time he can remember having such an intense desire for cocaine was when he used to snort the drug with his buddies while riding the trains in his hometown. He essentially generalized cocaine cravings (and use) to all subway trains.

By contrast, "discrimination" can be defined as the "learning of different responses to two or more similar but distinct stimuli because of the different consequences associated with each one" (Mehr, 1988, p. 153). The failure to discriminate contributes to many relapses during early recovery.

For example, let us suppose that an addict is discharged from an inpatient treatment facility. He has many new friends whom he has met through Narcotics Anonymous (NA), and many old friends with whom he used to get high. He insists that he can be with his old friends and not "pick up" or "slip." Unfortunately, he soon relapses, but he gradually learns that his old friends represent a stimulus condition that he must avoid. This gradual recognition is the process of "discriminative learning." This learning process is also important for understanding the dynamics of controlled drinking—an issue to be discussed later in the chapter.

Extinction

Another conditioning principle is "extinction," which is the absence or removal of a reinforcer. With regard to substance abuse, abstinence and treatment represent extinction procedures. Relapse can be considered evidence of an incomplete extinction procedure. However, the sheer availability of alcohol and drugs, and their ever-present potential for producing euphoria, make complete extinction of drug-seeking behavior difficult. Thus, from a behavioral perspective, a return to drug use (i.e., relapse) is always a possibility.

INITIATION OF ALCOHOL AND DRUG ABUSE

From a behavioristic perspective, the initiation of substance use is related to three factors: (1) availability, (2) lack of reinforcement for alternative behavior, and (3) lack of punishment for experimenting with alcohol or another drug. Clearly, use cannot begin if a substance is not available; this simple fact is the basis for the federal government's drug interdiction efforts. The second factor, lack of reinforcement, becomes operative when socially approved behavior (e.g., studying, working, attending church, and family recreational activities) that could take the place of drug-using behaviors is not sufficiently rewarded. In such cases, individuals are likely to engage in drug-taking behavior, which is accompanied by more potent or alluring reinforcers. Third, and perhaps most important, many people who experiment with a substance do not receive immediate punishment. Following the first use of a substance, few people get arrested, suffer an adverse physical reaction, lose a job, fail an exam, or receive harsh criticism from peers. The negative consequences of drug use are almost always delayed, sometimes for years or even decades (particularly with alcoholism and nicotine addiction). Not only are people unpunished immediately; they are usually quickly reinforced by euphoria and peer acceptance. Initiation, then, is the result of the combination of availability, reinforcers, and punishers in the social environment.

ADDICTION

McAuliffe and Gordon (1980) have offered the following behavioral definition of "addiction": an operantly conditioned response whose tendency
becomes stronger as a function of the quality, number, and size of reinforcements that follow each drug ingestion. Each addict experiences his/her own
set of multiple reinforcers. According to McAuliffe and Gordon (1980),
there are three classes of reinforcers: (1) euphoria, (2) social variables, and
(3) elimination of withdrawal sickness. The combination of these effects
will vary for each individual and each type of drug. For example, elimination of withdrawal sickness may be a more potent reinforcer for the heroin
addict than for the PCP addict. In addition, relief from withdrawal may be
a stronger reinforcer for the physically dependent heroin addict than for
one who is not physically dependent.

Euphoria is also important. For example, the euphoric consequence of
cocaine ingestion may be more important to the maintenance of cocaine
addiction than the euphoria that results from drinking alcohol. Furthermore, "peer acceptance," a social variable, may be a more potent reinforcer
for the adolescent marijuana smoker than for the 40-year-old marijuana
user. Thus, the specific combination of reinforcing effects is that which
"drives" each addiction.

For behaviorists, the inability to refrain from using a drug (i.e., loss of
control) merely indicates that a sufficient history of reinforcement has
probably been acquired to impel a high rate of use (McAuliffe & Gordon,
1980). Behaviorists do not believe that there is a single point at which an
individual suddenly becomes "addicted." Rather, the word "addiction" is
simply a term used to describe an operantly conditioned behavior that
occurs at a relatively high rate. The individual's addiction develops gradually and varies continually in response to drug-related contingencies. An
"addict" is merely a person who engages in a high rate of drug use and who
has a sufficient history of reinforced drug taking to outweigh the more
socially acceptable rewards of life (career accomplishments, family interests, marital sex, material possessions, etc.).

RELATIONSHIP BETWEEN ADDICTION
AND PHYSICAL DEPENDENCE

For behaviorists, physical dependence on a drug is neither a necessary nor a
sufficient condition for the development of an addiction (McAuliffe &
Gordon, 1980). This is consistent with criteria of the text revision of the
fourth edition of the *Diagnostic and Statistical Manual of Mental Disorders*
(DSM-IV-TR; American Psychiatric Association, 2000). Physical depend-

ence is simply a side effect of using certain classes of drugs at a high rate over a sufficient period of time. It merely sets the stage for experiencing withdrawal sickness and its relief. The relief is but one possible reinforcing effect that maintains addictive behavior. Euphoria and peer acceptance are equally potent, and in some cases, more potent, reinforcers. Again, this is especially true of drugs that do not produce physical dependence or do so only minimally (hallucinogens, inhalants, marijuana, etc.)

It may be readily apparent that some addictions are not driven by the reinforcing effects of relief from withdrawal sickness (e.g., marijuana dependence). However, it should also be pointed out that physical dependence can exist in the absence of addiction. The most common example involves hospitalized patients recovering from surgery. Such patients are sometimes administered large doses of narcotic analgesics after surgery, over an extended period of time. When the patients are gradually weaned off the drug, they may experience some symptoms of withdrawal (irritability, diarrhea, headache, muscle ache, depression, etc.). However, because they are not "addicted," they typically do not engage in drug-seeking behavior or verbalize cravings for the drug. In fact, in many cases they do not even recognize the symptoms as those of withdrawal but simply as those of recovery from surgery.

Even in heroin addiction, relief from withdrawal is sometimes not an important reinforcing effect. Three situations involving heroin addicts illustrate the distinction between addiction and physical dependence:

1. Some heroin addicts have been described as having "ice cream habits" because when administered a narcotic antagonist they are discovered to have no physical dependence on the drug (Ray & Ksir, 1999). They claim they cannot stop using heroin, even though they want to, and are adamant about continuing their use despite the known risks.

2. Many compulsive, long-term heroin addicts go for months, sometimes even years, without ever interrupting their use long enough to experience withdrawal. This indicates that physical dependence (i.e., relief from withdrawal) is not the reinforcer driving their addictive behavior.

3. Many detoxified heroin addicts continue to report that they still feel addicted to the drug many months after last using it. They often continue to express strong desires for heroin.

CESSATION AND RELAPSE

From a behavioristic perspective, cessation of alcohol and drug abuse occurs when the punishers that follow ingestion become less temporally remote (McAuliffe & Gordon, 1980). The immediate severity of punishment effects gradually builds over months or years of abusing a drug. Typically, alcoholics and addicts experience repeated brushes with the law, including perhaps longer and longer jail sentences; their sources of money become scarce, jobs become harder to find and keep, family members and friends become increasingly hostile, medical problems worsen, and so on. As these contingencies become more closely linked in time to the substance use, its rate gradually, or in some cases abruptly, ceases.

Behaviorists expect relapses to occur at relatively high rates among persons in early recovery, because drugs are widely available in our society, and because they always retain their ability to cause euphoria. Combined with these factors is the reality that many of the rewards (i.e., reinforcement) that come with abstinence and recovery are delayed. In fact, some abstinence-related reinforcers come only after months or years of sobriety. For example, to regain the trust and respect of family members and coworkers, addicts may have to maintain a year or more of abstinence. Some cocaine addicts have not been able to stabilize their financial affairs for years as a result of the debt they have incurred while using the drug. Drug dealers may not be able to make progress toward life or career goals because of jail time, or simply as a result of their convictions. Whenever reinforcers such as these are delayed to some distant point in the future, their effectiveness in maintaining behavior consistent with recovery is diminished. For these reasons, relapses are always a possibility, especially during early stages of recovery.

PRINCIPLES OF CONTINGENCY MANAGEMENT

The application of learning principles to the helping process is called "behavioral counseling," "behavior therapy," "behavioral contracting," "contingency management," or simply "contingency contracting." Based on the premise that alcohol and drug use (and addiction) are learned, a helping professional's role is to assist clients in learning more effective ways of behaving so that clients reach *their* goals. According to Ullman and Krasner (1965), contingency contracting begins with a functional analysis of behavior that asks the following questions:

1. What behavior is maladaptive? Specifically, what behaviors should be increased or decreased?
2. What environmental contingencies currently maintain or support the behavior? As applied to addiction, what are the rewards that maintain the drug use? Are there punishers associated with avoiding use?
3. What environmental changes can be manipulated to alter the behavior?

In behavioral counseling, the development and maintenance of addiction are the same as the development and maintenance of any other behavior. This view has two important implications. First, drug use is not inherently maladaptive; rather, it becomes inappropriate as the result of labels that significant others assign to it. For instance, an alcoholic is simply a person whose drinking behavior has adversely affected a family member, friend, or coworker. The second implication is that drinking or drug use is maintained because other, more adaptive behaviors are not reinforced or not possible. A typical example would include an alcoholic man in early recovery and his nonsupportive wife. As a result of several months of abstinence, he begins to demonstrate appropriate parenting behavior (e.g., helps his son with homework), which his wife criticizes. The lack of reinforcement for these new behaviors soon leads him back to drinking.

According to Dustin and George (1973), behavioral counseling is based on four assumptions about human nature and the change process. As applied to substance abusers, these assumptions are often questioned by laypeople and mental health professionals who feel that substance dependence is driven by unique dynamics. The four assumptions are as follows:

1. Humans are viewed as being neither intrinsically good nor bad, but as an experiencing organism who has potential for all kinds of behavior.
2. Humans are able to conceptualize and control their own behavior.
3. Humans are able to acquire new behaviors.
4. Humans are able to influence others' behavior as well as to be influenced by others in their own behavior. (p. 12)

Dustin and George (1973) identified three phases of contingency contracting. The first phase can be described as *problem specification*. With emphathetic understanding, the helping professional assists clients in identifying their problems in behavioral terms. For example, addicts who say that they are lonely and depressed may lack the kind of social skills necessary for meeting someone new. In teaching such skills, the helper would assist in identifying the necessary stimulus and reinforcing conditions for meeting someone new. The second phase consists of helping clients to *make a commitment to change*. There are many barriers to achieving this commitment, particularly with substance-dependent clients. The use of incentives to generate and maintain motivation for change is critical. Ignoring this phase or giving it little attention is a major reason that clients drop out of counseling or treatment. The third phase is *specifying goals*. Here it is important that the counselor work toward the clients' goals; the helper should not impose goals on clients.

APPLICATIONS OF CONTINGENCY MANAGEMENT

The following discussion shows how contingency contracting has been applied to a number of treatment issues. These include efforts to (1) establish and maintain controlled drinking; (2) initiate and maintain abstinence, and encourage the adoption of recovery behaviors (taking an Antabuse [disulfiram] tablet, attending AA each day, etc.); (3) promote positive change in a client's vocational, recreational, social, and familial functioning; (4) motivate the reluctant alcoholic to seek treatment; (5) reduce cocaine and other illicit drug use; (6) enhance compliance with methadone maintenance; and (7) engage couples in marital therapy.

Controlled Drinking

With a subset of problem drinkers, perhaps 15–25%, controlled drinking, managed by contingency contracting, is a viable alternative to abstinence (Miller, 1982). It should be emphasized that controlled drinking is not an effort to encourage recovering alcoholics to "try drinking again." With selected candidates, it is one of many options at the *onset of treatment.*

There is a large body of empirical evidence to suggest that there should be an expansion of the use of controlled drinking in the United States (see Sobell, Wilkinson, & Sobell, 1990). Controlled drinking appears to be a frequent outcome of both moderation-focused and abstinence-focused treatments; Sanchez-Craig and Lei (1986) found that the overwhelming majority of clients with positive outcomes adopted moderation in both goal conditions. Many successful clients benefit from abstinence-oriented treatment but apparently reject its basic goal and practice controlled use instead.

As a treatment strategy, controlled drinking is usually denounced in the United States (Goode, 1993). Yet, in Canada, Britain, and the Scandinavian countries it has much greater acceptance (see review in Rosenberg, Melville, Levell, & Hodge, 1994). For instance, a survey of treatment agencies in England, Scotland, and Wales found that about 75% of service providers reported controlled drinking to be an acceptable treatment goal (Rosenberg et al., 1994). About one-half of these providers thought it to be acceptable for 1–25% of their clients. The providers most frequently reported that their position on controlled drinking was based on their own professional experience, rather than on research or agency policy.

Heather and Robertson (1983) identified six possible advantages of a controlled-drinking strategy:

1. In our society, abstinence from alcohol is deviant behavior. This is unfortunate. However, the stigma and the label of "alcoholic" pose significant adjustment problems for some people.
2. Among some alcoholics, abstinence may lead to overwhelming states of anxiety or depression that are unlikely to be managed in other ways.
3. Sometimes, overall improvement in life functioning does not result from abstinence.
4. In some alcoholics, abstinence is associated with severe psychosocial problems that lead to frequent relapse.
5. Abstinence during treatment rules out the possibility for changes in drinking behavior.
6. The demand placed on alcoholics to abstain deters many from seeking help until their problem is quite severe.

Miller and Hester (1980) designed a model for controlled drinking based on behavioral principles: *behavioral self-control training* (BSCT). With selected candidates, Miller and Hester (1980) demonstrated an effectiveness rate for BSCT of 60–80%. In another study, Harris and Miller (1990) reported that 78% of problem drinkers in a self-directed BSCT group and 63% of those in a therapist-directed BSCT group were rated as maintaining improvement 15 months after initiating treatment. The improved group consisted of abstainers (confirmed by collateral reports) and controlled drinkers. The criteria for being classified as "improved" included (1) on average, no more than 20 standard drinks weekly; (2) not exceeding blood alcohol levels of .08–.10 on any occasion (verified by collateral reports); and for those who failed to meet the criteria for controlled drinking (3) succeeding in reducing their weekly alcohol intake by 30% or more (confirmed by collateral reports).

BSCT consists of the following components (Miller & Hester, 1980):

1. A functional analysis of the drinking behavior is conducted. Together, the client and the helping professional determine specific and appropriate limits for alcohol consumption; these depend upon body weight and safety concerns. Typically, limits for consumption range from two drinks to perhaps four on one occasion.
2. The client monitors and records consumption.
3. Clients are trained to control the rate of their drinking.
4. Self-reinforcement procedures are created to maintain gains.
5. Emphasis is placed on stimulus control training.
6. In place of alcohol, clients are taught a variety of coping skills for obtaining those outcomes they no longer derive from excessive alcohol use.

Numerous studies have demonstrated the effectiveness of BSCT in helping abusive drinkers to control their drinking. Unfortunately, it is probably not possible to apply BSCT to the broad spectrum of alcoholic clients who appear for treatment. In addition to not being appropriate for clients with certain medical conditions (discussed later), it may be ineffective for the large number of coerced clients (those who are more or less "forced" into treatment by employers, family members, the courts, etc.). Such clients often seek treatment to escape even more aversive sanctions and frequently have little interest in learning to modify their drinking behavior. The limited appeal of BSCT among many abusive drinkers is highlighted by the fact that many controlled-drinking studies have found it difficult to recruit clients (Cameron & Spence, 1976; Robertson, Heather, Dzialdowski, Crawford, & Winton, 1986). Harris and Miller (1990) solicited clients in the Albuquerque, New Mexico, metropolitan area for 6 months via the local news media. Despite the fact that the program was advertised as free of charge, they were able to recruit only 34 clients for their BSCT study.

It should be noted that even the proponents of controlled drinking do not believe that it is a viable strategy for most alcoholics (Miller, 1982). Good candidates are generally young, motivated clients who have no biomedical impairment from alcohol abuse. Lewis, Dana, and Blevins (1988) developed criteria for ruling out controlled-drinking candidates. Those who should not attempt it include the following:

1. clients with liver dysfunction, stomach problems, an ulcer, any other disease of the gastrointestinal tract;
2. clients who have cardiac problems that would be adversely affected by alcohol;
3. clients who have any physical illness or condition that would be negatively affected by alcohol;
4. clients who have a diagnosis of alcohol idiosyncratic disorder intoxication (American Psychiatric Association, 1980, p. 132);
5. clients who are committed to abstinence;
6. clients who have strong external demands for abstinence;
7. female clients who are pregnant or considering pregnancy;
8. clients who lose control of their behavior while drinking;
9. clients who have been physically addicted to alcohol;
10. clients using any medication or drug that is dangerous when combined with alcohol;
11. clients who are abstaining from alcohol;
12. those people with the following history: over 40, divorced and not in a supportive relationship, out of work, or with a family history of alcoholism; and
13. clients who have tried a competently administered moderation-oriented treatment and have failed. (p. 153)

Contracting for the Initiation and Maintenance of Abstinence

When abstinence has been chosen and initiated, certain behaviors are conducive to the maintenance of what is commonly called "recovery." They include the following:

1. Attending AA/NA meetings.
2. Calling one's sponsor.
3. Reading self-help literature.
4. Getting to work on time.
5. Avoiding "slipping places."
6. Taking Antabuse as prescribed.
7. Socializing with fellow recovering addicts.
8. Practicing relaxation exercises or other coping skills.
9. Attending to one's family responsibilities.

Contingency contracting can be used to help clients initiate and maintain these behaviors and any others found to be conducive to recovery. Reinforcers and punishers are linked to the occurrence and absence of specified behaviors, as outlined in a written contract. Of course, the contract is not legally binding; however, both client and counselor should sign it, and the client should receive a photocopy. Again, it is not forced on a client but, rather, is an agreement that a helping professional and client develop together.

Typically, contracts outline the rewards that clients give themselves if they engage in the specified behaviors. For example, if a client attends five AA meetings a week, he/she can go out for dinner on the weekend. If the client fails to make it to five meetings in a particular week, then he/she must forgo the restaurant outing. Likewise, a client may decide to "punish" him/ herself for neglecting to take Antabuse on a particular day. Such oversights can be self-penalized by arranging for donations (perhaps $5 or $10) to be given to a disliked political or religious organization.

There are a number of important principles involved in effective contingency contracting. Two of these are the temporal proximity of the reinforcer or punisher to the specified behavior and the potency of the contingency (Miller, 1980). First, in brief, reinforcers and punishers are most effective when they occur immediately after the specified behavior; those that are delayed are generally less effective. Second, individuals differ considerably in regard to rewards and punishers. For instance, ice cream might be a potent reinforcer for some recovering clients but completely ineffective for others. Thus, effective contracts will rely on contingencies that have special significance for the particular client.

Stitzer and Bigelow (1978) examined the desirability of reinforcers among a group of methadone maintenance patients ($n = 53$). Using a questionnaire, they found that the methadone "take-home" privilege was the most effective incentive available to methadone maintenance clinics. The second most effective reinforcer among this group was $30 per week, followed in descending order of desirability by $20 per week, opportunity to self-select methadone dose, fewer urinalyses, availability of a client representative/advocate, elimination of mandatory counseling, a monthly party, and finally the opportunity to play pool.

The Community Reinforcement Approach

Behavioral therapists have recognized that the application of contingency management procedures to isolated aspects of substance abuse is a narrow approach. To enhance the effectiveness of behavioral treatment, Hunt and Azrin (1973) and Azrin (1976) developed a multicomponent treatment strategy that makes reinforcement in the patient's community contingent upon abstinence from alcohol and/or drugs. A system of contingencies is created for four areas of a client's life: vocational, recreational, social, and familial. As long as abstinence is maintained, the recovering client receives reinforcers in these areas. Typically, the client's significant others are involved in these contingency contracts, and his/her behavior may be shaped as well.

In an early study in this area, Hunt and Azrin (1973) compared a community reinforcement program for alcoholism to a standard hospital treatment program and found that the former approach produced significantly better patient outcomes over a 6-month period. Compared to patients in the standard hospital program, those in the community reinforcement program spent less time drinking alcohol, were less likely to be unemployed, and were less likely to be readmitted for treatment. In a second study, Azrin (1976) was able to replicate these findings using a 2-year follow-up assessment.

Motivating the Alcoholic to Seek Treatment

Community reinforcement training (CRT) has been applied to the problem of motivating the violent, alcoholic husband to seek treatment (Sisson & Azrin, 1993). The focus of the training is the wife of the alcoholic. There were four objectives to the CRT program: (1) reduce physical abuse to the wife, (2) encourage sobriety in the husband, (3) increase the likelihood that the husband would seek treatment, and (4) teach the wife to assist in the treatment process. The basic premise of the program was that family members learn, by negative reinforcement, to personally avoid the negative consequences of the drinker's behavior. In the alcoholic family, the aversive stimuli are anticipated negative events such as the alcoholic losing his job, obvious drunkenness at a public event, or even physical brutality. From a behavioral perspective, spouses (typically wives) engage in a variety of behaviors to escape from these consequences. A potentially controversial aspect of this perspective is that the spouse's behavior is thought not to be so much an effort to protect the alcoholic, but to protect self.

The CRT program emphasizes the didactic training of specific skills (Sisson & Azrin, 1993). Wives are taught to be nice to their husband when he avoids alcohol. They are coached to talk about those topics their husband enjoys. This is often difficult for wives to carry out because of built-up resentment over past events. The wife is taught how to tell her husband that she likes him sober. The instruction guides her not to be pleasant when her husband is drinking and not to allow him to escape the consequences of drunkenness, if possible. She also learns to recognize the series of events that lead up to a violent episode and ways to prevent it. Finally, she is taught to take advantage of her husband's saying he would like to cut down or stop drinking. When this happens, she is prepared to act immediately. In the CRT program, the couple would be seen by a mental health professional the next day.

Before the husband actually begins treatment, the wife is "prepped" to participate in an "Antabuse contract" with her husband (Sisson & Azrin, 1993). The following is explained to the wife:

> "When he comes into counseling we are going to want him to take a pill called Antabuse. Antabuse is a small white pill that, if taken daily, prevents an individual from drinking even small amounts of alcohol. If a person drinks on Antabuse, they become violently ill. An important characteristic of Antabuse that can really help you is that once your husband is taking Antabuse regularly, even if he decides to stop taking it and go back to drinking, he can't for approximately 5 to 14 days because it stays in his system. We'll set up a procedure where you dissolve the pill in a small amount of water and watch him take it. You will know far ahead of time if he's going to drink so you won't have to worry daily if he is going to drink and become violent again. In addition, we have marriage counseling to help you learn to communicate better, and we have a job program to help your husband find a better job." (Sisson & Azrin, 1993, p. 41)

Once in counseling, the couple rehearses a procedure for administering the Antabuse on a daily basis. In addition, the couple practices "Antabuse refusal" procedures in preparation for the possibility that the husband will balk at taking the medication sometime in the future.

In an evaluation of CRT, Sisson and Azrin (1986) found that the program was superior to traditional counseling that relied on Al-Anon.

Training of the nonalcoholic family members resulted in a 50% reduction in drinking before the alcoholic entered treatment. The CRT program was much more likely to result in the alcoholic initiating treatment than the traditional approach. Furthermore, abstinence from alcohol was significantly greater for the husbands whose wives received reinforcement training.

Behavioral Treatment for Cocaine Dependence

During the 1990s, the failure to adequately treat cocaine dependence, based on pharmacological and psychosocial interventions, led to a resurgence of interest in research based on reinforcement principles (Higgins et al., 2004). Much of this research has relied on a voucher-based incentives approach, which involves "the delivery of vouchers exchangeable for retail items contingent on patients meeting a predetermined therapeutic target" (Higgins, Alessi, & Dantona, 2002, p. 888). Biochemically verified abstinence from recent cocaine use has usually been that target. The voucher-based approach has been found to increase treatment retention because clients must remain in the program to receive incentives. This is important because retention has been associated with positive treatment outcomes. In addition, a great deal of the research in this area has coupled the use of vouchers with CRT.

Higgins et al. (1991) conducted the first study testing the voucher incentive approach as a means to establish an initial period of abstinence in cocaine addicts in an outpatient setting. The investigation compared the efficacy of behavioral treatment to that of a traditional Twelve-Step drug counseling program. A total of 28 patients participated in the study. The first 13 cocaine-dependent patients were offered the behavioral treatment program; all 13 accepted it. The following 15 patients were offered the Twelve-Step drug counseling program. The authors note that 3 of the 15 patients refused this program option.

The two treatment regimens were quite different. In the behavioral program, patients and therapists jointly selected material reinforcers (Higgins et al., 1991). The goal of the behavioral program was specifically to achieve abstinence from cocaine. The program's contingencies pertained only to cocaine use. Urine specimens were collected four times a week, and patients were breathalyzed at these times as well; however, patients were not penalized for positive test results for drugs other than cocaine. The patients were informed of their urine test results immediately after providing their specimens.

The urine specimens testing negative for cocaine metabolites were rewarded with points that were recorded on vouchers and given to the patient (Higgins et al., 1991). Each point was worth 15 cents. Money was never given directly to patients; rather, it was used to make retail purchases in the community. Staff members actually made the purchases and gave the items to the patients. The first negative urine specimen earned 10 points (i.e., $1.50). The second specimen was worth 15 points ($2.25). The third one earned 20 points ($3). The value of each subsequent negative urine specimen increased by 5 points. Furthermore, to bolster the probability of continuous abstinence from cocaine, patients were rewarded with a $10 bonus each time they provided four consecutive negative urine specimens. Patients who remained continuously abstinent throughout the entire 12-week treatment program earned points worth $1,038, or $12.35 per day.

When the patient tested positive for cocaine or failed to provide a specimen, the value of the vouchers dropped back to 10 points (i.e., $1.50). Items that had previously been purchased did not have to be returned. Higgins et al. (1991) reported that the items purchased were "quite diverse and included ski-lift passes, fishing licenses, camera equipment, bicycle equipment, and continuing education materials" (p. 1220). In the program, counselors retained the right to veto purchases. Purchases were approved only if their use was consistent with treatment goals.

The community reinforcement procedures focused on four broad issues: (1) reciprocal relationship counseling, (2) identification of the antecedents and consequences of cocaine use, (3) employment counseling, and (4) development of recreational activities. These issues were addressed in twice-weekly 1-hour counseling sessions throughout the 12-week program. The emphasis appeared to be placed on the first issue, relationship counseling. Eight of the 13 patients in the behavioral program participated in reciprocal relationship counseling. This counseling consisted of procedures "for instructing people how to negotiate for positive changes in their relationship" (p. 1220). The authors describe how this worked as follows:

> To integrate the community reinforcement approach and contingency management procedures, the patient's significant other was telephoned immediately following each urinalysis test and informed of the results. If the specimen was negative for cocaine, the spouse, friends, or relative engaged in positive activities with the patients that had been agreed upon beforehand. If the result was positive for cocaine use, he or she refrained from the agreed upon positive activities but offered the patient assistance in dealing with difficulties in achieving abstinence. (Higgins et al., 1991, p. 1220)

The Twelve-Step drug treatment consisted of either twice-weekly 2-hour group therapy sessions or once-weekly group sessions combined with 1-hour individual therapy sessions (Higgins et al., 1991). In both formats, the Twelve Steps of NA were emphasized. The patients were informed that cocaine addiction was a treatable but incurable disease. They were required to attend at least one self-help meeting a week and to have a sponsor by the final week of treatment. The counseling sessions provided both supportive and confrontive therapy, as well as didactic lectures and videos on vital recovery topics. In the ninth week of treatment, attempts were made to involve family members in the treatment process. Finally, aftercare plans based on Twelve-Step principles were created in the latter weeks of treatment.

After 12 weeks, the two groups (i.e., behavioral treatment vs. Twelve-Step drug counseling) were compared on a variety of outcomes. Across all these measures, the patients in the behavioral treatment showed better outcomes than those in the Twelve-Step group (Higgins et al., 1991). For example, 11 of the 13 patients in the behavioral treatment completed the 12-week program, compared to just 5 of 12 in the Twelve-Step treatment. In the behavioral treatment group, one patient dropped out at week 9 and returned to cocaine use, and the other one had to be admitted to an inpatient unit because of "bingeing." The seven unsuccessful patients in the Twelve-Step treatment were terminated for the following reasons: (1) lack of regular attendance; (2) refused group counseling; (3) refused to abstain from marijuana; (4) did not return after being denied a prescription for antianxiety medication; (5) following a relapse, entered inpatient rehabilitation; (6) decided no longer needed treatment; and (7) was murdered.

Patients in behavioral treatment were also more likely than those in the Twelve-Step treatment to have longer periods of continuous abstinence from cocaine (Higgins et al., 1991). Of 13 behavior therapy patients, 10 achieved 4-week periods of continuous abstinence; of the Twelve-Step patients, only 3 of 12 did the same. Furthermore, six of the behavioral therapy patients achieved 8-week periods of continuous abstinence, whereas none of the Twelve-Step patients accomplished the same. In the behavioral treatment group, 92% of all collected urine specimens were cocaine-free, whereas 78% were "clean" in the Twelve-Step group. This occurred even though many more urine specimens were collected from the behavioral treatment group ($n = 552$) than from the Twelve-Step group ($n = 312$).

The results from this initial study were provocative for a number of reasons. First, the findings suggested that reinforcers could be found to compete with cocaine's intoxicating effects. At the time, the popular perception was that cocaine is so rewarding that food, sex, and all other sources of reinforcement could not compete with the drug; the Higgins et al. (1991) study suggested that money (in the form of vouchers) could be an effective alternative reward. Second, the findings suggest that polydrug abusers need not be required to stop use of all drugs at the same time. Contrary to traditional drug treatment philosophy, perhaps it is possible, even preferable, to work on eliminating use of one drug at a time. Finally, the

Higgins et al. study demonstrated how important incentives are in motivating clients to stay in treatment and to adopt and maintain abstinence. It appeared that many clients drop out of traditional Twelve-Step programs too early (i.e., before completing 3 months) because they either do not receive or do not anticipate receiving significant rewards for staying in treatment. Thus, the initial Higgins study raised the possibility that incentives may be the key to providing effective treatment for cocaine dependence.

Higgins and colleagues then conducted a series of randomized clinical trials to further test the efficacy of the combined CRT/voucher intervention (see Higgins et al., 1993; Higgins et al., 1994; Higgins et al., 1995; Higgins, Wong, Badger, Haug-Ogden, & Dantona, 2000; Higgins et al., 2003). Three of these trials were designed to assess the independent ability of specific intervention features to produce positive treatment outcomes (Higgins et al., 1994; Higgins et al., 2000; Higgins et al., 2003). The purpose of attempting to decompose the intervention was to possibly make the treatment more efficient to aid in its transfer to conventional treatment settings.

The first trial tested CRT in combination with voucher incentives against CRT alone (Higgins et al., 1994). Retention in treatment and abstinence from cocaine were significantly greater in the CRT/vouchers condition than in CRT alone. This finding indicates that the voucher component of the intervention made an active contribution to the positive outcomes produced by the combined CRT/vouchers treatment. In addition, these intervention effects were observed 6 months after the termination of treatment (Higgins et al., 1995). The second trial in this research program (1) provided further support for the active contribution of the voucher program to cocaine abstinence and (2) demonstrated that the positive effects of the voucher incentives could be detected 1 year following treatment termination (Higgins et al., 2000). The purpose of the third trial was to determine whether CRT combined with voucher incentives improves treatment outcomes above and beyond that produced by voucher incentives alone (Higgins et al., 2003). Compared to voucher incentives alone, the CRT/voucher combination was found to independently contribute to improved treatment retention and decreased cocaine use, but only during the treatment period. Thus, it appears that posttreatment abstinence from cocaine is more closely associated with the voucher incentives than with the CRT.

The CRT/voucher-based research presented here suggests that drug dependence is essentially a "reinforcement disorder" (Higgins et al., 2002, p. 907). Although the approach is clearly supported by evidence, the major obstacle to its widespread dissemination as a treatment option is how to cover program costs. The pioneering work done by Higgins and colleagues and other research groups is typically supported by federal research grants.

Thus, the unresolved issue is how a funding mechanism can be created to support incentive-driven treatment programs for persons with substance use disorders. In the public policy arena, this issue certainly would generate a great deal of controversy.

Enhancing Compliance with Methadone Maintenance

Methadone is a relatively long-lasting synthetic opiate that prevents opiate withdrawal symptoms for 24 to 36 hours (NIDA, 1987). In proper doses, methadone does not produce sedation or euphoria and therefore has been used for several decades as a treatment for heroin addiction. Though there are positive outcomes to methadone maintenance (Mueller & Wyman, 1997), one common problem is that many clients continue to use a variety of illicit drugs while receiving methadone from a clinic (NIDA, 1987).

Contingency contracting has been found to be an effective approach to this problem. A variety of contingencies have been used to increase the rate at which methadone clients produce drug-free urine samples. Money and program privileges have been used as positive reinforcers (e.g., Stitzer, Bigelow, & Liebson, 1980). Aversive consequences, such as contracting for the termination of methadone treatment, also have been found to be effective in reducing positive urine samples (Dolan, Black, Penk, Robinowitz, & DeFord, 1985). Another effective approach has been to make access to methadone maintenance contingent upon cocaine-free urine samples during the initial phase of treatment (Kidorf & Stitzer, 1993).

The combination of a "take-home" incentive (a positive reinforcer) and a "split-dosing" contingency (an aversive consequence) appears to boost the rate of drug-free urine samples among chronic polysubstance abusers who do not comply with conventional methadone treatment (Kidorf & Stitzer, 1996). A take-home incentive allows a client to leave the clinic with a dose of methadone. This is a convenience for the client because it reduces the frequency with which he/she must travel to the clinic. A split-dosing contingency requires clients to make two daily visits to the clinic to receive their full dose of methadone. Kidrof and Stitzer (1996) implemented split dosing following a positive urine test. They found that the combined use of positive reinforcers and aversive consequences had a marked effect on 28% of a previously noncompliant sample.

Behavioral Marital Therapy for Alcoholism

Research suggests that behavioral marital therapy is an effective way to treat married alcoholics (Noel & McCrady, 1993). Investigation into the role of spouse involvement in alcoholism found that the optimal treatment approach has three components: (1) behavioral treatment for the alcoholic, (2) interventions for the spouse to alter behavior that trigger or reinforce drinking, and (3) behavioral marital therapy.

Behavioral treatment for the alcoholic begins with a functional assessment of the alcoholic's drinking behavior and identification of the alcohol use goal. Noel and McCrady (1993) believe that while abstinence is the most realistic goal for most couples, it should not be imposed on them. However, they do request that couples establish an initial period of abstinence—usually 6 months. If reduced drinking is the long-term goal, the couple is asked to specify the parameters of controlled alcohol use. The aims of the behavioral treatment are to teach both the alcoholic and the spouse to (1) control the stimuli that provoke drinking urges and consumption, (2) rearrange the contingencies that prompt drinking, (3) restructure unproductive thoughts, and (4) develop alternatives to drinking.

The spouse intervention also uses stimulus control, contingency management, cognitive restructuring, and alternatives to drinking. Only here they are used to modify those behaviors that trigger or reinforce the spouse's drinking. Noel and McCrady (1993) indicate that cognitive restructuring is especially helpful for teaching the nonalcoholic spouse how to reinforce behavior that supports abstinence and when to ignore drinking behavior or be less alarmed by its consequences for self.

Behavioral marital therapy seeks to improve the couple's ability to communicate and to enhance the relationship. Cognitive restructuring is used here. In addition, the therapy helps couples plan for fun, communicate their needs better, negotiate conflict, and solve problems.

Compared to other forms of alcoholism treatment involving spouses, behavioral marital therapy has better outcomes (Noel & McCrady, 1993). The approach described previously increased marital stability and satisfaction and reduced drinking behavior. There was even evidence that after the 1-year follow-up, couples continued to improve even though active treatment had ended.

EFFECTIVENESS OF CONTINGENCY MANAGEMENT APPROACHES

An examination of the findings from behaviorally oriented treatment indicates that contingency contracting is an effective strategy for helping those with alcohol and drug problems. The strength of interventions based on operant principles is that they are grounded in *science*. Indeed, this is a principal concern of behaviorally oriented practitioners. Another strength is that these procedures rely on *incentives* to motivate clients. Many conventional treatment programs have failed to incorporate incentives into their intervention strategies as a means of enhancing client motivation. This is understandable because cost considerations make it a very challenging proposition.

Interest in behaviorally based interventions is likely to remain strong as long as public officials demand to know "what works." This emphasis on accountability, evidence, and outcomes is inherent to the behavior technology approach.

REVIEW QUESTIONS

1. What are some of the basic characteristics of behaviorism?
2. According to Skinner, who can be faulted for addiction and other problem behaviors?
3. How do respondent and operant conditioning differ?
4. What is the difference between positive reinforcement and negative reinforcement?
5. What is the difference between negative reinforcement and punishment?
6. What relevance do generalization and discrimination have for explaining relapse?
7. From a behavioristic perspective, what three factors predict initiation of substance use?
8. What are the three general classes of reinforcers in addiction? How do they vary across type of drug and characteristics of the user?
9. Why is physical dependence neither a necessary nor a sufficient condition for the development of an addiction?
10. When does cessation from substance abuse usually occur?
11. Why should relapse be expected among those in early recovery (in behavioral terms)?
12. What are the assumptions of behavioral counseling? What are the three phases of it as described by Dustin and George?
13. What is behavioral self-control training (BSCT)? Who are good candidates?
14. How can contingency contracting be used to structure and support abstinence?
15. What is community reinforcement training (CRT)?
16. How has CRT been used to help wives of violent alcoholics?
17. How did Higgins and colleagues treat cocaine dependence with CRT and voucher incentives?

18. Can cocaine dependence be effectively treated with an incentive-based approach?

19. What is the practical obstacle blocking widespread dissemination of the treatment approach devised and tested by Higgins and colleagues?

20. What contingency management procedures have been used to increase compliance with methadone maintenance?

21. What are the features of behavioral marital therapy for alcoholism?

22. What are the strengths of contingency management as a strategy for helping substance abuse clients?

CHAPTER 7

Cognitive Models

Substance use and abuse can be explained within a cognitive-behavioral framework. "Cognitive" in this context refers to covert mental processes that are described by a number of diverse terms, including "thinking," "self-talk," "internal dialogue," "expectancies," "beliefs," "schemas," and so on. These "hidden" variables mediate the influence of external stimuli in the production of observable human behavior. Because they represent "behaviors" that are not readily observable, cognitive models are usually distinguished from those that are strictly behavioral. This chapter draws on constructs from a number of cognitive-behavioral approaches including self-efficacy theory (Bandura, 1997) and alcohol expectancy theory (Goldman, Brown, & Christiansen, 1987). The discussion shows how cognitive constructs have been used to explain the initiation and maintenance of addictive behavior; they have also been used to guide the development of relapse prevention strategies based on enhancement of coping and social skills.

BASIC SOCIAL-COGNITIVE CONCEPTS

Albert Bandura is recognized as a leader in cognitive psychology. In his early work, he used the term "social learning theory" (SLT). As the theory became increasingly focused on cognition, he adopted the term "social-cognitive theory." As the theory continued to evolve, the construct of self-efficacy became central, sometimes leading to use of the term "self-efficacy theory." These propositions about human behavior grew out of dissatisfaction with the deterministic views of human beings as expressed by both psychoanalysis and behaviorism several decades ago. In the orthodox psychoanalytic perspective, humans are considered to be under the control of the unconscious, whereas in the behaviorist camp, behavior is controlled by external contingencies (i.e., rewards). In both of those theoretical systems, self-regulation plays no part. Bandura (1977) rejects this view and insists that humans can create and administer reinforcements (rewards and punishers) for themselves and to themselves. He describes it this way:

> Social learning theory approaches the explanation of human behavior in terms of a continuous reciprocal interaction between cognitive, behavioral, and environmental determinants. Within the process of reciprocal determination lies the opportunity for people to influence their destiny as well as the limits of self-direction. This conception of human functioning then neither casts people into the role of powerless objects controlled by environmental forces nor free agents who can become whatever they choose. Both people and their environments are reciprocal determinants of each other. (p. vii)

Note that Bandura indicates that self-direction is possible within limits. These limits vary by both person and environment. For example, a cocaine addict in early recovery who lives in a suburban neighborhood is probably going to have much more control over drug-taking behavior than a similar addict who lives in an inner-city, cocaine-ridden neighborhood. Bandura's (1977) reasoning is apparent in the following passage:

> If actions were determined solely by external rewards and punishments, people would behave like weathervanes, constantly shifting in different directions to conform to the momentary influences impinging upon them. They would act corruptly with unprincipled individuals and honorably with righteous ones, and liberally with libertarians and dogmatically with authoritarians. (p. 128)

In SLT, the consequences of behavior (i.e., reinforcements and punishments) do not act automatically to shape behavior in a mechanistic manner. Rather, these external, environmental contingencies influence the acquisition and regulation of behavior. Internal cognitive processes are also important; they mediate the influence of environmental contingencies. Wilson (1988) states that cognitive processes are based on prior experience and serve to determine (1) which environmental influences are attended to, (2) how these influences are perceived (e.g., as "good" or "bad"), (3) whether they will be remembered, and (4) how they may affect future behavior.

SLT stresses that individuals are actively involved in appraising environmental events. The acquisition and maintenance of behavior are not passive processes. Furthermore, Bandura (1977) maintains that the conditions for learning are facilitated by making rules and consequences known to potential participants. By observing the consequences of someone else's behavior, an individual can learn appropriate actions for particular situations. Bandura (1977) indicates that people create symbolic representations from these observations and rely on them to anticipate the future outcomes that will result from their own behavior. This cognitive process (i.e., symbolic representation) assists in generating motivation to initiate and sustain behavior.

Self-Regulation

Another central concept in SLT, and one of particular importance to the problem of substance use, is "self-regulation" (Abrams & Niaura, 1987). This concept refers to the capability of humans to regulate their own behavior via internal standards and self-evaluative assessments. The concept helps explain how human behavior can be maintained in the absence of external environmental rewards. In the process of self-regulation, humans make self-rewards (and self-punishments) contingent upon the achievement of some specific internal standard of performance. If a discrepancy develops between one's internal standards and one's behavioral performance, the individual will be motivated to change standards, behavior, or both. The internal standards are thought to be the result of one's history of modeling influences and differential reinforcement (Wilson, 1988).

In SLT, alcoholism and addiction are not thought to be conditions characterized by a lack of self-regulation but, rather, forms of self-regulation that are deemed problematic by society (and possibly the family). In other words, the disease model's concept of "loss of control" is disputed by SLT. The alcoholic's or addict's lifestyle is seen as regulated (i.e., organized) around the consumption of alcohol or drugs. The person's behavior is not random or unpredictable; it is purposeful and goal directed. The high degree of self-regulation is clear when consideration is given to the amount of time and effort needed (often daily) to obtain the drug, use the drug, conceal its use, interact with other users, and recover from its effects. Many persons with substance use disorders manage these lifestyles for years, even while holding jobs and having families.

In this context, it should be noted that "self-regulation" does not imply "healthy." This is a value-laden term, which by definition is subjective. Furthermore, SLT maintains that in some cases addiction may be a means of coping (i.e., regulating the self) with internal performance standards that are too extreme or unrealistic. For example, an alcoholic may cope with long work hours by consuming many martinis. For other addicts, their evaluation of self is not "activated" by other persons' opinions of their substance use; that is, criticism from others has little impact on how they perceive themselves. Thus, they easily engage in behavior (alcohol/drug abuse) for which there is little external reward and perhaps much punishment (social/family ostracism, arrests, financial debt, health problems, etc.).

Reciprocal Determinism

In Bandura's (1977) view, person, behavior, and environment are continually engaged in a type of interaction called "reciprocal determinism." That is, each of the components is capable of changing the nature of the interaction at any time. Individuals are thought to be capable of reassessing their behavior, its impact on the environment, and the environment's impact on themselves and their behavior. In a given situation, one of the three components may gain momentary dominance. Figure 7.1 diagrams the relationship among these components, where it can be seen that persons are not driven by internal forces alone, nor do they passively respond to external forces. Instead, a set of interlocking forces is involved. Wilson (1988) describes it this way: "a person is both the agent and the object of environmental influence. Behavior is a function of interdependent factors. Thus, cognitions do not operate independently. In a complete analysis of the cognitive control of behavior, mediating processes must be tied to observable action" (pp. 242–243).

MODELING AND SUBSTANCE USE

"Modeling," which is vicarious or observational learning, is an important concept in social cognitive paradigms. Wilson (1988) defines it in the following manner:

> In this form of learning people acquire new knowledge and behavior by observing other people and events, without engaging in the behavior themselves and without any direct consequences to themselves. Vicarious learning may occur when people watch what others ("models") do, or when they attend to the physical environment, to events, and to symbols such as words and pictures. (pp. 240–241)

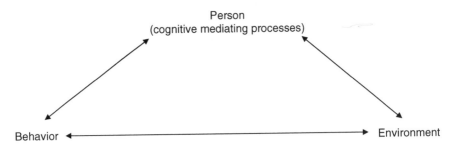

FIGURE 7.1. Interactive schema of person, behavior, and environment.

Bandura (1977) identified three types of effects on behavior that can result from observing a model:

1. *Observational learning effects.* These refer to behaviors acquired through observation of a model that did not previously exist in the individual's behavioral repertoire (e.g., smoking marijuana from a "bong").

2. *Inhibitory–disinhibitory effects.* These refer to increases or decreases in the intensity of a previously learned inhibition. Such behaviors usually result from observing a model's being rewarded or punished for some specific action. Thus a teenage boy may drink a beer—an action he had previously inhibited—when he observes an admired friend (i.e., a model) receive a reward for doing so. In this case, the "reward" may be any number of social consequences (e.g., other peers voice their approval; the admired friend becomes more sociable, funny, or easy to talk to; etc.).

3. *Response facilitation effects.* These refer to the appearance of behaviors that are not novel and were not previously inhibited. Examples of such behaviors are as follows: "People applaud when others clap; they look up when they see others gazing skyward; they adopt fads that others display; and in countless other situations their behavior is prompted and channeled by the actions of others" (Bandura, 1971, p. 6).

The pace at which a small group of friends drink beer is another example of a response facilitation effect. In such a group, drinking beer is not a new behavior and it is not inhibited, but the pace of an individual's drinking is influenced by that of the group. If the group is sipping slowly, it is also likely that a particular individual will match that pace. Consider a wine-tasting event in which small amounts are consumed for taste and food is eaten to cleanse the mouth. In such cases, individuals rarely become drunk, as models of such behavior do not normally exist at such events. In contrast, consider a typical college fraternity party, in which models of heavy drinking abound. Again, SLT asserts that the models in both of these two drinking situations facilitate the pace of the group's drinking behavior. The models do not cause or require others to increase or decrease their drinking; they simply influence it.

Controlled experiments using a bogus "taste-rating task" have systematically examined the influence of modeling on alcohol consumption. In this procedure, participants are manipulated by the investigator's deception. They are deceived into believing that they are participating in a procedure to evaluate the *taste* of alcoholic beverages. The story is concocted to provide study participants with a rationale for consuming alcoholic beverages in a laboratory setting.

In one such study, Caudill and Marlatt (1975) assigned heavy drinking, male college students ($n = 48$) to one of six groups in a 3×2 design.

Without their knowledge, the participants were exposed to different types of "confederate" models who had been trained by the investigators. The participants were exposed to one of three types of drinker models: heavy, light, or nondrinker. In addition, prior to the taste-rating task, they had a brief interaction with a model that was trained to act either "warm" or "cold" toward the participant. The findings showed that participants exposed to heavy drinking models consumed significantly more alcohol than those exposed to light drinking and no drinking models. The latter two groups did not differ from one another. Though the prior social interaction conditions (warm vs. cold) did not influence consumption, these experimental findings indicate that modeling can be an important social determinant of alcohol consumption (Caudill & Marlatt, 1975).

Collins, Parks, and Marlatt (1985) conducted two similar experiments to study modeling effects. Using male undergraduates who were moderate and heavy drinkers, students were recruited under the pretense of assessing the realism of an on-campus barroom laboratory. They were told that the assessment would involve consumption of alcohol. In one experiment, confederates, under the control of the investigators, acted in a sociable or unsociable fashion while modeling either light or heavy alcohol consumption. Heavy drinking was produced in the participants by exposure to three types of models: sociable heavy drinking, unsociable heavy drinking, and unsociable light drinking. The sociable light drinking models tended to produce light drinking in confederates. The investigators interpreted these findings in context of the camaraderie and rivalry that exist among young men under differing social conditions. In the second study, the confederates adopted different roles indicating three levels of social status: "transient laborer," "typical college student," and "30-year-old medical resident." Whereas the alcohol consumption of the participants matched that of the confederates, level of status did not influence drinking behavior (Collins et al., 1985).

SELF-EFFICACY AND TREATMENT OUTCOMES

Self-efficacy has become the unifying construct of the social-cognitive framework (Bandura, 1997). Previously, it tended to be described as a minitheory within the larger framework of SLT (e.g., Wilson, 1988). Regardless, self-efficacy has been defined as "a perception or judgement of one's capability to execute a particular course of action required to deal effectively with an impending situation" (Abrams & Niaura, 1987, p. 134). Efficacy beliefs have been shown to play an influential role in many classes of human behavior including coping with stress (Jerusalem & Mittag,

1995), educational attainment (Zimmerman, 1995), career development (Hackett, 1995), health-related behavior (Schwarzer & Fuchs, 1995), and addictive behavior (Marlatt, Baer, & Quigley, 1995).

The two components of self-efficacy are *outcome expectations* and *efficacy expectations*. An outcome expectation is a person's estimate that a particular outcome will occur. In other words, an individual assesses the situation and the various factors involved in his/her own performance and formulates an expectation of the probability that a specific course of action will lead to a particular outcome (Monte, 1980). Of particular relevance here are alcohol and drug expectancies. The next section of this chapter discusses these beliefs more fully.

An efficacy expectation is a person's belief that he/she can carry out the necessary course of action to obtain the anticipated outcome (Bandura, 1997). Thus, an outcome expectation is knowledge of what to do and what will be obtained, whereas an efficacy expectation is the belief (or doubt) that one can do it. Bandura (1995, 1997) contends that people who are healthy, personally effective, and successful tend to have a high sense of perceived self-efficacy. In other words, they believe that they can achieve what they set out to do. Furthermore, people with high self-efficacy are likely to interpret life problems as challenges rather than as threats or unmanageable situations.

Research has demonstrated that psychological treatments alter behavior to the extent that they affect efficacy expectations (Wilson, 1988). Treatment services that enhance a person's sense of personal competence are likely to lead to improved functioning. According to Wilson (1988):

> Unless treatment creates strong expectations of efficacy, coping behaviors may be easily extinguished following the termination of therapy. The phenomenon of relapse is a problem for all methods of psychological treatment, including behavior therapy. Self-efficacy theory is a means of conceptualizing the relapse process and suggests procedures for facilitating the long-term maintenance of behavior change, especially in the addictive disorders. (p. 243)

According to Bandura (1977), efficacy expectations are based on (and can be altered by) four sources of information. The most powerful influence is thought to be that of *performance accomplishments* in previous mastery situations. Past failure experiences will undermine efficacy beliefs, whereas success will boost them. The second source of efficacy expectations consists of *vicarious experiences*—that is, observation of others' success and failures. A third source is *verbal persuasion*; here, a person is told that he/she can master a task. This source has a relatively weak influence on efficacy expectations because it provides no personal experience of success or failure. The fourth and last source of efficacy expectations is the *emotional arousal* that stems from attempting a demanding task. The experience of anxiety is a powerful cue to people regarding their possibilities for success (or failure) and the amount of effort they will have to exert to achieve mastery. High levels of anxiety and fear are likely to have a debilitating effect on a person's attempts at mastery.

As applied specifically to substance use, Marlatt et al. (1995) identified five specific types of self-efficacy. *Resistance self-efficacy* has to do with judgments about one's ability to avoid the initial use of a substance. This type is important for understanding the onset of substance use, particularly in adolescents. *Harm-reduction self-efficacy* involves perceptions of one's ability to avoid harm following initial use of a substance. *Action self-efficacy* pertains to one's perceived ability to achieve abstinence or controlled use. This type is important for understanding initial behavior change efforts among people who have intensified involvement with substance use. *Coping self-efficacy* is concerned with one's anticipated ability to cope with relapse crises. Finally, *recovery self-efficacy* has to do with judgments about one's ability to return to recovery following lapses and relapses.

Efficacy expectations are particularly important in relapse prevention. Persons with substance dependence who doubt that they can maintain the tasks necessary for recovery (i.e., coping self-efficacy) are likely to relapse. Furthermore, the sources of efficacy expectations suggest specific relapse prevention strategies. Successful efforts will be those designed to ensure success (i.e., performance accomplishments) by first providing simple tasks and gradually building to more difficult ones. Successful efforts will also expose an addict to other successfully recovering addicts (i.e., vicarious experiences) and will teach ways to cope with negative affective states (emotional arousal). Finally, the sources of efficacy expectations suggest that "verbal persuasion" (e.g., "I know you can do it") is an inadequate intervention by itself.

Outcome studies have examined the associations between self-efficacy and drinking/drug use status at follow-up and to participation in treatment. Burling, Reilly, Moltzen, and Ziff (1989) examined the relation between self-efficacy and relapse among 81 inpatient substance abuse clients. In general, self-efficacy increased during treatment and at a 6-month follow-up was higher among abstainers than relapsers. Interestingly, they found that low self-efficacy at intake was related to longer stays in treatment and a more positive status at discharge. Self-efficacy ratings at the end of treatment were not related to alcohol and drug use. The investigators speculate that some substance abusers may minimize the severity of their problems and, as a result, report inflated levels of self-efficacy. In such cases, there may be an underestimation of the difficulties facing them in recovery and, hence, less willingness to learn new coping behaviors (Burling et al., 1989). When pressured into treatment by the criminal justice system, an employer, or one's family, clients might exaggerate reports of self-efficacy.

Rychtarik, Prue, Rapp, and King (1992) tracked changes in self-efficacy among a male alcoholic population in treatment and for the 12 months following discharge. They found that clients who had high self-efficacy and actively participated in aftercare had significantly better outcomes than did other groups of clients. Intake self-efficacy ratings were predictive of relapse status at both 6- and 12-month follow-ups, but discharge self-efficacy was not related to relapse at either of these two time intervals. Rychtarik et al. (1992) also conclude that many clients report greatly inflated levels of self-efficacy at the time of discharge from treatment. They speculate that in some cases this may result from genuinely unrealistic expectations about the challenges of recovery, whereas other clients may be actively involved in "impression management."

Findings from a recent study of cocaine-dependent clients in an outpatient setting ($n = 126$) indicate that prior abstinence (a past "performance accomplishment") is the best predictor of treatment success (Wong et al., 2004). Structural equation models revealed that the establishment of cocaine abstinence periods during treatment independently predicted abstinence and coping self-efficacy at 6-month follow-up. There was no evidence of a bidirectional (reciprocal) relationship between coping self-efficacy and abstinence, as would be predicted by SLT. Thus, baseline coping self-efficacy was not a predictor of posttreatment abstinence from cocaine after accounting for abstinence during treatment (Wong et al., 2004). These findings suggest that at least under some conditions, self-efficacy could be simply an artifact of existing behavior (in this case cocaine use). More research is needed in this area.

ROLE OF OUTCOME EXPECTANCY IN ALCOHOL AND DRUG USE

Cognitive models of substance abuse rely heavily on the "outcome expectancy" and "efficacy expectancy" constructs. The former concept has been used to predict and explain drinking behavior and other drug use, whereas both play a role in relapse (and its prevention). This section provides a detailed discussion of both alcohol and other drug outcome expectancies.

There is no widely accepted definition of the term "expectancy." Usually the term refers to a cognitive variable that intervenes between a stimulus and a response. Goldman et al. (1987) define outcome expectancy as the "anticipation of a systematic relationship between events or objects in some upcoming situation" (p. 183). The construction implies an "if–then" relationship between a behavior and an anticipated outcome.

Many models of substance abuse and dependence have focused on biological differences among individuals that make some people more susceptible to excessive use than others (e.g., Goodwin, 1990). Other theories have scrutinized the pharmacological effects of drugs (e.g., Koob, 1992). Although it does not completely ignore the biomedical and pharmacological aspects of substance use and abuse, expectancy theory comes close to doing so (Goldman et al., 1987). The theory asserts that drug self-administration is largely determined by the reinforcements an individual expects to obtain as a consequence of putting the substance into one's body. Hence, expectancy theory focuses on the *anticipated* reinforcement of drug use.

Alcohol and other drug expectancies vary in strength from person to person; they are greatly influenced by one's family, peer group, and culture, and perhaps even by the mass media (e.g., alcohol advertising). Goldman et al. (1987) indicate that a lack of positive alcohol expectancies should lead one to abstain from alcohol, whereas heavy drinking can be predicted by a variety of strongly held expectancies. Thus, those drinkers who consume abusively may strongly expect alcohol to make them more relaxed, more sexy, or possibly more aggressive. Moderate and light drinkers may hold weaker expectancies in these areas or expect no positive outcomes in some of them. Other drug expectancies operate in much the same manner.

The intriguing aspect of alcohol expectancy theory in particular is that it is not necessary to assume that the outcomes of drinking (tension reduction, enhanced sexuality, aggression, etc.) are related to the pharmacological qualities of ethanol. According to Goldman et al. (1987):

> All this model requires is a belief in a relationship between stimuli and outcomes or between behaviors and outcomes. The model operates even if these beliefs are not based on reality. For example, if a person in a typical drinking environment believed they had consumed alcohol, they might produce covert and overt alcohol-related responses (which appear to observers as pharmacologic effects), not because the drug action of alcohol made them do it, but instead because they believed desired outcomes were available if they behaved in this way in this context. (p. 139)

The essence of alcohol expectancy theory, then, is that alcohol's ability to transform an individual's behavior is not attributable so much to the action of ethanol as it is to the anticipated outcomes of consuming alcohol.

Whether the same can be said to be true for drugs such as marijuana and cocaine is less clear; there has been little hypothesis testing of illegal drug expectancies.

Laboratory Research

Empirical support for the alcohol expectancy hypothesis comes from laboratory research using placebo and balanced-placebo designs. In early laboratory research on alcohol use, placebo designs were used to control for the effects of expectancy. This was done for the most part as a control formality, following customary practice in pharmacological research (Goldman et al., 1987). It was not hoped that the placebo condition would produce effects similar to that of the actual condition.

One early placebo study tested the disease model's concept of loss of control (Merry, 1966). According to this concept (which was discussed in detail in Chapter 2), alcoholics experience intense, probably biologically induced cravings for alcohol after having consumed just a small amount; this intense need for alcohol (once consumed) leads to a loss of control over drinking behavior. Merry (1966) tested this hypothesis by administering alcohol to nine inpatient alcoholics without their knowledge. During an 18-day period, each patient was given an orange-flavored beverage at breakfast. The patients were told that the beverage contained a mixture of vitamins that would help them remain abstinent from alcohol. The beverage was alternated every 2 days such that the patients received either a totally nonalcoholic drink or one that contained 1 ounce of vodka. As a routine part of their treatment regimen, patients were asked to rate their level of alcohol craving later each morning. There was no relationship between their ratings and the beverage consumed, indicating that the basis for alcohol cravings was not pharmacological. Other studies have yielded consistent findings.

In the 1970s, the placebo effects themselves increasingly became the focus of research. Investigators expanded the placebo design. They developed a balanced design that included four cells:

I. Told alcohol, given alcohol.
II. Told alcohol, given only tonic.
III. Told no alcohol, given alcohol.
IV. Told no alcohol, given only tonic.

In this balanced-placebo design, an "antiplacebo" condition (III) is added; this condition assesses alcohol effects in the absence of the usual drinking mind-set (Goldman et al., 1987).

Using the balanced-placebo design, Marlatt and his colleagues conducted pioneering research on the relationship between alcohol expectancies and drinking behavior. In one landmark study, Marlatt, Demming, and Reid (1973) investigated the loss-of-control hypothesis by presenting separate groups of male alcoholics and social drinkers with the bogus alcohol taste-rating task (as described in the discussion of modeling in this chapter). Both drinker groups had 32 members. The alcoholics (mean age = 47) were actively drinking with no intention to quit. They met at least one of the following criteria: (1) history of alcoholism treatment, (2) five or more arrests for "drunk and disorderly conduct," (3) previous membership in AA or a vocational rehabilitation program for alcoholics. Most of the alcoholics (25 of 32) met more than one of these criteria. The social drinkers (mean age = 37) did not meet the aforementioned criteria and they were screened out if they described themselves as "heavy" or "problem" drinkers (Marlatt et al., 1973).

The subjects were told that the beverages were either vodka and tonic or tonic only. The actual beverage contents were systematically varied to be either consistent or inconsistent with the instructional set. It was found that both alcoholic and nonalcoholic men drank significantly more when they thought their drinks contained alcohol, regardless of the actual contents. This finding seriously challenges the loss-of-control hypothesis of the disease models, which holds that alcoholic drinking is mediated by a physiological mechanism that can be triggered by the introduction of alcohol to the body. Rather, it appears that the subjects' beliefs (expectancies) about beverage content were the crucial factors in determining amount of alcohol consumed.

Survey Research

The results of survey research also provide strong support for the alcohol expectancy theory. Much of this survey work was initiated by Sandra Brown and her colleagues, who developed the Alcohol Expectancy Questionnaire (AEQ). This 90-item self-report questionnaire assesses whether alcohol, when consumed in moderate quantities, produces specific positive effects (Brown, Christiansen, & Goldman, 1987a). The AEQ was derived from an initial pool of 216 verbatim statements collected from 125 people, who were interviewed individually and in groups. They ranged in age from 15 to 60, and their drinking behavior varied from total abstinence to chronic alcoholism. When the items were factor-analyzed, the following six alcohol expectancy factors emerged:

1. Global-positive change.
2. Sexual enhancement.

3. Physical and social pleasure.
4. Increased social assertiveness.
5. Relaxation and tension reduction.
6. Arousal with power.

These factors represent relatively distinct domains of anticipated drinking outcomes. The factors were subsequently used in a large number of survey research studies as variables to predict various drinking practices. In general, the research has consistently linked these expected consumption outcomes to actual use, abuse, and related problem behavior. For example, Brown, Creamer, and Stetson (1987b) found that alcohol abusers expected more positive outcomes from drinking than did their nonabusing peers. Similarly, Critchlow (1987) found that heavy drinkers held stronger expectations of positive consequences of alcohol use than did light drinkers, and that they generally evaluated all drinking outcomes more positively. Furthermore, Brown (1985) and Thombs (1991) reported that alcohol expectancies were better predictors of heavy and problem drinking than a set of demographic variables.

Among young adolescents, alcohol expectancies have been shown to predict the onset of the initiation of drinking behavior 1 year later (Christiansen, Roehling, Smith, & Goldman, 1989). Among college students, one study found that problem drinkers expected more relaxation/tension reduction than did social drinkers, while the latter group expected more social enhancement (Brown, 1985). Another college student study found that the expectancy profile that distinguished female problem drinkers from female nonproblem drinkers was relatively distinct from the profile that separated these drinker types among males (Thombs, 1993). In this same study, the AEQ factor that had the strongest discriminating value among the women problem drinkers (and thus provided the clearest indication of what they sought through drinking) was arousal with power, whereas for the men it was physical and social pleasure (Thombs, 1993). Finally, one study examined cross-cultural differences in alcohol expectancies (Brown et al., 1987a). A group of Irish (Dublin) adolescents was compared to a group of American (Detroit) adolescents. The groups were matched by age and gender. Results indicated that there were no differences between the two groups on total AEQ scores. However, there were significant differences on subscale scores: The Irish teens expected more arousal and aggression and less sexual enhancement from drinking than did the American teens (Brown et al., 1987a). Irish youth also had significantly lower expectations for enhanced social and cognitive-motor functioning compared to American youth.

Survey research also has identified the outcome expectancies associated with some illegal drugs. In a sample of 704 college students, Schafer and Brown (1991) used factor analysis to identify the anticipated outcomes of marijuana and cocaine use. Six marijuana expectancy factors were identified:

1. Cognitive and behavioral impairment.
2. Relaxation and tension reduction.
3. Social and sexual facilitation.
4. Perceptual and cognitive enhancement.
5. Global negative effects.
6. Craving and physical effects.

Though the six sets of items (each factor) had weak to modest internal consistency, multivariate analysis revealed that there were significant correlations between the expectancy measures and patterns of marijuana use and nonuse in college students (Schafer & Brown, 1991). On some of the scales, such as cognitive-behavioral impairment and global negative effects, the nonusers of marijuana had the strongest expectancies, compared to infrequent, recreational, and regular users of the drug. On relaxation and tension reduction measure, the regular users had the greatest score of the four groups. This finding suggests that the perceived negative consequences of marijuana use act as a deterrent to experimentation with the drug, but once use is initiated, strong positive expectations may spur a high level of involvement with marijuana.

Schafer and Brown (1991) identified five cocaine expectancy factors as well:

1. Global positive effects.
2. Global negative effects.
3. General arousal.
4. Anxiety
5. Relaxation and tension reduction.

The internal consistency for the items comprising global positive effects was good. The other item sets had more modest interitem equivalence. Again, multivariate analysis found significant correlations between the expectancy measures, as a set, and patterns of cocaine use in college students (Schafer & Brown, 1991). Parallel to the marijuana relationships, scores on global positive effects were highest in the frequent cocaine users, whereas scores for global negative effects were highest among the nonusers of cocaine.

The investigators noted that the identification of relaxation and tension reduction as an anticipated outcome of using cocaine, a stimulant, seems counterintuitive. In all four cocaine user groups, scores on this measure were relatively low. Furthermore, there was little variation across the groups (Schafer & Brown, 1991).

Drug Expectancy: Precursor or Consequence of Drug Use?

A challenge facing the drug expectancy research has been to demonstrate that the construct is not an epiphenomenal correlate of drug use. The basic question is: Does expectancy influence drug use or is it merely an artifact of existing drug-taking behavior? This question has important implications for primary prevention and early intervention. A number of studies have examined the question as it pertains to both alcohol and marijuana expectancies.

Miller, Smith, and Goldman (1990) sought to determine whether alcohol expectancies could be detected in a sample of 114 elementary school children, grades 1–5. The investigators developed an assessment procedure which relied on hand puppets to collect expectancy data from the first to third graders. For fourth and fifth graders, the adolescent version of the AEQ was administered in addition to the use of handpuppets. Though they were less differentiated than those of adolescents and adults, it was found that alcohol expectancies were present in this age group. As age increased, expectancies about drinking tended to increase as well. Most of the increase occurred during third and fourth grades (children ages 8½–10 years). Because these children presumably had little or no personal drinking experience, it can be assumed that their expectations were the result of exposure to family drinking models, commercial advertising, and other media messages.

In a prospective study, a sample of 422 preteens and teens (mean age at baseline = 12.8 years) were assessed twice at a 12-month interval (Reese, Chassin, & Molina, 1994). Baseline alcohol expectancies were found to prospectively predict drinking consequences (problems) 12 months later. This relationship was observed even after the effects of the following variables were controlled for: baseline drinking consequences, parental alcoholism, and age. However, expectancies did not predict alcohol use, perhaps because of the relatively high number of abstainers and light drinkers among younger participants.

Another prospective study assessed 461 participants, ages 12–14, over a 2-year period (Smith, Goldman, Greenbaum, & Christiansen, 1995). A baseline assessment was followed by two 12-month follow-ups. The purpose of the study was to examine the relationship between expectancy for social facilitation and alcohol use. The investigators found that teenagers' expectations for social facilitation had a reciprocal relationship with their past drinking behavior. In other words, the greater their expectation for social facilitation, the greater their drinking level, followed then by the greater expectations, and so on. Two other directional models were not supported by the data: (1) expectancy influences alcohol use and (2) alcohol use influences expectancy.

In a third prospective study, Stacy, Newcomb, and Bentler (1991) assessed alcohol and marijuana expectancies among 584 participants as they moved from adolescence to young adulthood. Their primary purpose was to determine the nature of the relationship between drug expectancy and drug use. Three possibilities were tested by structural equation models: (1) expectancies predict future drug-taking behavior; (2) expectancies result from drug use, that is, they merely reflect personal experience with a substance; and (3) the relationship between expectancy and drug use is reciprocal.

Stacy et al. (1991) assessed their sample twice at a 9-year interval. At the first assessment interval, the cohort's mean age was about 18. The investigators found that the adolescent measures of expectancy were predictive of adult drug-taking behavior. Furthermore, the data suggested that expectancy is not a consequence or artifact of existing drug use but, rather, the antecedent of these behaviors. Little evidence was found to support the social learning proposition that expectancy and drug use have a reciprocal relationship (Stacy et al., 1991).

Alcohol Expectancy as a Function of Memory

Theories of human memory have proposed that "expectancy" is a name given to information stored in memory (Bolles, 1972). This information consists of associations between cues and consequences and behaviors and consequences. These two types of associations may combine to influence decision making when cues in the environment match those stored in the predictive relations of memory, which suggests that the structure and function of memory may play a role in drinking behavior.

Studies have attempted to link the alcohol expectancy construct more explicitly to cognition and memory (Dunn & Goldman, 1996; Rather & Goldman, 1994; Rather, Goldman, Roehrich, & Brannick, 1992). The conceptualization of Goldman and colleagues is that alcohol expectancies are stored in memory networks. These networks are collections of memories about the predictive relations between drinking and its outcomes. Such information may influence the decision-making process about alcohol use.

Rather et al. (1992) identified a preliminary alcohol expectancy semantic network in college students. They found that though all study participants tended to associate positive/prosocial outcomes with drinking, heavier drinkers tended to expect arousal from alcohol consumption. In contrast, lighter drinkers were more likely to expect sedation. Rather and Goldman (1994) replicated this semantic memory network in a separate sample of college students. They also found that compared to lighter drinkers, the expectancy networks of heavier drinkers were more "tightly configured," meaning more packed with information. By comparison, the networks of lighter drinkers were spatially diffuse, which suggests that when exposed to an alcohol stimulus, heavier drinkers may rapidly associate many positive and arousing effects to alcohol use but be "cognitively insulated" from the sedating and negative outcomes. In lighter drinkers, the network of associations may consolidate more slowly and thereby inhibit alcohol use.

In a sample of 470 second- to fifth-grade children, Dunn and Goldman (1996) found that alcohol expectancy information was organized in memory networks similar to that of adults, even though presumably there was little or no personal drinking experience; they tended to perceive that alcohol generates either arousal or sedation. It also was discovered that older children were more likely to anticipate positive and arousing outcomes from alcohol use. Dunn and Goldman (1996) speculate that as children move through elementary school, they become "cognitively prepared" to drink as a result of being exposed to parental and older peer drinking models, and to the commercial advertising. These findings suggest that prevention strategies should seek to undermine the expectation that alcohol produces positive and arousing effects.

Expectancy and Treatment Outcomes

Research by Jones and McMahon (1994) indicates that specific types of expectancy predict abstinence rates among alcoholic men in residential treatment. The investigators administered the AEQ and the Negative Alcohol Expectancy Questionnaire to 53 clients at admission and again at 1- and 3-month follow-ups after treatment. The AEQ assessed the immediate, expected, positive outcomes of drinking and the second instrument measured expectations of "same-day," "next-day," and "continued-drinking" negative consequences. Expectancies did not predict 1-month abstinence rates, but at 3 months both Global Positive Change (AEQ subscale) and continued-drinking negative expectancy were predictive of abstinence. The same-day and next-day negative consequences were not as closely related to abstinence. Jones and McMahon (1994) conclude that global positive expectancies combine with long-term negative expectations to influence drinking decisions following treatment.

Caudill and Hoffman (1994) assessed expectancies among a sample of cocaine-dependent clients in treatment. Most of the clients were crack smokers (86%), male (62%), African American (94%), and self-referred to treatment (92%). The investigators found that clients with strong cocaine expectancies overall tended to remain in treatment longer. However, the expectancy measures were not predictive of long-term treatment outcomes. They speculated that clinical outcomes were related more to coexisting psychiatric disorders than to cocaine expectancies (Caudill & Hoffman, 1994).

ALCOHOL AND STRESS: COGNITION AS A MEDIATING PROCESS

When alcoholics are asked, "Does drinking reduce tension and stress?," the overwhelming majority answer "yes." Stockwell (1985) found that 93% of a sample of 2,300 alcoholics in treatment reported that they drank to relax. For some time, numerous other studies, using a variety of assessment methodologies, have arrived at similar conclusions for both nonproblem and problem drinkers (Brown, 1985; Masserman, Jacques, & Nicholson, 1945; Wanberg, 1969). Yet the "tension reduction hypothesis" (TRH) has been a long-standing source of controversy in the alcoholism field. There have been two principal reasons for this debate. First, the TRH deviates from some of the tenets of the disease model (e.g., loss of control) and has treatment implications (e.g., the possibility of controlled drinking) that are inconsistent with it (Langenbucher & Nathan, 1990). Second, the findings from studies of the TRH have inconsistently supported its validity (Cappell & Greeley, 1987).

The TRH relies on principles of operant conditioning. As a theory, it is rather simple, straightforward, and readily testable. Furthermore, it is consistent with both folklore and clinical observations. According to Langenbucher and Nathan (1990), "the theory presumes that alcoholic drinking is a product of escape learning; alcoholics drink because they have been negatively reinforced for drinking in the face of life stress" (p. 133). Essentially, the relief from stress (whether it be anxiety, depression, frustration, fear, etc.) maintains high levels of consumption. The relief from these negative emotional states is the reward provided by drinking.

The TRH model actually consists of two subhypotheses, which have been tested in a number of studies. These are as follows: (1) in the presence of stress, alcoholic drinking will increase; and (2) the stress of alcoholics will be relieved by drinking (Cappell & Greeley, 1987; Langenbucher & Nathan, 1990). Before the evidence for and against these subhypotheses is discussed, some of the early work in this area is examined.

According to a review of the TRH by Cappell and Greeley (1987), the pioneering alcoholism researcher of the 1940s, E. M. Jellinek, was among the first to link alcoholic drinking to tension reduction. Jellinek (1945) proposed that as modern society evolves, it becomes more complex and more difficult for the individual to cope with. As a result, "individuals are more likely to experience increases in frustration, anger, anxiety, and tension. Individual releases are sought. Since there is a substance which can give the desired relief, harassed man will want to take recourse to it" (p. 19). Jellinek was careful to avoid suggesting that all alcohol use is driven by a desire to find relief from tension; rather, he felt that this desire is one important motivation for drinking, especially for problem drinking.

Jellinek did not formally coin the phrase "tension reduction hypothesis," however. About a decade later, Conger (1956), in a seminal study on the relationship between alcohol use and tension, first used the term. Conger was an experimental psychologist who relied on laboratory data from animal studies. In the early 1950s, Conger made use of an approach–avoidance conflict procedure using rats. He trained his rats to run down an alley for food (the reward or reinforcer). As they began to eat, he would electrify the grid upon which they rested. Obviously, this produced conflict for the hungry rats! They were being reinforced and punished at the same time.

Over time, Conger (1951) adjusted both the food deprivation level (making the food a stronger or weaker reinforcer) and the electric shock level. Eventually, the rats "learned" to run part way down the alley but not to touch the food. Conger found that when one group of rats was injected with alcohol, they would approach and eat the food almost immediately, despite the electric shock. By contrast, a group of rats that only received a placebo injection required many more trials before they would approach and eat the food on an electrified grid. In essence, the alcohol ameliorated the conflict between eating and receiving a shock. Conger (1951) concluded that these findings supported an important element of the TRH—that is, that alcohol mitigates aversive states such as fear or tension.

Since Conger's (1951) early work, numerous TRH studies have been conducted, and several comprehensive reviews of this body of research exist. Each one reaches slightly different conclusions about the validity of the TRH. The most recent review, by Langenbucher and Nathan (1990), indicates that empirical evidence generally supports the validity of the TRH. Specifically, the authors conclude that (1) there is a statistically significant positive correlation between a study's year of publication and its methodological quality, and (2) the greater the methodological adequacy of a study, the more strongly its findings support the TRH (Langenbucher & Nathan, 1990).

A 1987 review of TRH studies is somewhat more cautious in its assessment of the research. Cappell and Greeley (1987) observe that studies relying on *conflict paradigms* (e.g., Conger's work) in both humans and animals "provide relatively consistent support for the TRH" (p. 44). However, these studies have not specified the exact elements of conflict that alcohol is able to ameliorate.

In contrast, *stress-induction paradigms* produce equivocal results. Under aversive stimuli, such as tension, individuals respond in different ways when given alcohol. It is possible that biological differences among individuals make some much more responsive to the tension-dampening effects of alcohol than others. Furthermore, some studies have suggested that low or moderate amounts of alcohol may dampen responses to stress, whereas high amounts may actually exacerbate it. Finally, studies that have made use of social stressors (those most similar to the "natural" ones most alcoholics would experience) have been least likely to produce findings in support of the TRH. Cappell and Greeley (1987) conclude that the inconsistencies in the "social stressor" class of TRH studies are difficult to explain. However, it is possible that individuals interpret and respond to identical, stressful social situations (e.g., interpersonal conflict) in varied ways, with or without alcohol. Thus, the complexity of the relationship may be especially pronounced. Powers and Kutash (1985) have neatly summarized these findings in the following passage:

> Alcohol use does not cause the relief of stress, in that alcohol is neither a necessary nor a sufficient condition for that occurrence. Alcohol is not a necessary condition for stress relief, for very often stress relief occurs without the presence of alcohol. Alcohol is not a sufficient condition, for at times alcohol use results in an increase in stress or no change. Alcohol is best considered as one of many possible contributors to stress relief. Many interactive factors determine whether alcohol use results in a reduction of stress. The most prominent factors identified thus far include: expectations regarding alcohol's effects, pharmacological effects of alcohol at varying dosages, individual differences in the appraisal of stressors and in coping behaviors, and the entire constellation of stressors and stress responses experienced by the individual. (p. 471)

The Stress Response Dampening Model

In response to the inconsistent findings of studies testing the TRH, Levenson, Sher, Grossman, Newman, and Newlin (1980) created the stress response dampening (SRD) model. The model builds on the TRH by *specifying the conditions under which alcohol will be used to reduce stress or tension*. The major propositions of the SRD model can be summarized as follows:

1. Alcohol is a drug that can dampen the physiological stress response.
2. Drinking behavior tends to be reinforced when alcohol is used in a stressful context.
3. Stress reduction is due to pharmacological mechanisms—not expectancy of alcohol effects.

4. Physiological arousal (i.e., the stress response) alone does not predict alcohol use.
5. Instead, alcohol use is likely in stressful situations when there are no negative consequences for drinking and when the individual possesses certain personality traits, particularly antisociality and impulsiveness (Sher, 1987).

Support for the SRD model is demonstrated by findings from an experimental study that compared the alcohol consumption of two groups of social drinkers; half were adult children of biological fathers who abused alcohol (Sayette, Breslin, Wilson, & Rosenblum, 1994). All participants were exposed to a social stressor (anticipation and delivery of a public speech) after consuming either a moderate dose of alcohol or tonic water. The instructional set was varied to be either consistent or inconsistent with the beverage they actually received in the experiment. It was found that alcohol intoxication reduced subjective anxiety and negative self-evaluation in response to the stressor. This was true for both men and women. Parental history and belief about whether they received alcohol or a placebo had no effects on response to the stressor. Furthermore, alcohol expectancies, as assessed by the AEQ, also had no correlation with stress reactivity (Sayette et al., 1994). The findings support the SRD model by showing that alcohol's ability to reduce stress rests primarily on its pharmacological action. Alcohol expectancies, from the psychological domain, appear to be relatively unimportant moderators of stress reactivity. Expectancy variables may have greater influence on other forms of behavior, particularly those involving social interaction, such as sexual risk taking (Dermen, Cooper, & Agocha, 1998).

Appraisal Disruption: Alcohol's Ability to Interfere with the Processing of Stressful Information

Further explication of the conditions under which alcohol will dampen stress is found in research conducted by Sayette (1993). The following propositions are the major components of his appraisal-disruption model:

1. The pharmacological actions of alcohol interfere with the *initial appraisal of stressful information* by diminishing the power of a stressor to activate associated memories and concepts in long-term memory.
2. Alcohol will be most likely to dampen stress when it is consumed *prior to appraisal of the stressor.*
3. When alcohol is consumed after appraisal of the stressor, *the stress response may be enhanced rather than reduced.*

The thrust of Sayette's appraisal-disruption model is that the *timing of the alcohol consumption*, in relation to the appearance of a stressor, is critical for understanding whether the stress response will be dampened or exacerbated by drinking; it certainly helps explain why negative emotional states are sometimes intensified by drinking (e.g., profound grief reactions among those drinking at an Irish wake).

TIFFANY'S MODEL OF DRUG URGES AND CRAVINGS

The construct of "urge" or "craving" is central to many explanations of addictive behavior. It is used to explain the maintenance of a high rate of use as well as relapse. The notion that urges or cravings prompt substance use seems to be taken for granted by laypersons, addicts themselves, and many professionals.

Marlatt (1985) has proposed a distinction between "urge" and "craving," noting that an urge is an *intention* that motivates use, whereas craving represents the *anticipation* of a positive drug effect (i.e., an outcome expectancy). Regardless of whether this distinction is accepted, Marlatt's conception represents a positive reinforcement model of urge/craving. In contrast, an earlier model by Jellinek (1955) proposed that cravings represented the anticipation of relief from withdrawal, in essence, a negative reinforcement model.

In a review of the empirical research, Tiffany (1990) contends that data do not support either Marlatt's or Jellinek's models. His case is based on an examination of the relationship between drug urge and actual use. Across both self-report and physiological measures, he found that the correlations between urges and drug use were only of modest or moderate magnitude. This suggests that *drug use occurs frequently without being prompted by urges.* Furthermore, Tiffany (1990) observed that *many relapses were not provoked by urges and cravings.* In such cases, he concluded that these episodes could be characterized as "absentminded relapses" (p. 163). To account for these observations, Tiffany created the following cognitive model to explain drug urges and cravings.

Human cognitive processing includes both *automatic* and *nonautomatic* processes (Shiffrin & Schneider, 1977). According to Tiffany (1990), an automatic cognitive process is "a relatively permanent sequence of tightly integrated associative connections in long-term memory that always become active in response to a particular input configuration" (p. 152). Among humans, across many classes of behavior, automatic processes are revealed by the following: (1) speed in task performance; (2) the behavior is executed without intention and is elicited by specific stimuli; (3) under eliciting stimuli, the behavior is difficult to inhibit or curtail; (4) the behavior is easy and nondemanding to carry out; and (5) the behavior can be conducted without much conscious awareness. The common example of automatic cognitive process is driving a motor vehicle to a familiar destination, such as work. Operation of the vehicle occurs automatically and without much conscious awareness.

The same processes may guide compulsive drug self-administration, whether it be smoking, alcohol consumption, or drug injection. Tiffany (1990) asserts that with repeated practice, drug acquisition and consumption become behavior produced by automatic processes. He employs the concept of *drug use action plans* to emphasize that over time, the sequence of behaviors involved in using alcohol and/or drugs becomes integrated, efficient, and effortless. In typical situations in which drug use occurs unimpeded, urges do *not* accompany the process. It is on this point that Tiffany's model departs significantly from traditional views of urges/cravings. To explain how urges are generated, Tiffany points to an opposite set of cognitive processes. Nonautomatic cognitive processing is slow, and it depends on careful attention and effort. Other features of nonautomatic processing include (1) identification of strategies, (2) conscious decision making, (3) planning, and (4) monitoring of task performance.

In Tiffany's (1990) model, *both* abstinence-avoidance and abstinence-promotion urges are produced by nonautomatic processes. Abstinence-avoidance urges occur when drug use action plans are blocked or obstructed by external barriers (e.g., run out of cigarettes late at night), whereas abstinence-promotion urges are produced when the individual is attempting to change drug use or to maintain abstinence (e.g., while in treatment). Tiffany (1990) hypothesizes that stress and other negative emotional states give rise to both types of urges, which generate competing nonautomatic processes that can influence drug use action plans. This competition tends to inhibit the impact of abstinence-promotion urges and thereby increases the likelihood of individuals executing their automatic drug use action plans.

RELAPSE

A "relapse" can be defined as a return to excessive alcohol and/or drug use following a period of sustained abstinence. It is probably the most significant issue in treating chemically dependent clients. It is often puzzling that individuals who seem to recognize the seriousness of their addiction, who appear committed to recovery, and who have gained some mastery over their drinking or drug-taking behavior often have tremendous difficulty in remaining abstinent.

Historically, views on relapse have tended to be moralistic. Such views still predominate in many segments of our society. Relapsed alcoholics or addicts are scorned: They are thought of as lazy, irresponsible, or possibly weak-willed. Essentially, they are viewed as having a defect of character. Unfortunately, such views, especially when held by legislators, government officials, and other key decision makers, impede progress in treatment approaches by depriving treatment and research centers of much-needed financial support.

Interestingly, the disease model of addiction has traditionally had little to say about relapse prevention. AA folklore, and especially its slogans, provides various messages of caution about "slippery places" and directs members to call their sponsors, but little is provided in the way of skills. Moreover, the disease model has not elaborated on the meaning of relapse. The loss-of-control concept in alcoholism has, in fact, been cited for inadvertently contributing to full-blown relapses. The assertion that alcoholics cannot stop drinking once alcohol enters their bodies seems to establish an expectation that 1 drink must lead to 20. Thus, when many alcoholics and other drug addicts do relapse, they often seem to go on extended binges.

Stress as an Impetus for Relapse

Stress is frequently associated with relapse among recovering persons (Hunter & Salmone, 1986; Milkman, Weiner, & Sunderwith, 1984; Marlatt & Gordon, 1979). A review of the research literature indicates that it is the most frequently cited explanation for relapse (Milkman et al., 1984). For instance, of the 20 conditions that Hunter and Salmone (1986) described as being associated with relapse, 12 are stress related. One prominent study collected data on 137 relapse episodes reported by groups of alcoholics, cigarette smokers, and heroin addicts (Marlatt & Gordon, 1979). All subjects had completed treatment programs with complete abstinence as the goal. Results revealed that 76% of the relapses studied occurred in three contexts: (1) intrapersonal negative emotional states (37%), (2) social pressure (24%), and (3) interpersonal conflict (15%).

In general, it appears that relapsers evaluate more life situations as threatening than do nonrelapsers. Those who relapse seem to have greater difficulty in coping with unpleasant emotions, frustrating events, and unsatisfactory relations with others. In other words, they have lesser tolerance for life's frustrations and disappointments (Ellis, McInerney, DiGuiseppe, & Yeager, 1988). Persons who do not relapse seem to learn more effective strategies for coping with problems. This seems to apply to the gamut of addictions. The cognitive dynamics appear similar in cigarette smoking, overeating, alcoholism, and heroin and cocaine addiction.

An Analysis of Relapse and Its Prevention

SLT offers a perspective on relapse that differs from the one put forth by the traditional disease model. According to Lewis et al. (1988), "The social learning perspective . . . looks at a return to substance use as a learning experience that can be successfully used to bolster gains previously made in treatment" (p. 200). In fact, clients are taught to view "slips" in just this way. Relapse is not viewed as something that is "awful" or "terrible," and clients are not taught to fear it. Instead, they are encouraged to understand it as a response to environmental cues that constantly impinge upon them. It is not evidence that they are incompetent, stupid, or worthless. The experience of relapse can provide clients with the opportunity to learn about their high-risk situations or "triggers," and to identify strategies that they can use to prevent them.

Much of the work done in relapse prevention has been carried out by Marlatt and Gordon (1985). They view relapse as the result of *high-risk situations* combined with the tendency to engage in *self-defeating thinking*. High-risk situations are those that may trigger a "slip"; they may include visiting a friend at a bar, attending a wedding reception, returning to an old neighborhood, or the like. In AA parlance, they are referred to as "slippery places." Relapse prevention strategies teach clients how to cope better with high-risk situations. Thus, this approach can be viewed as an attempt to enhance coping skills. Client self-efficacy is a critical factor.

Marlatt and Gordon (1985) believe that self-defeating thinking emerges from lifestyle imbalances. These lifestyle imbalances occur when the external demands on an individual's time and energy interfere with his/her ability to satisfy desires for pleasure and self-fulfillment. In this imbalance, recovering clients feel pressure to "catch up" for lost time and thus feel *deprived* of pleasure, enjoyment, fun, and so on. As a result, they come to feel that they deserve indulgence and gratification. During this state of perceived deprivation, cravings for their preferred substance tend to arise, and they begin to think very positively about the immediate effects of the drug. In other words, they generate positive alcohol or drug expectancies in which substance use is anticipated to make their immediate situation better. At the same time, they deny or selectively forget about all the negative consequences that go along with a reinitiation of use. There is often the tendency to rationalize the return to using (e.g., "I owe myself this drink").

Apparently Irrelevant Decisions

In this process of covert cognitive change, recovering persons may find themselves in more and more high-risk situations prior to the first "slip."

As this movement begins, they start making "apparently irrelevant decisions" (AIDs, Marlatt & Gordon, 1985). According to Lewis et al. (1988):

> These AIDs are thought to be a product of rationalization ("What I'm doing is OK") and denial ("This behavior is acceptable and has no relationship to relapse") that manifest themselves as certain choices that lead inevitably to a relapse. In this respect AIDs are best conceptualized as "minidecisions" that are made over time and that, when combined, lead the client closer and closer to the brink of the triggering high-risk situation. (p. 203)

Figure 7.2 illustrates the sequence of covert, cognitive events that precede a relapse.

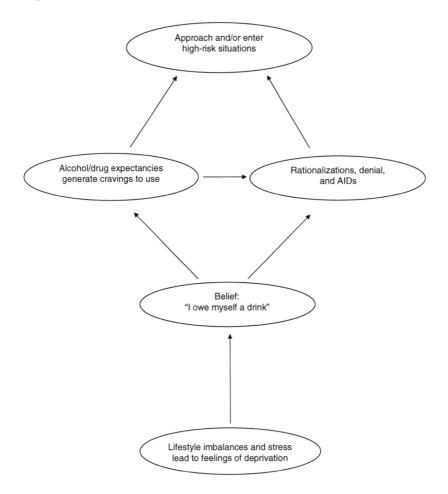

FIGURE 7.2. Covert (cognitive) events leading to a relapse.

Examples of AIDs abound. Following is a list of typical ones as they apply to recovery:

1. A recovering alcoholic begins to purchase his cigarettes at liquor stores. He insists that the liquor stores are more conveniently located than other sales outlets.
2. A recovering alcoholic begins taking a new route home from work. She says she is bored with the old way. The new route is somewhat longer; it also has several liquor stores along the way.
3. A husband in early recovery begins to offer to run to the store for groceries. His wife is pleased. He regularly goes to the supermarket with a liquor store next door, even though it is further from home. He says that this market has better prices.
4. A recovering substance abuser goes to an old drug buddy's house to borrow a hammer.
5. A recovering alcoholic offers to go alone on out-of-town business trips. Her supervisor says that it's not necessary that she always go, but she says she likes to travel by herself.
6. A recovering alcoholic refuses to get rid of his liquor cabinet. He says he needs it when entertaining friends and relatives.
7. A recovering substance abuser transfers to a new job within the company. It is not a promotion, but it happens to have little direct supervision.

The Abstinence Violation Effect

In the SLT perspective, there is a significant difference between a "lapse" (or a "slip") and a full-blown relapse (Abrams & Niaura, 1987). A lapse is seen as a return to drinking that is brief, involves ingesting a small amount of alcohol or another drug, and has no other adverse consequences. By contrast, a relapse involves a return to heavy use (perhaps a prolonged binge) and is accompanied by a host of emotional and physical complications. The aim of relapse prevention is to prevent lapses from turning into relapses (Abrams & Niaura, 1987).

The "abstinence violation effect" is the experience of intense shame, guilt, and embarrassment that frequently occurs following a lapse or a slip (Marlatt & Gordon, 1985). It increases the likelihood that a slip will turn into a full-blown relapse. Among those recovering persons who are committed to abstinence, the slip may be interpreted as evidence of personal inadequacy or incompetence. The person can be overwhelmed by intense negative emotion directed at self. One recovering alcoholic told this author that he recalls saying this to himself after he slipped: "I can't believe I did this. I'm so stupid. What I've done is horrible. My wife will have no respect for me. This shows that I really am nothing but a no-good drunk—just a piece of shit. I might just as well keep drinking. It don't matter no more."

Early in treatment, prior to lapses, clients need to be educated about the meaning of slips and relapses. It is important that they not think of relapse as personal failure. This type of cognitive restructuring teaches that a slip is only a mistake, not evidence of inadequacy or worthlessness. Furthermore, it is helpful for the clients to attribute the slips to environmental cues rather than to themselves. By doing this, they place the focus properly on dealing effectively with the trigger situations. Such a focus tends to build self-efficacy as the clients learn skills for coping with high-risk situations.

PROJECT MATCH: A TEST OF COGNITIVE THERAPY

In 1989, the National Institute on Alcohol Abuse and Alcoholism initiated a study entitled *Matching Alcoholism Treatments to Client Heterogeneity* (Project MATCH). The project was a national, multisite, randomized clinical trial designed to assess the benefits of matching alcoholic clients to three different psychosocial treatments while accounting for 10 client characteristics (Project MATCH Research Group, 1997). Project MATCH was the largest and most statistically powerful trial of psychotherapy outcomes ever carried out.

Details about the findings of the trial are not fully discussed here. However, in a review of cognitive models it is important to mention that cognitive-behavioral coping skills therapy was one of the tested treatments. The other two were motivational enhancement therapy and Twelve-Step facilitation therapy (Project MATCH Research Group, 1997).

All three therapies, delivered in either aftercare or outpatient settings, had substantial positive effects on measures of "percent days abstinent" and "drinks per drinking day." However, the study yielded little evidence to support the value of matching clients to different treatments. Hence, cognitive-behavioral coping skills therapy was not superior to the other forms of therapy offered in the trial. In fact, there was evidence to suggest that in outpatient settings specifically, Twelve-Step facilitation therapy produced better outcomes than the cognitive therapy in clients with low psychiatric severity. Neither therapy was superior for clients with high psychiatric severity (Project MATCH Research Group, 1997).

SUMMARY

The cognitive-behavioral models provide a sound conceptual base for understanding substance use. The initiation of substance use is influenced by outcome expectancies and by modeling. Young people initiate substance use as a result of observing others. They imitate parents, peers, media figures, and others, because they anticipate deriving the same rewards they observe others obtain.

Alcohol and drug abuse are self-regulated behaviors. The high degree of self-regulation is demonstrated by the time and effort required to maintain a lifestyle centered around drinking and/or drug use. Viewing such behavior as "out of control" is probably inaccurate.

The concept of "self-efficacy" is an extremely important one in assisting persons with substance use disorders. Evidence suggests that a crucial determinant in whether treatment will be successful is the client's belief in his/her ability to master the various tasks of recovery. Without this belief, treatment is likely to fail. In addition, research indicates that self-efficacy is most likely to be enhanced by "performance accomplishments." Thus, it is imperative that clients initially be given small tasks at which success is virtually assured, before they attempt more difficult ones.

Recent cognitive models have shed light on how drug outcome expectancies influence drug use and related behavior, including treatment outcomes. Some of this work has attempted to tie expectancy formation to human memory and cognitive processing. These important advances in cognitive science have added precision to our understanding of such nebulous topics as alcohol use and stress and drug urges and cravings.

Relapse is often related to an inability to cope with environmental stressors (i.e., high-risk situations). It often appears to result from negative emotional states, social pressure, and interpersonal conflicts, rather than being evidence of a character flaw. Effective relapse prevention strategies will anticipate these events by teaching clients specific coping skills tailored to their individual needs.

Finally, cognitive-behavioral relapse prevention considers lapses (and even relapses) to be opportunities for learning. Instead of viewing them as events to be fearful of, and as evidence of treatment failure, treatment providers should assist clients in analyzing their high-risk situations and covert cognitive processes. Helping clients to think differently about the meaning of relapse can result in a reduction of the abstinence violation effect and thus in fewer subsequent full-blown relapses.

REVIEW QUESTIONS

1. As it relates to determinism, how does social learning theory (SLT) differ from both psychoanalysis and conditioning theory?

2. How are expectancies and modeling related to one another?

3. How can alcohol and drug use be influenced by modeling?

4. What is the significance of "self-regulation" and "reciprocal determinism" for understanding substance use?

5. What is "self-efficacy"? How is it influenced?

6. With respect to substance use, what types of self-efficacy exist? Has research found self-efficacy to be related to treatment outcomes?

7. What are "alcohol and drug expectancies"?

8. How are placebo conditions used to study alcohol expectancies?

9. What is the bogus taste-rating task?

10. How does "sociability" moderate modeling effects on drinking?

11. Has survey research been able to link expectancies to substance use? What are the anticipated outcomes of marijuana and cocaine use?

12. Does the evidence indicate that drug expectancies are the precursors or consequences of substance use?

13. What role does memory play in drinking behavior? How are the memory networks of heavy drinkers different from those of lighter drinkers?

14. What is the role of drug expectancy in psychiatric comorbidity?

15. What types of alcohol expectancies are linked to treatment outcome?

16. What is the tension reduction hypothesis (TRH)? Do existing data support its validity?

17. What are the propositions of the SRD model?

18. Under what conditions does alcohol disrupt the initial appraisal of stressful information?

19. In Tiffany's model, when do drug urges appear in cognitive processing?

20. How has relapse been viewed historically?

21. What is the most frequently cited explanation for relapse in the professional literature?

22. What are the cognitive patterns that lead to relapse? What is the significance of feeling deprived?

23. In SLT, how are recovering clients taught to view relapse?

24. What are "apparently irrelevant decisions" (AIDs)? How do they lead to relapses?

25. What is the "abstinence violation effect"?

26. What were the outcomes of Project MATCH?

C H A P T E R   8

The Family System

Systems theory and family therapy have been linked with each other for several decades; however, the two are not synonymous. In "systems theory," the unit of analysis is the social system. Relatively little consideration is given to intrapsychic factors. The determinants of behavior are thought to be the "ongoing dynamics and demands of the key interpersonal system(s) within which the individual interacts" (Pearlman, 1988, p. 290). The emphasis is on social roles that are carried out within the context of the organizations to which one belongs. In this culture, the family is usually the dominant influence on behavior, though the workplace, the neighborhood community, and the church can also be considered influential systems.

The literature on addiction and the family has evolved from two sources: (1) the clinical experience of family therapists and (2) empirical research. According to Sher (1997), two bodies of knowledge have been created that are relatively distinct from one another. This chapter first presents key concepts from the clinically focused literature, followed by a review of findings generated from research studies.

CLINICALLY GENERATED CONCEPTS

Social systems, such as families, are complex organizations that are hierarchical in nature. Their dynamics consist of stable, predictable patterns of relationships. Rules (which are often unspoken, but known to members) guide these relationship patterns. Whenever one element in the system is changed (e.g., an alcoholic family member stops drinking), all other elements are affected. The entire system attempts to compensate for the change. Thus, systems theory stresses the wholeness of the social unit, and the interdependence of all the members of the system is emphasized. Again, psychological factors are not usually scrutinized. According to Steinglass (1978), the significance assigned to "wholeness" and interdependent relationships is that which distinguishes systems theory from most other perspectives on addictive behavior.

Boundaries

In a family system (as well as other systems), there is organization. Several systems concepts are typically used to describe the nature of the organization. One such concept is referred to as "boundaries." Boundaries exist to

> distinguish those elements contained within the system from other elements within the broader environment. Boundaries are significant within a system framework since they not only define membership within a given system or subsystem but also characterize the quality of the relationship between the system per se and its surrounding milieu. This latter property of a boundary is referred to as its permeability and describes the ease of exchange of information with other systems. (Pearlman, 1988, p. 290)

Boundaries have also been described as "rules of interaction" and "methods of functioning," which fall on a continuum from "very diffuse" to "very rigid"; in the middle of this continuum lie "clear" boundaries (see Figure 8.1). Within most family systems, boundaries lie at some point in the middle, though they may be closer to one extreme or the other. Optimally functioning family relationships are characterized by clear boundaries. That is, they allow for individuality yet maintain intimacy; they are based on mutual respect; the members show genuine love and concern for one

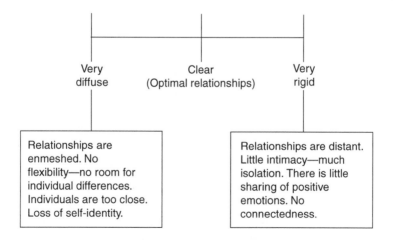

FIGURE 8.1. Family boundaries continuum.

another without attempting to control one another, freedom and flexibility are evident, and communication patterns are clear and direct.

Where very diffuse boundaries exist, relationships are characterized by overinvolvement. There is no room for separateness or individual uniqueness; an overemphasis is placed on sameness and unity (Lawson & Lawson, 1998). Families with very diffuse or enmeshed boundaries do not allow adolescents to pull away from the family. They discourage the development of exceptional or unique talents. Some adolescents may rebel against this "smothering" by abusing alcohol or drugs. When marital relationships are characterized by overinvolvement, the individuality of each spouse is "sacrificed" for the "sake of the marriage" (Lawson & Lawson, 1998, p. 58).

In other chemically dependent families, boundaries may be very rigid or disengaged. Individual members of the family (particularly the alcoholic or addict) may be isolated, or, at other times, the entire family may be isolated from the community. According to Lawson and Lawson (1998), alcoholic families have three rules:

1. "do not talk about the alcoholism,"
2. "do not confront drinking behavior," and
3. "protect and shelter the alcoholic so that things don't become worse." (p. 58)

Unfortunately, such rules enable an alcoholic or addict to keep drinking or using drugs and inadvertently contribute to the progression of addictive behavior. A vicious cycle develops in which the isolation imposed by the three rules perpetuates the alcohol or drug abuse, and, in turn, the substance abuse maintains the need for isolation (see Figure 8.2).

When one spouse is an alcoholic or addict, the marital relationship may be disengaged at a fixed distance. That is, the partners may remain

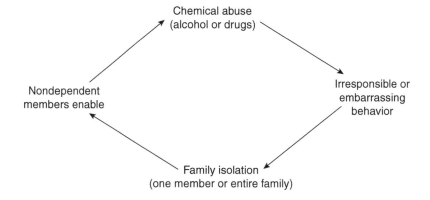

FIGURE 8.2. Reciprocal relationship between family isolation and chemical abuse.

married, but they lead relatively separate lives. The alcoholic or addict may work and spend much time with drinking or drug-using buddies rather than at home. The nondependent spouse may carry the full parenting load and pursue other interests without the chemically dependent spouse. Children of these disengaged families typically feel rejected and unloved. They may develop emotional problems or "act out." Either way, their maladaptive behavior represents a plea for help.

Subsystems and Hierarchies

"Subsystems" and "hierarchies" also contribute to the organization of the family system. There are several subsystems within the family. The original subsystem is the marital one. Within the marital subsystem, certain privileges, communication patterns, and behaviors are appropriate (financial decisions, career decisions, sexual relations, etc.). The birth of the first child creates a new subsystem (the parental subsystem). Within this subsystem, the decisions about how to raise the children are made. This power rests with the parents; thus, a hierarchy appears in which parents have more power than the children. In chemically dependent families where the alcoholic or addict is a parent, the nondependent spouse typically assumes most of the parental power. The addicted spouse gives up or turns over power as a parent. This shift in role obligations places a heavy burden on the nondependent spouse and usually creates feelings of resentment. Sometimes a grandparent or older sibling may assume some parental power (as demonstrated by cooking meals, shopping, doing laundry, etc.); in this way, subsystem boundaries may become blurred.

A sibling subsystem also evolves. Its complexity depends on the number of children, their age differences, their gender, and their common interests (Lawson & Lawson, 1998). Sibling subsystems may distinguish the sons from the daughters, the oldest from the youngest, or the athletic from the nonathletic. In functional families, these subsystems remain somewhat fluid and dynamic as time passes and the children mature. In dysfunctional families, the subsystems may remain static as the children are required to assume inappropriate roles, such as that of a parent. Allowing a child into the marital subsystem (e.g., incest) is another example in which subsystems are likely to remain static (Lawson & Lawson, 1998).

Family Rules

Another characteristic of family organization pertains to the rules that govern interactions between and among members. Often these rules are implicit rather than explicit; however, most or all members somehow seem to know them. They define appropriate conduct within the family system. They function to provide order, stability, consistency, and predictability in family affairs. They also serve to restrict behavioral options (e.g., "incest is unacceptable"). Families usually have rules governing the manner in which different emotions are expressed. In some families anger is not allowed, whereas in others shouting is permissible. In some families affection is demonstrated with hugs and kisses, while in others physical contact is minimized.

Barnard (1981) has noted six areas in which families usually formulate rules:

1. To what extent, when, and how family members may comment on what they see, feel, and think.
2. Who can speak to whom and about what.
3. How a member can be different.
4. How sexuality can be expressed.
5. What it means to be male or female.
6. How a person can acquire self-worth, and how much self-worth is appropriate to possess.

In chemically dependent families, certain family rules are typical. For example, it is usually prohibited to talk openly about the substance abuse: the "conspiracy of silence" (Deutsch, 1982). There often exists a "don't feel, don't trust, don't talk" rule in such families as well. A rule often found in alcoholic families is that "anger can only be expressed when the alcoholic is drinking" (Lawson & Lawson, 1998). The family's alcoholic sometimes operates according to this rule: "I am comfortable expressing my affection for you only after I have been drinking."

Causality in Family Systems

Systems theory emphasizes reciprocal rather than linear causality. That is, relationships between and among variables or elements in systems include feedback loops. Simple cause-and-effect relationships are viewed as too reductionistic and as incapable of capturing the complexity of family interactions. Thus, behaviors that are stimulated by one element themselves become stimuli for other behaviors. Pearlman (1988) notes that most family therapists have firsthand knowledge of the reciprocal patterns in family relationship problems. As an example, Figure 8.3 represents the most common marital pattern in alcoholism.

Homeostasis

"Homeostasis," a metaphor borrowed from the physiological sciences, has long been an important concept in systems theory (Pearlman, 1988). According to Stanton (1980), homeostasis in a family with an alcoholic or

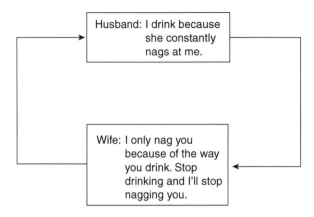

FIGURE 8.3. Reciprocal relationship between husband's abusive drinking and wife's nagging.

addict is a pathological equilibrium in which the nondependent family members have an emotional investment in the chemically dependent member's maintaining his/her addiction. It explains "the family's tenacity in holding onto existing behavioral repertoires, resisting change, and exerting pressure to minimize or reverse change when it occurs" (Pearlman, 1988, p. 292).

The application of the homeostasis metaphor to alcoholic- or drug-dependent families is at odds with the conventional view that these problems "tear families apart." In the majority of such families, the impact of alcohol and drug use is much more subtle. Alcohol and drug abuse usually do not evoke immediate separation or divorce. According to Steinglass (1981), the more common situation is that "most families seem to work out a compromise in which the family remains economically and structurally intact despite the presence of a member with chronic alcoholism in its midst" (p. 578).

Rather, the abuse of alcohol and/or drugs may be thought of as an effort to maintain family balance. If the drinking or drug use is stopped (e.g., an attempt at recovery), the family is thrown out of balance. These transition periods typically involve heightened interpersonal interaction that can be uncomfortable for members (Steinglass, 1981). To reestablish greater emotional distance, nondependent family members often (unconsciously) attempt to sabotage the member's recovery effort and thereby return the family to rigid stability. Some treatment programs that work with families are aware of these dynamics and make efforts to help members cope with the anxieties of transitioning from active use to sobriety (Laundergan & Williams, 1993).

The sabotaging behavior of the nondependent members may take many forms. For example, let us suppose that a 40-year-old male alcoholic makes good progress in an aftercare program. After several months of abstinence and frequent Alcoholics Anonymous (AA) attendance, his wife begins to complain bitterly that they never "go out" any more because he is always at "those" meetings. Her nagging eventually prompts him to relapse. She did not intend for him to slip, but her behavior has nevertheless had that result. Another example of sabotaging involves a husband of a female cocaine addict in early recovery. Upon her leaving inpatient rehabilitation, he agrees to care for the kids while she attends aftercare and Twelve-Step meetings. After a few weeks, he protests that he feels too "tied down" and refuses to continue babysitting. She soon relapses. Other spouses have been known to complain that their recovering spouses are "not the same person"; often, they have ambivalent feelings about the behavioral and personality changes. They may feel that their mates are now too assertive, "kind of boring," or less sociable than when they were drinking or abusing drugs.

Not only will the newfound sobriety throw the marital relationship into turmoil, but the children are also affected. The following excerpt highlights typical reactions of children to a father in early recovery: "Mother is not needed as the overly responsible martyr when Dad returns to take over running the household. Brother has no reason to stay away from home and must reevaluate his relationship with Dad. The family suddenly notices little sister's hyperactive mannerisms." (Lawson & Lawson, 1998, p. 54)

From a systems point of view, the abusive drinking or drug use has adaptive consequences. That is, it functions to keep the family "in balance"—not a "healthy" balance, but a relatively stable one nevertheless. This pathological equilibrium is preferred over continual chaos and crisis. In essence, such families opt for low-level discomfort and "put up" with the substance abuse in order to avoid grappling with even more painful and sensitive issues.

Alcohol or drug abuse can stabilize a family (i.e., keep it in balance) in a number of ways. It can divert attention from marital problems and allow angry or hurtful feelings to go unexpressed. For example, among married male alcoholics, abusive drinking is often a way to avoid intimacy with their wives. It establishes an emotional distance that can become fixed over time. Frequently, such men feel much ambivalence about their marriages and their children. They may love them but at the same time may believe that their wives and kids are responsible for their lost opportunities. This may be particularly true of men who married and had children relatively young. The family is often seen as a financial and emotional burden, one that many men fear they will not be able to support. In such cases, men feel a loss of freedom, especially when the perceive themselves to be trapped in jobs that they dislike. Excessive drinking is one way to cope with these pressures. It serves as an analgesic for the family pain; it also prevents crises that could lead to family breakup if they were faced squarely.

Homeostatic mechanisms, such as drinking, regulate the amount of change to which a family can adapt at any one time. Change can occur in the family, but the need for balance slows it by relying on compensatory measures. In functional families, change is incorporated relatively easily via compensatory efforts that allow all members to get their needs met. If young Johnnie starts Little League baseball, for instance, Dad makes an effort to adjust his work schedule to get him to practice. However, in dysfunctional families, adaptation to the evolving needs of the members is more resistant and less fluid. All members are less likely to get their needs fulfilled.

Pearlman (1988) notes that these family regulatory processes are maintained by feedback loops, which can be points of intervention in family systems therapy. He states:

> Positive feedback loops introduce change into the system. Negative feedback loops, on the other hand, promote a steady state and diminish the impact of change that is introduced into the system. Negative feedback loops are, therefore, closely associated with a system's homeostatic tendencies, and have become an important focal point for the systems therapist in attempting to identify and ultimately overcome a family's seemingly inherent tendency to resist change. (p. 292)

It should be noted that dysfunctional families are not forever locked into maladaptive patterns of interaction. The concept of homeostasis only describes the tendency to regulate change; it does not describe an unalterable pattern of maladaptive interaction.

The Impact of One's Family of Origin

How are dysfunctional marriages and families created? Is the development of such a union predictable, or is it simply the result of choosing the wrong mate? Framo (1976) believes that individuals select mates in an attempt to fill voids they experienced in their own families of origin. This is an unconscious effort for the most part, and it involves bargaining: "I will be your conscience if you act out my impulse" (Framo, 1976, p. 194). In this way, one spouse (typically the woman) seeks to control the other, while the other (typically the man) expresses the rebellion that the first dares not reveal (Lawson & Lawson, 1998). This may partly explain why some women are attracted to men who engage in risky behavior (drinking abusively, using drugs, driving fast, fighting, etc.), and why such men often find restrained, traditional women desirable in turn.

Lawson and Lawson (1998) describe in the following passage how alcoholic marriages become increasingly problematic:

> The two personalities become dependent on each other and increasingly inter-twined, making it difficult for either to leave regardless of the dysfunction of the relationship. Marital partners enmeshed in these relationships (based on the inability to function as an individual) can manifest dysfunctions leading to superficial relationships, emotional upheaval, and possible drinking behavior (if this drinking model was present in their family of origin). Often these mari-tal partners reach out to each other for identity and fuse into a single entity in the marriage. To achieve some separateness the marital partners must set up emotional distance. One spouse may take the dominant position in the rela-tionship with the remaining spouse adapting to the other and further losing identity. (p. 34)

A marital relationship usually consists of an "emotional pursuer" and an "emotional distancer" (Fogarty, 1976). In U.S. culture (and probably other Western cultures as well), the woman is the pursuer, and the man is the distancer. Typically, as the woman strives for intimacy, the man backs away. In healthy marriages, both individuals will at least occasionally be pursuers and thus will establish intimacy. In dysfunctional marriages, over time, a fixed emotional distance may occur; that is, neither spouse strives for emotional intimacy. Such is often the case when one spouse abuses alco-hol or drugs (or when both do). This underinvolvement often leads the nonabusing spouse to become overinvolved with the children (when there are children). The nonabusing spouse may get some of their emotional needs met through the children. In addition, the children may become overly dependent on the nonabusing parent (typically the mother) because of the other parent's distance.

The Teen's Fear of Separation

Dysfunctional marital relationships can have deleterious effects on the teen-age children of such unions. Adolescent alcohol or drug abuse is one of the negative consequences of problems between the parents. Stanton (1980) has explored the family dynamics that give rise to substance abuse among teens who are children of alcoholics or addicts. He suggests that an overinvolvement with the nonabusing parent creates an intense "fear of separation." At the same time, the teen has normal developmental needs to begin separating from the family of origin. Thus, drug abuse becomes a way in which the teen demonstrates a "pseudoindividuation"—that is, a false independence from the family. The act of abusing drugs or alcohol represents rebellion and autonomy, but, according to Stanton (1980), it is only an "illusory independence." Such a teen establishes a link to the drug subculture (which outwardly suggests adulthood) but also maintains a foothold in the family.

Stanton (1980) cites his own research for evidence of pseudo-individuation among teens and young adults. He found that 66% of heroin addicts, for example, lived with or saw their mothers daily. This may not seem particularly unusual, until consideration is given to the fact that their average age was 28. Considering U.S. cultural norms, this suggests prolonged overdependence on their mothers. Thus, it appears that some young, unmarried addicts will vacillate between their families of origin and the drug subculture. They want to appear strong and independent, but they also fear separation from an overinvolved relationship with a parent.

Triads

Bowen (1976), Stanton (1980), and others maintain that dysfunctional families form triadic patterns of interaction, which contribute to the development of addiction in children. "Triads" are family subsystems that consist of three members. Typically, this interactive pattern in a case of chemical dependence involves a young adult (or adolescent) addict and the parents. However, other triads can develop as well, especially in extended families. For example, a triadic subsystem may consist of a young adult male alcoholic, his wife, and his mother (with whom they reside).

In the most common triad, one parent is intensely involved with the addict, while the other parent is underinvolved and perhaps punitive. Usually the overinvolved parent is pampering and indulgent of the addicted child. This parent is usually of the opposite sex from the child; thus, the emotionally distant parent is often a father, the overinvolved parent is the mother, and the addict is male.

The triad forms as a means of protecting the marriage and the family. In essence, the triad serves a protective function: It helps maintain the family structure by distracting the parents from their own marital difficulties. The child's drug problem provides a focal point around which they can unify, instead of focusing on their own problems. The drug problem gives them a reason for remaining together. All their emotional energies are directed toward the child, rather than toward each other. Thus, the child's drug problem functions to suppress marital conflict.

Stanton (1980) asserts that it is no accident that alcohol or drug abuse typically begins in early or middle adolescence. Parents in a dysfunctional marriage may be threatened by the fact that their child is growing up. They may fear losing the child (to a girlfriend or boyfriend, to military service, to higher education or a career, to a move to a geographically distant area, etc.). This parental anxiety, according to Stanton (1980), stems from the deeper fear that they will have to face their relationship problems. They anticipate that the void in their marriage will no longer be filled by their child. Such parents often feel threatened and incapable of overcoming long-standing marital problems. They only see two options: (1) staying permanently in an unsatisfying relationship, or (2) divorce.

The Dance

Stanton (1980) has noted that triads become "stuck" in a chronic, repetitive pattern of interaction. He uses the metaphor of the "dance" to describe the process. This is more than simply a description; the "dance" metaphor explains, from a systems viewpoint, how relapse occurs. The dance consists of the various forms of repetitive, consistent, and predictable displays of behavior (Stanton, 1980). One of the steps in the dance is the act of abusing drugs or alcohol. Box 8.1 describes the experience of one 23-year-old polydrug addict who was engaged in a triadic relationship with his parents.

The concept of the dance provides insight into the dynamics behind relapse. Stanton (1980) indicates that these dynamics often go unrecognized and that those who relapse are labeled "unmotivated" or perhaps "emotionally unstable." From a systems perspective, such assessments are superficial; they overlook the addict's enmeshment in the family system. Thus, effective relapse prevention should include intervention with the family rather than just focusing narrowly on intrapsychic factors within the addict.

BOX 8.1. Billy and His Parents

For as long as Billy can remember, his parents argued. Sometimes their fights became violent, with many household items being broken. Billy began using drugs in his early teens; by his senior year in high school, he could be described as a drug addict. His drug use came to the attention of his parents because he was "busted" at school. Previously, they had been too involved with their own problems to notice.

Billy's parents reacted in distinctively different ways. His father was enraged and very condemning of Billy; he threatened him with all kinds of consequences. Mom, on the other hand, was very reassuring and protective. She attempted to shield him from his father and to make excuses for him. It appeared that his parents unconsciously welcomed the drug problem because it gave them relief from their own conflict. As a result, they focused much energy on disciplining Billy and helping him with his prob-

lem. They arranged for him to be admitted to a drug rehabilitation program.

Upon Billy's discharge, he remained abstinent for several weeks. His
parents were on their best behavior during this time. Gradually (and as a
result of Billy's abstinence), Mom and Dad began to argue again. Their
conflict resurfaced without Billy's "problem" to distract them. In turn,
Billy relapsed. It was as if they were in a dance: When Mom and Dad's
arguing flared up, so did Billy's drug abuse; when Billy's drug abuse sub-
sided a bit as a result of their efforts and attention, Mom and Dad's arguing again resumed. They were right in step with each other. This pattern
continued for 5 years, with four attempts at inpatient rehabilitation. After
his fourth discharge, Billy managed to obtain a good-paying job. He
remained clean and sober, and he established a relationship with a woman
he met through work. Everything was going well until his mother began to
harangue him about not visiting and calling. One night she called him
while she was drunk and accused him of not really caring for her, and not
being appreciative of all of the things she and his father had done for him
through the years.

In an aftercare group, Billy reported that he was "shaky" and anxious, and had suddenly begun having drug cravings. He had difficulty linking these symptoms to his conversation with his mother, though he felt her
trying to "pull" him back home. Mom was threatened by Billy's increasing
independence and maturity.

This story has a happy ending for Billy. He did not relapse, and is
doing well in his job and marriage. Mom and Dad are now divorced.

BOWEN'S FAMILY SYSTEMS THEORY

A relatively large number of family systems theories exist. Each one emphasizes different aspects of the family, though most share common elements as
described previously (Pearlman, 1988). Among the most prominent of
these theories is the work of Murray Bowen. The Bowen theory is presented here as the prototypical family systems theory. It should be noted
that this is not specifically a theory of addiction but, rather, one of family
dysfunction. Addiction is considered an example of dysfunction in the family unit.

Differentiation of Self

Bowen (1976) considers "differentiation of self" to be the central concept
of his theory. This concept classifies people on a continuum. On one end

of the continuum are people whose lives are extremely dominated by automatic emotional reaction. They are said to be "fused" (Bowen, 1976); that is, no differentiation exists between the emotional and the intellectual self. Emotion, at this extreme, completely dominates the self. According to Bowen (1976), "These are people who are less flexible, less adaptable, and more emotionally dependent on those about them. They are easily stressed into dysfunction, and it is difficult for them to recover from dysfunction. They inherit a high percentage of all human problems" (p. 65).

On the other end of the continuum are those persons who are highly differentiated. That is, they possess a balance between emotional and intellectual responding, and these two processes are more clearly separated. Bowen (1976) maintains that complete differentiation of self is impossible. However, people whose emotional functioning and intellectual functioning are relatively well separated will be more autonomous, more flexible, and better able to cope with stress; they will also demonstrate more independence of emotions. In essence, they possess a high level of emotional maturity. Bowen (1976) states that "their life courses are more orderly and successful, and they are remarkably free of human problems" (pp. 65–66) (see Figure 8.4).

Of those persons on the low end of the continuum (scores = 0–25), Bowen (1976) writes:

> The intellect is so flooded by emotionality that the total life course is determined by the emotional process and by what "feels right," rather than by beliefs or opinions. The intellect exists as an appendage of the feeling system. It may function reasonably well in mathematics or physics, or in impersonal areas, but on personal subjects its functioning is controlled by the emotions. (p. 66)

This insight may explain, at least partly, the resistance that many families (and individuals) demonstrate when offered help or therapeutic feedback. The assistance is usually principled; that is, it is formed from reason. It is rational. Thus, it is often rejected because of the overreliance on emotional functioning.

It should be noted here that Bowen does not discount the emotional dimension of human experience. He does not advocate human development that is cold, distant, or uncaring. Rather, he emphasizes that the poorly differentiated individual is "trapped within a feeling world" (Bowen, 1976, p. 67). They have no options in responding; they simply react in an automatic fashion. In contrast, a highly differentiated person can express emotion (both positive and negative) in appropriate, productive ways.

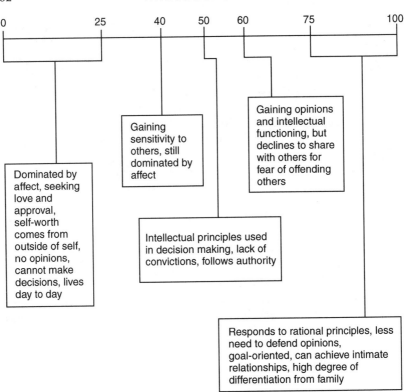

FIGURE 8.4. Bowen's scale of differentiation.

Poorly differentiated persons are "totally relationship oriented" (Bowen, 1976, p. 69). Most of their energy goes into pleasing others and keeping their relationships, especially with family members, in harmony. Conflict is avoided. Typically, these persons say "I feel . . . " when expressing their views. They are unable to form personal beliefs and thus avoid saying "I think . . . " or "I believe . . . " (Bowen, 1976).

Persons with low levels of differentiation have other difficulties as well. They find it difficult to make plans and carry them out. Long-term goals are almost impossible to form for these individuals. They tend to live from day to day and remain overly dependent on their parents well into adulthood. They are preoccupied with making others happy. Sometimes employers find such characteristics useful, so poorly differentiated individuals may remain in the same low-level positions for many years. Extremely low-functioning individuals in this group may be institutionalized and labeled "psychotic," "schizophrenic," or "mentally ill."

Bowen (1976) describes individuals whose level of differentiation is a bit higher (scores = 25–50) in the following passage:

> Lives are guided by the emotional system, but the life styles are more flexible than the lower levels of differentiation. The flexibility provides a better view of the interplay between emotionality and intellect. When anxiety is low, functioning can resemble good levels of differentiation. When anxiety is high, functioning can resemble that of low levels of differentiation. Lives are relationship oriented, and major life energy goes to loving and being loved, and seeking approval from others. Feelings are more openly expressed than in lower level people. Life energy is directed more to what others think and to winning friends and approval than to goal-directed activity. Self-esteem is dependent on others. It can soar to heights with a compliment or be crushed by criticism. Success in school is oriented more to learning the system and to pleasing the teacher than to the primary goal of learning. . . . They may have enough free-functioning intellect to have mastered academic knowledge about impersonal things; they use this knowledge in the relationship system. However, intellect about personal matters is lacking, and their personal lives are in chaos. (pp. 70–71)

Bowen (1976) indicates that scores of 50–75 on his continuum represent moderate levels of self-differentiation. Among this group, the two systems, intellect and emotion, function cooperatively; neither system dominates the other. In particularly stressful situations, the intellectual system may be overwhelmed, but for the most part these individuals lead satisfying lives. The intellectual system learns that discipline is required to obtain long-term gains. Thus, persons in this group are capable to some degree of delaying gratification and planning for the future. They are also somewhat more able to think for themselves. They are aware of differences between thinking and feeling and at least occasionally are able to state unpopular beliefs or opinions.

The highly differentiated person (scores = 75–100) is "more hypothetical, than real," according to Bowen (1976, p. 73). Few individuals reach such a level of development. Such persons are aware of the relationships around them, but they do not become mired in emotional "stuck-togetherness." They are aware of various response options available to them. They presumably choose how to act, instead of automatically reacting to a situation. Again, highly differentiated persons are not emotionally cold or distant; in fact, they welcome and express sincere, authentic emotion. However, they avoid the various insincere expressions of emotion that are often required by unwritten family rules or by social conventions.

Triangles

A triangle (or triad) is thought to consist of a comfortably close twosome and an uncomfortable outsider. To avoid separation, the partners in the twosome work to achieve closeness; often they are overinvolved with each other. The uncomfortable outsider seeks closeness to one of the twosome. These attempts at maneuvering have been described earlier in the chapter as the "dance." Bowen (1976) notes that the constant motion within the triangle results from moderate levels of tension in the twosome, which are felt by only one of them. The other is oblivious to the conflict in the pair. The "uncomfortable other" mediates or diverts some of the tension to him-herself by engaging the twosome and thus initiates a new equilibrium within the triangle.

During periods of great stress and tension, the "outsider" position is sought by each member of the triangle. In times of stress, this is the least uncomfortable position. Obviously, all three individuals cannot shift to the outside position. When such shifts are prevented, one of the twosome involves a new outsider, and a new triangle is formed. Bowen (1976) believes that these shifting dynamics often result in all family members being "triangled" at different points in time. Furthermore, when all available family triangles have been exhausted, the family typically seeks to form triangles with people outside itself (members of the clergy, police officers, mental health professionals, social service agencies, school officials, etc.).

Bowen (1976) describes the typical triangle in the following passage:

> The best example of this is the father–mother–child triangle. Patterns vary, but one of the most common is basic tension between the parents, with the father's gaining the outside position—often being called passive, weak, and distant-leaving the conflict between the mother and child. The mother—often called aggressive, dominating, and castrating—wins over the child, who moves another step toward chronic functional impairment. . . . Families replay the same triangular game over and over for years, as though the winner were in doubt, but the final result is always the same. Over the years the child accepts the always-lose outcome more easily, even to volunteering for this position. (pp. 76–77)

The Emotional System in the Nuclear Family

In each generation of a family, certain patterns of emotional functioning appear. These patterns, involving parents and children, are replicated from the mother's and father's separate families of origin. According to Bowen (1976), families transmit these patterns of emotional responding from generation to generation. These patterns are readily observable in most families.

Typically, the nuclear family begins with a marriage. Bowen (1976) maintains that individuals of similar levels of differentiation will be attracted to each other. The lower their level of differentiation, the more intense the emotional fusion in the marriage. In most marriages, one spouse becomes more dominant in decision making for the couple. The other spouse adapts to the arrangement. Bowen (1976) describes the fusion that occurs among most couples in the following passage:

> One [spouse] may assume the dominant role and force the other to be adaptive, or one [spouse] may assume the adaptive role and force the other to be dominant. Both may try for the dominant role, which results in conflict; or both may try for the adaptive role, which results in decision paralysis. The dominant one gains self at the expense of the more adaptive one, who loses self. More differentiated spouses have lesser degrees of fusion, and fewer of the complications. The dominant and adaptive positions are not directly related to the sex of the spouse. They are determined by the position that each had in their families of origin. From my experience, there are as many dominant females as males, and as many adaptive males as females. These characteristics played a major role in their original choice of each other as partners. (p. 79)

When there is a high degree of fusion in the relationship, spouses are preoccupied with the behavior of the other and as a result tension increases to high levels. Spouses with relatively high degrees of differentiation make minor adjustments to cope with the anxiety that results from emotional fusion. Less differentiated spouses develop more problematic symptoms. Bowen (1976) describes four common manifestations of marital fusion:

1. Emotional distancing.
2. Marital conflict.
3. Dysfunction in one spouse.
4. Impairment of one or more children.

The first symptom, emotional distancing, occurs among couples of moderate levels of self-differentiation, as well as among those who are highly fused (and anxious about being so). It is extremely common among most couples, almost universal. Few couples want to maintain the degree of fusion that they experienced during their courtship and the early days of their marriage. The loss of self (adaptive role) and the burden of decision making (dominant role) exact too great an emotional cost over prolonged periods of time. Thus, emotional distancing occurs to various degrees in most marital relationships.

Marital conflict results when neither spouse is willing to "give in" to the other—that is, neither spouse is willing to assume the adaptive role. Bowen (1976) indicates that marital conflict does not involve the children. The spouses are intensely involved with each other, with occasional periods of emotional distancing.

Dysfunction in one spouse results when one spouse absorbs a large amount of undifferentiation into him/herself while assuming the adaptive role (Bowen, 1976). In this situation, the dysfunctional spouse strains to adapt to the other over prolonged periods of time.

There is a loss of self. The adaptive spouse develops such symptoms as physical illness, substance abuse, mental disorders, or irresponsible behavior. These disorders become chronic. Bowen (1976) notes that such marriages tend to be enduring, for this reason: "The underfunctioning one is grateful for the care and attention, and the overfunctioning one does not complain" (p. 81).

When the parents project their undifferentiation onto one or more of the children, they are likely to become emotionally impaired as well. According to Bowen (1976), the intensity of the parents' projection is related to two variables. The first variable has to do with the degree of emotional isolation of the family—that is, the degree to which the family is withdrawn from their extended family, their church, their community, and so on. The second variable pertains to the level of tension in the family: The greater the levels of anxiety (and isolation), the more pronounced the parental projection. Bowen (1976) considers this process of projection to be fundamental to most human problems. As such, he more fully develops the concept by describing it as the "family projection process."

The Family Projection Process

The family projection process involves a father–mother–child triangle. The parents' undifferentiation is projected onto a child. Because the mother gives birth to the child and because she is usually the primary nurturer, Bowen (1976) believes that the process revolves around her emotional energy, which in turn originates in her family of origin. The family projection process can be the principal cause of a child's emotional impairment, or it can superimpose itself on a child's preexisting illness (e.g., leukemia) or disability (e.g., Down's syndrome, spina bifida, and muscular dystrophy). Bowen (1976) notes that "the process is so universal it is present to some degree in all families" (p. 81).

In Bowen's systems theory, the emotional energy arising from the parents' undifferentiation is expressed in one or more of the following ways: (1) marital conflict, (2) dysfunction in one spouse, and (3) projection to the children. The undifferentiation is also absorbed in these three ways. Family members typically shift the weight of the undifferentiation around so that no one member becomes too dysfunctional.

Thus, the children are sometimes projected onto in order to reduce marital conflict or spouse dysfunction. This homeostatic mechanism protects the marriage in the former case and the adaptive spouse in the latter. According to Bowen (1976), "I have never seen a family in which there was not some projection to a child. Most families use a combination of all three mechanisms" (p. 82).

The projection to the children is not equally distributed. For various unconscious reasons (discussed later), the projection first focuses on one child. If the focus becomes too intense (i.e., if the child becomes too impaired), it is often shifted to another child (a new father–mother–child triangle is created), and so forth. In this fashion, each child may become "triangulated" at some point in the life of the family.

Emotional Cutoff

The final concept in Bowen's theory to be presented here is "emotional cutoff." According to Bowen (1976), individuals with lower levels of differentiation have not separated emotionally from their parents. They have unresolved emotional attachments to their families of origin. "Emotional cutoff" describes the manner in which individuals separate from their parents. Some individuals separate by isolating themselves emotionally, though they continue to live close to their parents. Others may move to a geographically distant area but remain emotionally dependent on their parents. Still others may sever all communication but remain affected by unresolved attachments. Bowen (1976) notes that many people will use a combination of these methods to "cut off."

The more intense the emotional cutoff, the greater the likelihood that an individual will bring the "unfinished business" from the family of origin into his/her present marriage and family. It is also likely that the children of such individuals will cut off in a similar fashion. (Bowen, 1976). Again, parents tend to transmit their level of differentiation to their children.

The preceding discussion has provided a brief overview of the Bowen theory. The concepts provide insight into the ways families function.

CODEPENDENCY

The concept of "codependency" (also called "coalcoholism" when alcoholism is involved) refers to an unhealthy pattern of relating to others that results from being closely involved with an alcoholic or addict (Subby & Friel, 1984). "Codependency" is a generic term, and it has been defined in various ways, but all definitions describe unhealthy relationship patterns (Beattie, 1987). The chemical abuser in a codependent's life is usually a husband, but it can also be wife, a parent, a close friend, a child, or a coworker.

Koffinke (1991) indicates that the codependent is overly focused on (i.e., overinvolved with) the substance abuser. Their relationship is enmeshed and problem filled. The problems provide endless opportunities for the codependent to be preoccupied with the addict. Hypervigilance is the norm. For women who grew up in chemically dependent families, this behavior seems normal. In fact, some believe that women from such families learn codependent behavior early in life and are thus attracted to substance-abusing mates (Koffinke, 1991). They also find it very difficult, if not impossible, to leave dysfunctional relationships.

As a result of this emotional enmeshment, the codependent tends to lose all sense of "self" or identity and to become emotionally dependent on the addict. The addict's mood dictates the codependent's mood. In a sense, the codependent becomes an appendage to the addict and the substance abuse.

The codependent often protects the alcoholic or addict from the natural consequences of substance abuse (Koffinke, 1991). Such behavior is referred to as "enabling." Examples include calling in sick to a dependent spouse's employer when the spouse has been out drinking or using drugs all night, or cleaning up after a spouse who has vomited during the night from too much alcohol. Hence, codependency is considered an unhealthy relationship pattern, whereas enabling is a common behavior arising from it.

In addition, the codependent may purposely isolate him/herself (and the family) from the extended family and friends, in order to keep the "family secret" and save the family from embarrassment. Unfortunately, this isolation removes opportunities to release feelings of anger, hurt, fear, and frustration (Koffinke, 1991).

Chief Characteristics

Several writers have identified chief characteristics of codependency. Following is a descriptive list of the psychological distress codependents are reported to experience.

1. *Poor self-esteem.* Codependents suffer from low self-esteem; that is, they feel little personal worth and think poorly of themselves. This has many sources. They themselves may have grown up in alcoholic families, or families in which chemical dependency was not an issue but physical or emotional abuse was present nevertheless. It is also possible that they grew up in homes in which the parents were overprotective and domineering.

2. *Need to be needed.* Many codependents believe that their worth depends on how well they take care of loved ones. In our culture, women are especially socialized to be nurturers, so it may come easily for them. As a result, codependents may neglect their own emotional needs for security, love, and attention.

3. *Strong urge to change and control others.* Codependents usually develop the belief that they have the power to control the alcoholics or addicts and therefore must use this power to change them (i.e., get them to cut down or stop their drinking/drug use). Norwood (1985) notes that many codependents learned this notion as children. They may have been instructed by their mothers to "leave dad alone when he is drinking, or you could upset him" (Norwood, 1985); such instructions teach them that they can control others. An overdeveloped sense of responsibility develops, in which the codependents come to believe almost grandiosely that they are at the center of the universe and all-powerful in a very unhealthy sense. This may partly explain why some codependent women always seem to end up in dysfunctional relationships with addicted men, and why some women appear to take on unhealthy or impaired men as "rehabilitation projects."

4. *Willingness to suffer.* Norwood (1985) suggests that many co-dependents ask, "if I suffer for you, will you love me?" (p. 47). This is the tendency to become a martyr. It is as if some satisfaction or reward is gained from suffering. They may not be happy, but they can claim to be superior (i.e., morally, emotionally, or socially) to their impaired spouse (Norwood, 1985). They can also claim to be superior to others who desert the alcoholic/addict. Because many codependents grew up in chemically de-pendent families, they do not recognize that they are suffering emotionally. Depression and low self-worth have been experienced for so long that these conditions seem normal.

5. *Resistance to change.* Codependents typically are immobilized by their own sense of guilt. Leaving the alcoholic/addict is not an option, because they fear being overwhelmed by guilt feelings. These feelings make self-examination very painful; in fact, codependents may develop a great deal of secondary anxiety about feeling guilty. From a systems perspective, these beliefs and feelings preserve the family balance, but they blind the codependents from seeing how they contribute to the drinking and/or drug use.

6. *Fear of change.* Typically, codependents fear and resist change. Again, from a systems perspective, codependents may have an emotional investment in the alcoholic's/addict's continued drinking/drug use. These are almost always unconscious desires. They may fear change (i.e., absti-nence/recovery) because they (a) do not want assertive, sober loved ones; (b) may be financially dependent on the substance abuser, and fear that divorce or other disruption would come with sobriety; (c) may want to

avoid sexual relations, which could be expected to resume with sobriety; or (d) expect some family conflict or secret to emerge during sobriety.

Rewards Gained by Codependents

The rewards for staying in a codependent relationship are often not apparent to the outside observer. Many inexperienced professionals are amazed at the amount of suffering codependents are willing to endure, and they have a difficult time understanding why the codependent does not simply leave the alcoholic/addict. Yet a deeper, more thoughtful examination reveals that codependents do attain rewards by staying in dysfunctional relationships. Codependents come to affirm their self-worth by "carrying the cross" of other persons' addiction (or other destructive behavior)—by being a martyr. They may quietly believe that because they suffer, they are special and important. This self-perception represents a misguided grandiosity, which is essentially a shield against feelings, personal inadequacy, and low self-esteem.

CHILDREN IN ALCOHOLIC FAMILIES: CLINICAL ACCOUNTS

Despite skepticism about the usefulness of the ACOA (adult children of alcoholics) concept, it is quite true that children growing up in alcoholic families often experience emotional difficulties. Charles Deutsch (1982) describes what growing up in such a household is like from a child's point of view. He relies on extensive interviews with children from alcoholic homes. Deutsch (1982) pays particular attention to three conditions such children experience: (1) inconsistency, insecurity, and fear, (2) anger and hate, and (3) guilt and blame. Each one is described in turn.

Inconsistency, Insecurity, and Fear

According to Deutsch (1982), inconsistency is the hallmark of most actively alcoholic parents. They demonstrate it both when intoxicated and when sober. They can change moods dramatically, swinging from being warm, caring, and jovial to angry and frustrated within minutes. Because the children do not know what to anticipate, they tend to be insecure. The lack of parental predictability breeds distrust and uncertainty. As a result, many children adopt the "don't feel, don't trust, don't talk" rule. As Deutsch (1982) reports one child saying, "we learned to walk on eggshells without cracking a single one" (p. 42).

Domestic violence is reported in many alcoholic homes. A child's insecurity and fear are heightened considerably when an alcoholic parent acts out in a violent way. Deutsch (1982) indicates that the target of the violence does not seem to matter. The alcoholic who only destroys property instills as much fear as the alcoholic who strikes family members. Interestingly, a child often reports that the nonalcoholic spouse is the more violent and feared parent. In such a case, the nonalcoholic spouse may be attempting to force the alcoholic to stop drinking, or may be ventilating pent-up anger and frustration about the drinking problem. Deutsch (1982) quotes one child as saying:

> "She tried to kill us, actually kill us. We all had our turns fighting her. Everybody used to say, 'ignore her,' but you can't ignore her when she comes after you with a knife, you know? One time she choked me, I mean, she was on top of me, choking me, and I would have died; I felt like I was dying. My father came in—this was really great—he had a cigarette in his mouth, he came in and my little sister was screaming—it was just me and my little sister at home. My mother had me and she was, I mean, I was blue, I thought I was dying, and my sister was standing there screaming. My father came in and threw the cigarette on the floor. And 'cause we were in my mother's bedroom, it—started a fire and later our carpet had to be thrown out. My father came in and pulled my mother off me, and I just ran out of the house. When I came back five hours later, she told me, 'Now you're all right, you're all right.' " (p. 44)

Avoiding conflict becomes the primary concern of children in alcoholic homes. Children become preoccupied with not upsetting the alcoholic or violent parent. Conflict is avoided at all costs. One child quoted by Deutsch (1982) described it this way:

> "There were things we all did just to placate him, like eating together whether we were hungry or not. We were scared a good deal of the time. One time, he demanded his dinner and my mother threw cereal boxes at him. I sat there thinking, 'now that was stupid, why the hell did you do that?' I wished she hadn't done it because I knew I'd have to keep him off her." (p. 44)

Anger and Hate

Though it may not be difficult to understand why children from such homes hate their parents, the children themselves often find these feelings unacceptable. Just as the alcoholic may deny a drinking problem, the children may deny hateful feelings toward their parent. The denial is unconscious; many of these children are simply unaware of these feelings. The "unacceptableness" stems from cultural norms that prohibit children from hating their parents.

The children's anger and hate may be directed at others or at themselves. It is not usually directed at the alcoholic parents, because that would be too dangerous. Deutsch (1982) quotes one 7-year-old boy as saying, "Yeah, sometimes I yell at my teddy bear and sometimes I yell at my teacher when I'm angry at my father. And I know she doesn't like it" (p. 46). Many of these children develop guilt feelings about hating their alcoholic parents. They are unaware that their thoughts and feelings, given the family circumstances, are normal. They feel especially guilty about fantasies they may have in which the alcoholic is killed, dies, or just disappears. One adolescent girl confided to Deutsch (1982): "All the time, I used to lay in bed at night and plot how to kill her without getting caught and stuff. I was a mean kid" (p. 47).

Guilt and Blame

Young children are naturally egocentric. They tend to believe that they are the cause of all that goes on around them. Thus, they tend to blame themselves for their parents' problems; this is particularly true of parents' drinking problems. Alcoholic parents often reinforce the children's self-blame with such rationalizations as these:

> "I'll stop drinking when you behave the way you're supposed to."
> "Why do you think I drink so much in the first place?"
> "You kids drive me to drink."
> "I can't relax—you kids drive me crazy."

Nonalcoholic parents also teach these children to believe (falsely) that they cause their alcoholic parents to drink. Deutsch (1982) indicates that many children in alcoholic homes hear their nonalcoholic parent instruct them, "Please go with Daddy, it will make him happy," or "You have to be quiet today, Mom seems nervous." Implied in these instructions is the notion that the children have power over their parent's drinking—that they can increase it or decrease it through their actions. Deutsch (1982) believes that these children take this notion of personal power into adulthood. As adults, he believes they continue to feel possessed of power and capable of controlling others. These needs to dominate and control others are thought by some clinicians to lead to dysfunctional adult relationships at home and work. As noted earlier, many such people refer to themselves today as ACOAs. At ACOA self-help meetings, power and control issues are often the focus of group discussion.

ROLE BEHAVIOR

At several points in this chapter, the chemically dependent family has been described as a closed social system. The family tends to isolate itself, its boundaries are rigid, and outside influences are not allowed to penetrate. This kind of closed, rigid system fosters tension. The tension is managed, in part, by each family member's adopting a specific, predictable role. The roles serve to divert attention from the alcoholic/addict, or to reduce the family tension in total.

Family therapists have created a variety of schemes for classifying the types of role behavior in the chemically dependent family. Generally, they have been generated from the clinical experience of therapists, not from empirical studies. Thus, researchers (e.g., Sher, 1997) often question the validity of the classification schemes and the claims made of these typologies. Nevertheless, family role schemes are frequently relied on in clinical settings and the addictions practitioner should have an understanding of these concepts. The following discussion presents one of the common classification schemes. The players in this scheme are (1) the substance-dependent person, (2) the chief enabler, (3) the family hero, (4) the scapegoat, (5) the lost child, and (6) the mascot.

In this scheme, the family is assumed to be a nuclear one, with two parents and four or more children. Also, because one of the parents is assumed to be chemically dependent, the scheme emphasizes the adaptive roles of the children in the family. Furthermore, it should be noted that although some chemically dependent families have members who clearly fall into a specific role, other families have members who exhibit characteristics of more than one role; others have members who shift from role to role as time passes; and in the life of some families certain roles never appear. Thus, the roles are probably too "neat" for most chemically dependent families. However, for sake of discussion, each one is presented in its stereotypical form.

The Chemically Dependent Person

Within a family systems perspective, the chemically dependent member is not diseased but is playing a role, which is to act irresponsibly. This role has a homeostatic function. Typically, it serves to suppress more basic marital conflict, or to divert attention from more threatening family issues.

An important aspect of the chemically dependent role is emotional detachment from the spouse and the children. One consequence of this distancing is the abandonment of parental power. The power is often assumed by the nondependent spouse and an older child (to be described later). The "first love" of the alcoholic or addict becomes the bottle or the drug. Over time, the self-administration of the substance becomes the central activity in this person's life; family life diminishes in importance.

The Chief Enabler

The second role is often referred to as the "chief enabler," or simply the "enabler." Often, numerous enablers exist in the family; however, the chief enabler is usually the nondependent spouse. Enabling is a behavior that inadvertently supports the addiction process by helping an alcoholic or addict avoid the natural consequences of irresponsible behavior. Most addicts have at least one enabler in their lives, and many have three, four, or more to keep them going.

From a family systems perspective, the chief enabler reduces tension in the family (i.e., maintains family balance) by "smoothing things over"— that is, making things right. The enabler often faces a dilemma: If he/she (more often she) does not bail the alcoholic/addict out of a bad, sometimes dangerous situation (e.g., a drunk husband alone at a bar), the substance abuser could do serious harm to self or others. A wife of an alcoholic once told me that she knew she was enabling her husband by picking him up from their snow-covered yard but she had no choice, as otherwise he would have frozen to death.

In many cases, the chief enabler is unaware that the enabling behavior is contributing to the progression of the alcoholism or drug addiction. Enablers believe that they are simply being helpful and acting to hold their families together. Though well intended, their efforts often have destructive long-term consequences for their chemically dependent spouses (Deutsch, 1982).

The Family Hero

The role of the "family hero" is usually adopted by the oldest child. This role is also referred to as the "parental child," the "superstar," and the "goody two shoes" (Deutsch, 1982). This child attempts to do everything right. He/she is the family's high achiever, and as such appears quite ambitious and responsible. Given the family circumstances (i.e., a chemically dependent parent), the child is often admired for excelling under difficult conditions.

The family hero often takes on parental responsibilities that the chemically dependent parent gave up. He/she provides care for younger siblings by cooking for them, getting them ready for school, putting them to bed, doing laundry, and so on. The nondependent spouse (i.e., the chief enabler) usually does not have much time for these chores because his/her time is divided between working and caring for the alcoholic or addicted spouse.

Family heroes frequently do well in academic and athletic pursuits (Deutsch, 1982). They may be class presidents, honor students, starters on the basketball team, or the like. They are achievement oriented and frequently develop well-respected professional careers. Deutsch (1982) suggests that many of them later become "workaholics."

The family hero reduces tension in the family simply by doing everything "right." The hero is the source of pride for the family, inspiring desperately needed hope and giving the family something to feel good about. The hero's accomplishments are distinctions around which the family members can rally and say to themselves, "We're not so bad after all."

The Scapegoat

The "scapegoat" role is often adopted by the second oldest child. The scapegoat can be viewed as the alter ego of the family hero (Deutsch, 1982). This child does very little right and is quite rebellious, perhaps even antisocial. Scapegoats may be involved in fights, theft, or other trouble at school or in the community; they are often labeled "juvenile delinquents." Male scapegoats may be violent, while female scapegoats may express themselves by running away or engaging in promiscuous sexual activity. Scapegoats of both genders most often abuse alcohol and drugs themselves.

A child in the scapegoat role seems to identify with the chemically dependent parent, not only in terms of substance abuse but in other ways as well (attitude toward authority, attitude toward the opposite sex, vocational interests, etc.). The scapegoat typically feels inferior to the family hero; still, the two of them are usually very close emotionally, despite the differences in their behavior. This special bond may continue throughout adulthood.

This child is referred to as the "scapegoat" because he/she is the object of the chemically dependent parent's misdirected frustration and rage. The child may be abused both emotionally and physically by this parent. This is especially true when the chemically dependent parent is the father and the scapegoat his son. In effect, the scapegoat becomes, in common parlance, "his father's son." That is, the son, filled with his father's anger and rage, adopts his father's self-destructive and antisocial tendencies. He models himself after his father despite hating him.

The scapegoat expresses the family's frustration and anger. The child in this role maintains family balance by directing some of the blame from the chemically dependent parent to him/herself. This allows the chemically dependent parent to blame someone else for his/her own drinking and drug use. It also shields the chemically dependent parent from some of the blame and resentment that would have been directed at him/her; this process of diversion allows the addiction to progress further (Deutsch, 1982).

The Lost Child

Even in functional families, the middle children are thought to get less attention than their siblings, and they seem less certain of their contribution to the family. This tendency is exacerbated in chemically dependent families (Deutsch, 1982). The "lost child" may be a middle child but may also be the youngest. The chief characteristic of the lost child is seeking to avoid conflict at all costs. Such children tend to feel powerless and are described as "very quiet," "emotionally disturbed," "depressed," "isolated," "withdrawn," and so on. These children tend to be forgotten, as they are very shy. They are followers, not leaders. They engage in much fantasy. If they stand out in school in any way, it is by virtue of poor attendance (Deutsch, 1982). If asked to do something they fear doing, they may pretend not to have heard the instructions or claim not to understand them (Deutsch, 1982). These behaviors point to a great deal of insecurity.

According to Deutsch (1982), the lost child is probably the most difficult child in a dysfunctional family to help. He/she may not have close friends or other systems outside the family for emotional support. Also, the child's behavior is usually not disruptive in school; hence, teachers and counselors do not identify him/her as needy.

As adults, lost children exhibit a variety of mental health problems. They may complain of anxiety and/or depression and obtain psychotherapy. They have difficulty with developmental transitions because they fear taking risks. Thus, they may put off making decisions about careers or where to live. They may also back out of intimate relationships once someone starts to get too close. According to Deutsch (1982), lost children may or may not abuse alcohol and drugs. If they do, their drug of choice is usually different from that used by their chemically dependent parents.

The lost child helps maintain balance in the family by simply disappearing—that is, by not requiring any attention. In essence, the youngster in this role supports the family equilibrium by causing no new problems and requiring minimal attention.

The Mascot

The last commonly described role is that of the "mascot." This role is also referred to as the "family clown." The youngest child in the family often adopts the role of the mascot. Everyone in the family likes the mascot and is comfortable with having him/her around. The family usually views the mascot as the most fragile and vulnerable; thus, he/she tends to be the object of protection. Deutsch (1982) notes that even the chemically dependent parent treats the mascot with kindness most of the time.

Mascots often act silly and make jokes, even at their own expense. The clownish behavior acts as a defense against feelings of anxiety and inadequacy. They often have a dire need for approval from others. As adults, they are very likable but appear anxious. Deutsch (1982) believes that they may self-medicate with alcohol and/or tranquilizers.

The child in the mascot role helps maintain family homeostasis by bringing laughter and fun into the home. By "clowning around" and making jokes, he/she brightens the family atmosphere, becoming a counterbalance against the tension that is so prevalent and oppressive in dysfunctional families. The mascot may be the one family member about whom no one has a complaint.

FINDINGS FROM THE RESEARCH LITERATURE

Patterson's Parental Family Management Models

For two decades, Patterson (1986, 1996) has written extensively about his research on the development of antisocial behavior in children and adolescents. Patterson has relied on rigorous measurement procedures, including the use of structural equation modeling to test hypotheses. His work does not focus specifically on substance abuse, though his models do encompass the problem. Rather, Patterson provides a framework for understanding how adolescent drug and alcohol abuse emerges as one feature of a general pattern of deviant behavior. The assumption here is that early involvement in substance use and delinquency are somewhat different aspects of a unified pattern of antisocial behavior. This can be considered a reasonable assumption because antisocial personality disorder (ASPD) and substance use disorders often coexist in adults (Ross, Glaser, & Germanson, 1988). Importantly, the parental family management models explain how the family mediates between social conditions (e.g., economic cycles, unemployment, and disorganized communities) and the production of delinquency and crime (Patterson, 1996).

The main hypothesis of this research is that "chronic antisocial behavior is the direct outcome of a breakdown in parental family management" (Patterson, 1996, p. 88). Problem behavior in children and adolescents results from inadequate parenting, particularly a lack of monitoring and poor disciplinary practices. Furthermore, parental antisocial behavior plays an important role. One of Patterson's empirical models indicates that parental stress, as evidenced by single-parent homes, stepfamily arrangements, and multiple family transitions, is not enough to produce boys with an early onset of arrest. The mediating construct is parental antisocial behavior. Under times of stress, parents with antisocial tendencies tend to engage in *irritable discipline.*

Irritable discipline is a feature of a social interaction process that Patterson (1986) describes as *coercion.* The assumption of this model is that the failure of parents to effectively stop a child's relatively innocuous coercive behaviors sets into motion a series of interaction sequences that can be considered aggression training. The provocative idea here is that parent and child train each other to become increasingly aversive (Patterson, 1986). Relatively trivial child behaviors, such as refusing to comply with a simple request, whining, yelling, and so on, provide parents with opportunities to learn "high-amplitude aggressive behaviors" (Patterson, 1986, p. 436). As mentioned previously, parental stress and antisocial tendencies may initiate and exacerbate this coercion process, but other variables are important as well. The confluence of forces includes disorganized or high-risk neighborhoods, poor parenting skills, parental substance abuse, and a difficult temperament of the child.

Transition from simple noncompliance to aggression usually occurs in the older child. The transition appears when the child becomes conditioned by a three-step, escape–avoidant arrangement. This interaction sequence first involves an attack by a parent or other family member, followed by a counterattack from the child, which is followed by the attacker's withdrawal. The attacker may withdraw to reduce the tension of the interaction or to show rejection of the child. In either case, the attacker's withdrawal reinforces or rewards the child's counterattack. Based on observation data collected in homes, Patterson (1982) reports that this sequence may occur hundreds of times a day in some families. About 20% of the coercive behavior of antisocial children falls into the three-step pattern. About one-third of the child's coercive behaviors were provoked by an aversive attack on them, and perhaps most important, about 70% of the time the child's counterattack was successful—meaning the attacker withdrew. As a result of their work with parents of antisocial children, Patterson and colleagues have identified five critical family management skills: (1) discipline, (2) monitoring, (3) family problem solving, (4) parent involvement, and (5) positive reinforcement.

Other Family Influences on Adolescent Alcohol and Drug Use

A large number of studies have examined other family influences on the development of substance abuse. This review highlights some of the important findings from these studies.

It appears that family values are related to teenage substance abuse. Jessor and Jessor (1977) assessed mothers' religiosity, tolerance of deviance, and traditional beliefs. They found that adolescent problem behaviors, including abusive drinking and illegal drug abuse, were less prevalent in families in which the mothers were highly religious, conventional, and traditional. The teens with the greatest prevalence of problem behaviors (e.g., alcohol and drug abuse) had mothers whose ideology deemphasized religion and traditional social values.

Several studies have linked adolescent substance abuse to single-parent families. For example, Burnside, Baer, McLaughlin, and Pokorny (1986) asked a large number of high school students about both their drinking practices and their family structure. The study found that teens in single-parent and stepparent families reported greater alcohol consumption than did those in intact families. Furthermore, the parents in the nonintact families used more alcohol than the parents in the intact families, and the adolescents' alcohol use was positively correlated with that of their parents. The relative influence of nonintact family status versus parental alcohol use in predicting adolescent alcohol consumption was assessed as well; it was determined that nonintact status had an effect on teen drinking that was independent of parental alcohol use.

Family size, sibling spacing, and birth order are family structure variables that have been thought to be linked to the development of alcoholism. However, the findings in this area are equivocal. Barnes (1990), in a review of this literature, concludes that there is little evidence to support the notion that birth order influences alcoholism. The issue of sibling spacing has not been adequately addressed, either. Research findings regarding family size are somewhat clearer; it appears that a disproportionate number of alcoholics come from large families. Zucker (1976) has offered explanations for this relationship: Larger families may exhibit diluted socialization effects, more authoritarian discipline, looser parental controls, or greater sibling rivalries. Any one or a combination of these conditions may explain why a relatively large percentage of alcoholics come from larger families.

Convincing evidence exists that teenage drinking practices are linked with parental drinking behavior (Barnes, 1990). It appears that children and teens learn to drink (or not to drink) through the process of imitation. Young people tend to model their behavior (including drinking) after those whom they observe, especially those with whom they are close. Kandel, Kessler, and Marguiles (1978), for instance, found that parents' use of hard liquor was a moderately good predictor of their adolescents' initiation to the use of hard liquor. In other words, the heavier the parental consumption, the earlier the teens began to use it. Data from a study by Harburg,

Davis, and Caplan (1982) indicate that children tend to imitate their perception of their parents' drinking. Moreover, boys particularly imitate their perception of their fathers' drinking, as do girls with their mothers' drinking. However, when parental alcohol consumption was perceived to be extreme (i.e., unusual), imitation decreased; here, "extreme" meant either abstinence or heavy drinking by parents. This effect is consistent with that found by Barnes, Farrell, and Cairns (1986) in which abstaining parents had not only a high proportion of abstaining children but also a high proportion of heavy-drinking children. It appears that children of abstaining parents lack adult role models for sensible drinking. Thus, if they do initiate alcohol use, they have a tendency to drink in a binge-like manner. The reason why this heavy-drinking subgroup initiates use in the first place (when another subgroup of children of abstaining parents abstain) is unclear.

During the teenage years, it can be expected that the peer group will have more influence on adolescent behavior as the family (parental) influence diminishes somewhat. Numerous studies have examined the interaction between peer influences and family influences as they relate to teen drinking. For example, Barnes and Windle (1987) have collected data showing that adolescents who value peer opinions, as opposed to parental opinions, are at heightened risk for alcohol and drug abuse and for other problem behaviors. Kandel and Andrews (1987) found that parental closeness discouraged teen drug use and promoted the choice of non-drug-using friends. This finding is consistent with those of other studies, which have found that adolescents who are close to their parents are less likely to associate with deviant peers (Barnes, 1990). Similarly, Dishion and Loeber (1985) found that lack of parental monitoring had an indirect effect on teen substance abuse by increasing the probability that a teen would "hang out" with deviant peers.

According to Barnes (1990), one of the most neglected areas of research on the development of adolescent substance abuse is that of sibling influence. Though relatively few studies have been done, "siblings may constitute a potentially powerful combination of peer and family socialization agent" (Barnes, 1990, p. 151). In a sample of 9th- and 10th-grade students, Brook, Whiteman, Gordon, and Brenden (1983) investigated older brothers' influence on younger siblings' drug use. It was found that having an older brother who used marijuana had a significant effect on a younger sibling's substance use, even after nonfamily influence was controlled for. Needle et al. (1986) conducted a study in which information was obtained independently from both younger and older siblings. They found that the younger siblings' frequency of drug use was predicted by older siblings' and peers' substance use (each remained significant after the other variable was controlled for). In addition, older siblings, as well as peers, were sources of information about drugs and companions in the use of drugs with their younger siblings. Further research is needed in this area. Though this is not well substantiated at this point, it is not unreasonable to speculate that older siblings in the family may be a potent factor in determining whether younger siblings initiate the use of alcohol and drugs.

Day-to-Day Marital Interactions in Alcoholic Families

For 3 months, with eight couples, Dunn, Jacob, Hummon, and Seilhammer (1987) tracked the drinking behavior of alcoholic husbands and both spouse's daily marital satisfaction ratings and psychiatric symptoms. The husbands were of two subtypes: "in-home" drinkers and "out-of-home" drinkers. The findings of the study were distinct for these two groups.

Among the in-home drinkers, the husbands' alcohol consumption was interpreted to prompt positive marital ratings in most couples and decrease negative symptomatology in wives. The researchers concluded that this was particularly likely to occur when (1) the alcoholic's behavior is predictable and involves steady drinking (not binge drinking), (2) family stress is reduced during drinking times, and (3) the drinking has been accepted and incorporated into family life (Dunn et al., 1987).

In contrast, in the out-of-home drinkers, husbands' alcohol consumption was interpreted to have a negative impact on marital ratings and wives' psychiatric symptomatology. In the out-of-home group, there tended to be more binge drinking. This could not be readily anticipated by wives and thus was probably more disruptive to family life. Also, alcoholic husbands who mostly drink away from home may have more psychopathology (Dunn et al., 1987).

In another study of marital interaction, Haber and Jacob (1997), during three laboratory sessions, observed four groups of couples: (1) alcoholic male ($n = 50$), (2) alcoholic female ($n = 15$), (3) male and female alcoholic ($n = 16$), and (4) neither partner alcoholic ($n = 50$). During one of the interview sessions, alcohol was made available to the couples. Thus, there was a "drink"–"no drink" condition. The researchers found that compared to nonalcoholic couples, all alcoholic couple groups demonstrated greater negativity and lower positivity and congeniality toward one another. Furthermore, female alcoholic couples showed high negativity toward one another in the "no drink" situation, which was erased by the drink session. Couples with two alcoholic partners also demonstrated high negativity in the "no-drink" situation, but this effect was exacerbated by the drink session. These findings suggest that alcohol does have adaptive value for marital interaction, and that there may be unique features to these interactions when the alcoholic is female.

Children of Alcoholics: A Major Research Focus

The research literature on children of alcoholics (COAs) has grown enormously during the past 15 years. Four major findings can be gleaned from this work. Each is reviewed below.

First, there is a great deal of heterogeneity in families in which alcoholism is present (Chassin, Rogosch, & Barrera, 1991; Jacob & Leonard, 1986; Seilhammer & Jacob, 1990; Zucker, Ellis, Bingham, & Fitzgerald, 1996). Specifically, it appears that not all alcoholic families are equally problematic. Family subtypes exist and some are much more likely to produce adjustment problems and psychopathology in children than others.

Contrary to popular notions, the alcoholic father–child relationship is not always perceived to be unsatisfactory by sons and daughters. Seilhamer, Jacob, and Dunn (1993) found that when children of alcoholic fathers perceive their father as either more pleasant or unchanged when drinking, their daily satisfaction ratings of their relationship with him are positive. However, when children perceive that their father's drinking makes him act strange, become aggressive, spend money that the family needs, or generally causes chaos, then their perceptions of their relationship with him are negative.

Ellis, Zucker, and Fitzgerald (1997) have proposed a probabilistic–developmental model that identifies the biological/genetic, peer, community, and family risk factors that determine COA adjustment (see Table 8.1). The first risk factor is the child's exposure to parental drinking models. Zucker, Kincaid, Fitzgerald, and Bingham (1995) found that COAs as young as 3-5 years of age are more familiar with a wider range of alcoholic beverages and are better able to distinguish among them by smell than non-COAs. Furthermore, COAs may be likely to later imitate their parent's drinking if they admire that person. Modeling may not occur when the alcoholic parent is perceived by the child to be severely impaired by drinking or when the parent exhibits severe psychopathology, including aggression.

A second risk factor is the development of alcohol expectancies that may serve as the mediators between observations of parental drinking and decisions about one's own drinking (Reese et al., 1994). Alcohol expectancies appear to develop before the child has consumed any alcohol. COAs are inclined to develop positive expectations about drinking; that is, they tend to attribute positive affective changes to drinking. Such expectations may be acquired by observing how drinking transforms their parent(s). COAs' alcohol expectancies may be shaped by the family's cultural heritage as well.

Ellis et al. (1997) also have identified a number of family risk factors that influence COAs' overall psychosocial development rather than just

TABLE 8.1. Family Risk Factors Affecting Alcohol Attitudes and Psychopathology among COAs Compared to Non-COAs

Risk factor	Research finding
Modeling of drinking behavior	COAs are more familiar with a wider range of alcoholic beverages at a younger age and develop alcohol-use schemas earlier than do non-COAs.
Alcohol expectancies	COAs are more likely than non-COAs to expect that alcohol will make them feel good.
Ethnicity and drinking practices	COAs from certain ethnic groups are more likely to hold positive alcohol expectancies.
Parent psychopathology	Subgroups of COAs are raised in families where alcoholic parents have a coexisting psychiatric disorder.
Socioeconomic status	COAs are more likely than non-COAs to come from homes where there is financial stress.
Family dysfunction	Alcoholic families have less closeness or cohesion in relationships, more conflict, and poor problem-solving skills than do nonalcoholic families. COAs are more likely than non-COAs to come from broken homes.
Family aggression/ violence	COAs are more likely than non-COAs to be victims of physical abuse and to witness family violence.
Parental cognitive impairment	COAs are more likely than non-COAs to be raised by parents with poor cognitive abilities in environments which lack stimulation.

Note. Adapted from Ellis, Zucker, and Fitzgerald (1997).

drinking attitudes and behavior. When there is significant psychopathology coexisting with parental alcoholism, particularly ASPD and/or depression, COAs are at much greater risk for adjustment problems. As can be seen in Table 8.1. the other family risk factors associated with poor COA adjustment are low socioeconomic status, low family cohesion/high conflict, aggression and violence, and low intellectual capacity of parents.

In a longitudinal study, Zucker et al. (1996) found that the family risk factors (identified in Table 8.1) tend to aggregate in a nonrandom manner. In other words, they are nested within subtypes of alcoholic families. The subtyping is based on the presence or absence of ASPD in the father. Hence, Zucker et al. (1996) classified the familes they are tracking as (1) antisocial alcoholic families, (2) nonantisocial alcoholic families, or (3) control families (matched nonalcoholic families recruited from the same communities). Their findings indicate that antisocial alcoholic families represent a high-risk environment for COAs, ages 3–8. On all the assessed child risk indicators, children in the antisocial alcoholic families exhibited more problem behavior than did children in the nonantisocial alcoholic families and the control families. Children in the nonantisocial alcoholic families were similar to those in the nonalcoholic families (Ellis et al., 1997). Table 8.2 summarizes the child risk factors that cluster in antisocial alcoholic families.

A second major finding of COA research is that though COAs, as a group, do experience elevated levels of depression and anxiety and are more likely than non-COAs to have some type of conduct disorder, many of these children do not experience significant mental health or behavioral problems (Sher, 1997). A number of studies have found that the observed differences between COAs and non-COAs on cognitive, emotional, and behavioral measures are not great (e.g., Bennett, Wolin, & Reiss, 1988). Often scores for both groups fall in the normal range. The relatively small group differences may reflect the significant variability in the environments of the alcoholic families in which these children are raised.

The third major finding from COA research is that although ACOAs are at elevated risk for substance use disorders and ASPD, the majority show no evidence of significant mental health problems (Ellis et al., 1997; Searles & Windle, 1990; Sher, 1997). ACOAs are more likely than adult non-COAs to have an alcohol or other drug diagnosis, including tobacco dependence. However, this represents a minority of ACOAs. ASPD is more common in ACOAs than adult non-COAs, but this may be attributed to being offspring of antisocial alcoholics rather than a consequence of being raised in alcoholic families (Sher, 1991). There is little evidence that ACOAs are at high risk for other personality disorders other than ASPD. The literature on depression and anxiety disorders in ACOAs is equivocal and no firm conclusions can be drawn at this time (Sher, 1997). One study found that ACOAs, as a group, score somewhat higher on measures of

---

TABLE 8.2. Child Risk Factors That Tend to Aggregate in Antisocial Alcoholic Families

1. One parent has an alcohol or other drug use disorder *and* ASPD.
2. Both parents have an alcohol or other drug use disorder and/or other psychopathology (ASPD or depression).
3. Parental alcohol use is severe and/or problematic.
4. Dense family history of alcoholism; children are exposed to multiple extended family members with alcohol problems and have higher genetic risk for the disorder.
5. Parental intellect is relatively low.
6. There is a relatively high rate of aggression toward the children, including aggressive disciplinary practices.
7. Parents are verbally abusive with one another; there is violence between the parents.
8. Family socioeconomic status is relatively low.

Note. Adapted from Ellis, Zucker, and Fitzgerald (1997).

state and trait anxiety than do non-COAs, but most often the former group was in or near the normal range on these variables (Maynard, 1997). Hence, it is important that mental health professionals not make assumptions about clients' psychological health solely on the basis of being raised in an alcoholic family.

The final conclusion to be drawn from the COA research is that the portrayals of ACOAs and codependency in many clinical training texts are inconsistent with empirical studies (e.g., S. A. Brown, 1995; Doweiko, 1993; Fields, 1995; Stanton & Heath, 1995). Some clinical texts have attempted to balance descriptions of these constructs with cautions about their lack of empirical support (e.g., Doweiko, 1993). However, this is often not the case; one unfortunate outcome could be inaccurate stereotyping of COA clients. Thus, practitioners must be judicious in their application of the ACOA and codependency concepts.

The research literature indicates that it is difficult to make valid generalizations about COAs (Sher, 1997). A major reason for this is that many alcoholic parents have coexisting psychiatric disorders such as ASPD, major depression, phobia, and so on. Hence, alcoholics and the families they create are not homogenous. This is highlighted by the work of Zucker and colleagues (described earlier). As Sher (1997) pointed out:

> Thus, some COAs also are children of depressives, children of agoraphobics, children of people with antisocial personality disorder, and so forth. Given the many forms of psychopathology that are possible in parents of COAs, difficulties arise in attributing any apparent COA characteristic specifically to parental alcoholism. (p. 248)

Although the ACOA/codependency movement has maintained that ACOAs suffer from *unique* emotional patterns and problems, research to date has not supported this contention (Gotham & Sher, 1996; Seefeldt & Lyon, 1992). Alterman, Searles, and Hall (1989) found no differences between children of alcoholic fathers and control subjects on a variety of personality variables, mental health problems, and alcohol-related measures. Hence, researchers warned against stereotyping ACOAs as necessarily having a special set of characteristics or problems. Sher (1997) suggests that when COAs do report elevated levels of anxiety and depression, it may be the result of having been raised in a *disruptive home* rather than being exposed to an alcoholic parent.

Seefeldt and Lyon (1992) reached an interesting conclusion about the ACOA/codependency phenomenon. They examined three groups: non-ACOAs ($n = 93$), ACOAs not in treatment ($n = 36$), and ACOAs in treatment ($n = 18$). Subjects were assessed on 11 different personality variables that Woititz (1983) described as essential features of ACOAs. Seefeldt and

Lyon (1992) found no significant differences among the three groups on any of the variables. In fact, the ability of the 11 variables to correctly classify subjects into the three groups (by discriminant analysis) was only slightly better than random assignment.

Some researchers then have attributed the popularity of the ACOA/ codependency movement to a tendency known as the "Barnum effect" (Goodman, 1987; Seefeldt & Lyon, 1992). Named after the huckster P. T. Barnum, this is "the tendency to interpret a description that applies to everyone as being particularly valid to one's self" (Seefeldt & Lyon, 1992, p. 588). It is argued that many descriptions of ACOAs and codependents are similiar to those used by fortune tellers and astrologers. At first they seem specific, but in reality they are actually quite vague and applicable to almost all persons.

Child Maltreatment and Violence in the Home

Though popular lore has linked substance abuse, particularly alcohol abuse, with child maltreatment and domestic violence for hundreds of years, it has only been since the mid-1980s that the problem has begun to receive substantial attention in the research literature (Lee & Weinstein, 1997). Recent studies provide credibility to the anecdotes.

For example, Egami, Ford, Greenfield, and Crum (1996) analyzed self-report data from 9,841 respondents in three communities. About 1.5% of the sample admitted they had *abused* children and an additional 1.4% acknowledged *neglect* of a child. (We might suspect that these relatively low rates reflect an underreporting bias.) Multivariate analysis showed that lifetime history of an alcohol disorder was significantly associated with both child abuse and neglect (even after controlling for other factors). Thus, people with a past history of alcohol abuse and/or alcoholism appear to be at risk for abusing or neglecting children. Unfortunately, the study design could not directly link intoxication or other alcohol-related behavior to these incidents.

In a review of the impact of alcohol and drug abuse on the child welfare system, Young, Gardner, and Dennis (1998) concluded that 40–80% of parents with children in the child welfare system have alcohol or drug problems that interfere with caretaking. One government report has noted that in Los Angeles, New York City, and Philadelphia County, parental substance abuse was a factor for 78% of the children placed in foster care (U.S. General Accounting Office, 1994). A separate investigation found that 55% of families reported to child protective services had one or two caretakers who had a substance abuse problem (Wolock & Magura, 1996). It is important to note that the relationships identified here are correlational and not necessarily causal (NIAAA, 1994). In some cases, alcohol and drug use may facilitate child maltreatment among caretakers who had a prior proclivity for such behavior; in other cases, there may be mechanisms that mediate between substance use and maltreatment of a child. Regardless, Young et al. (1998) assert that these problems have not been adequately addressed because there are a lack of linkages between the child welfare system (i.e., child protective services, juvenile justice, delinquency and violence prevention, family counseling) and substance abuse treatment services.

Rivara et al. (1997) conducted a case-control study of the factors associated with 388 homicides and 438 suicides in three large metropolitan areas in the United States. Structured interviews of persons close to the decedents were used to collect information about the alcohol and drug use of the subject. The findings indicated that both homicide and suicide risks were associated with either alcohol or illegal drug abuse. Violent death, in particular, was linked to *chronic* alcohol abuse. Importantly, the researchers also found that nondrinkers and non-drug users living with substance abusers were at increased risk for homicide. This was particularly the case for non-drug-using persons residing in a home with a drug abuser. Rivara et al. (1997) conclude that it is not only the alcohol or drug abuser who is at risk for homicide but others in the home as well.

SUMMARY

It is imperative that practitioners be familiar with family systems concepts. As the primary social unit, the family exerts a powerful influence over an individual's drinking or drug use. The systems emphasis on reciprocal causality is unique among theories of addictive behavior. It proposes that substance abuse is functional in a certain sense; that it is a manifestation of deeper conflict; and that it helps the individual to minimize, distract from, or cope with interpersonal problems.

A word of caution about family systems concepts is also in order. Put simply, there is not much empirical support for the efficacy of the systems approach as a treatment for alcoholism and other addictions (Alexander & Barton, 1995; Collins, 1990). Relatively few well-designed studies have tested the effectiveness of family systems therapy. It has been shown to be as effective as individual treatment but less effective than a behavioral treatment (McCrady, Moreau, Paolino, & Longabaugh, 1982; McCrady, Paolino, Longabaugh, & Rossi, 1979). O'Farrell, Cutter, and Floyd (1985) reported that a brief family systems intervention is just as effective as more prolonged and intensive treatment. Collins (1990) concluded a review of this literature by stating that "while descriptions of systems approaches to treating alcoholic families abound, the body of methodologically sound empirical research on systems approaches is limited" (p. 296). Considering the reputation of family systems therapy in the substance abuse treatment field, the discrepancy between its prominence and its empirically established validity is conspicuous. Though more research is needed before firm conclusions can be reached, it appears that *behavioral approaches* to marital and family therapy may be effective treatments for substance use disorders (Noel & McGrady, 1993).

REVIEW QUESTIONS

1. What are the sources of literature on addiction and the family?

2. What are "boundaries," "subsystems," "hierarchies," "family rules," and "homeostasis"?

3. What is meant by "reciprocal causality"?

4. How does a person's family of origin affect the person's mate selection and manner of childrearing?

5. How does a teen's fear of separation contribute to his/her abusing drugs?

6. What are "triads"? How do they spur substance abuse?

7. What is the "dance"?

8. What does Bowen mean by "differentiation of self"? What are characteristics of poorly differentiated persons and highly differentiated persons?

9. What does Bowen mean by "triangles"?

10. How does Bowen describe the development of the emotional system in the nuclear family?

11. What does Bowen mean by "family projection process"?

12. What does Bowen mean by "emotional cutoff"?

13. What is "codependency"? What are its chief characteristics?

14. What rewards are gained in a codependent relationship?

15. What three emotional conditions are prevalent in the lives of children living with alcoholic parents?

16. What are the six roles that sometimes develop in chemically dependent families? How does each reduce family tension?

17. What are the components of Patterson's parental family management models?

18. What family factors are linked to adolescent substance abuse?

19. How does "in-home" versus "out-of-home" drinking affect marital satisfaction? How are the marital interactions of alcoholic couples different from those of nonalcoholic couples?

20. What are the major findings from the COA research?

21. What are the alcohol-specific risk factors and family risk factors that influence COA adjustment?

22. Does research support the links between substance use and child abuse and domestic violence?

CHAPTER 9

Social and Cultural Foundations

This chapter examines the "macroenvironment" of substance use and abuse (Connors & Tarbox, 1985). Macroenvironmental factors include trends in drug use over time; the role of government regulation, laws, and tax policy (on alcoholic beverages); attempts by professions to make claims for controlling the problem of substance abuse; drug subcultures and crime; and, in general, the social values, beliefs, and norms that influence drug use. These concepts are the social and cultural foundations of addictive behavior.

THE INFLUENCE OF CULTURE ON DIAGNOSTIC DETERMINATIONS

From a sociological perspective, the problems of excessive drinking and drug abuse have become "medicalized" (Schwartz & Kart, 1978); that is, because of its vested interests, the medical and mental health communities have redefined the problem as one of "illness" or "disease." According to sociologists, this labeling process functions as a means of social control (Schwartz & Kart, 1978). It gives credibility to physicians' and mental health professionals' efforts to control, manage, and supervise the care given to persons with substance abuse problems. It makes legitimate such potentially lucrative endeavors as hospital admissions, insurance company billings, expansion of the client pool, consulting fees, and so forth. It also serves to restrict the number and type of practitioners who are permitted to assist person with these problems. In fact, the acceptance of the term "treatment" in the substance abuse field reflects the dominant influence of medicine and the medical model.

The social process of labeling also functions to restrict alcohol consumption in the community. It defines, for the average citizen, appropriate and inappropriate drinking practices. For example, in our culture, conduct norms typically discourage obvious drunkenness, drinking before noon, drinking at work, impaired driving, and binge drinking. It is interesting to note that many of these popular, "man-on-the-street" notions of alcoholism have found their way into widely used "clinical" assessment instruments, such as the Michigan Alcoholism Screening Test (MAST).

A "diagnosis" is the formal label of problem behaviors applied by medicine and the mental health professions. To justify this labeling process, the helping professions have created elaborate sets of criteria based mostly on clinical experience. Of course, the most prominent example in the mental health arena is the text revision of the fourth edition of the *Diagnostic and Statistical Manual of Mental Disorders* (DSM-IV-TR; American Psychiatric Association, 2000). Labeling theorists have described these professional practices as the *medicalization of deviant behavior* (Conrad, 1992; Conrad & Schneider, 1992). From a sociological perspective, it is an attempt by modern medicine to redefine deviance from "badness" to "sickness." Thus, the control of deviance shifts from the criminal justice system to medicine and the substance abuse treatment system.

In the sociological perspective, clinical diagnostic criteria for substance dependence are derived largely from cultural norms. Thus, those drinking and drug use practices that are considered "alcoholic" or "addictive" are those that deviate from socially acceptable standards. Alcoholism and other drug addictions are considered social deviance rather than a medical problem. Sociologically, treatment is an effort to force the alcoholic to conform to socially "correct" standards of conduct.

The cultural foundations of alcoholism diagnoses have been recognized by Vaillant (1990, 1995), a proponent of the disease conception. Vaillant (1990) has stated: "Normal drinking merges imperceptibly with pathological drinking. Culture and idiosyncratic viewpoints will always determine where the line is drawn" (p. 5). The sociocultural origins of diagnoses force us to consider certain possibilities. First, a diagnosis, as applied to a particular client, may not be very different from a personal opinion: It may be based not so much on scientific evidence as on the values and beliefs of the addictions practitioner. The practitioner's own history, relative to his/her use of alcohol and drugs, clearly influences the opinion.

It is also possible that drinking that is considered "alcoholic" in one period of time or place may not be viewed similarly in another temporal or geographic context. Heath (1988) noted that 150 years ago, Americans consumed three times more alcohol (per capita) than they consume today. Clearly, the notion of what an alcoholic was then would have differed substantially from our conception today.

These cultural factors also should sensitize substance abuse counselors as to the consequences, both positive and negative, of applying the diagnosis (i.e., label) of alcoholism or drug addiction to a particular client. In the best of cases, the diagnosis will motivate the client to adopt abstinence. However, a positive diagnosis also could lead to overly intrusive treatment, social stigma, estrangement from family members, loss of employment, feelings of worthlessness and humiliation, or even exacerbation of existing drinking problems. Obviously, the addiction diagnosis should be made with caution. One can legitimately question the value of making a positive diagnosis (even when one is clearly appropriate) if there is reason to believe that it will have an adverse effect on a client.

SOCIOLOGICAL FUNCTIONS OF SUBSTANCE ABUSE

From a sociocultural vantage point, abuse of alcohol and drugs can be described as having four broad functions. One is the facilitation of social interaction. That is, the use of alcohol (and often illegal drugs as well) enhances social bonds. It makes communication involving self-disclosure easier. Interpersonal trust is strengthened, whereas barriers or guards are diminished. In addition, the intoxicated state and the attending rituals and jargon allow users the opportunity of a shared experience.

A second function is to provide a release from normal social obligations. Alcohol and drug abuse have been characterized as "time-out" periods (Heath, 1988). The purpose of intoxication is to permit people to withdraw from responsibilities that society normally expects teenagers and adults to carry out. In this view, substance abuse is an effort to escape temporarily from the roles thrust upon individuals (parent, spouse, employee, student, etc.) Intoxication allows for a temporary respite from the stresses and strains inherent in these roles.

A third function of alcohol and drug abuse is to promote cohesion and solidarity among the members of a social or ethnic group. The use or nonuse of a drug can be viewed as a means of group identification. It also establishes group boundaries. That is, substance abuse serves as a social boundary marker, defining who "we" are and who "they" are.

A fourth function of substance abuse, from a sociocultural perspective, is the repudiation of middle-class or "establishment" values. A substance abuse subculture consists of abusers of a particular drug that all hold similar antiestablishment values. In essence, members of drug subcultures "thumb their nose" at conventional mores and norms, particularly those related to morality and economic productivity. Lifestyles are characterized by hedonistic pursuits, spontaneity, and freedom from family responsibilities. This is a value structure at odds with that of working- or middle-class America.

SOCIAL FACILITATION

Some illicit drug use (e.g., LSD) is associated with motivations unrelated to increased sociability. Alcohol, in contrast to the illegal substances, has a distinctive social function. Because its consumption is legal, alcohol is more closely associated with good times, parties, and fun with others.

Distinctive Social Function of Alcohol

The use of alcohol to facilitate social pleasure and interactions with others has been reported for thousands of years among most of the cultures of the world. For example, the Hammurabi Code, the earliest known legal code (promulgated circa 1758 B.C. in Babylon), contains laws governing the operation and management of drinking establishments (McKim, 1986). At another time, the Greek philosopher Plato expressed concern about the drinking of his countrymen, so he established rules for conduct at "symposia," which in reality were drinking parties. He directed that at each symposium a "master of the feast" must be present. This person was to be completely sober. His responsibilities included deciding how much water should be added to the wine and when to bring on the dancing girls (McKim, 1986). Plato observed:

> When a man drinks wine he begins to feel better pleased with himself and the more he drinks the more he is filled full of brave hopes, and conceit of his powers, and at last the string of his tongue is loosened, and fancying himself wise, he is brimming over with lawlessness and has no more fear or respect and is ready to do or say anything. (Jowett, 1931, p. 28)

"Drinking" has been thoroughly integrated into mainstream U.S. culture today. Alcoholic drinks have come to be known simply as a "drink." If a person invites a neighbor "to come over for a drink," everyone usually recognizes that alcohol is being offered. Alcohol consumption is expected behavior at various social, family, and business gatherings, both formal and informal. Though individuals are not usually directly pressured to take a drink in such gatherings, a subtle pressure to do so often exists. A blunt refusal often invites puzzlement, covert speculation, or even suspicion as to one's motives.

Frequently, refusing to drink is interpreted as passing on an opportunity to meet and talk in an informal way. This is particularly true in busi-

ness or other work settings characterized by formal or professional relationships. In such settings, people often desire to escape from the restrictive
confines of stiff or rigid professional roles. Drinking together is seen as the
way to "loosen up."

The Social Context of Adolescent Drinking

Research conducted by Kenneth Beck and Thombs confirms that convivial
drinking practices are well established in adolescence. They have developed
a social context model to explain adolescent alcohol use. Derived from
factor-analytic studies, this model contends that the adolescent's motivation
to drink arises not just from intrapersonal characteristics, such as expectancies or sensation seeking traits, but from situational and temporal aspects
of the immediate social environment as well (Thombs & Beck, 1994). Findings suggest that these three sources of drinking motivation (psychological,
situational, and temporal) tend to cluster in unique ways to form distin-
guishable patterns of *social context*. Furthermore, this body of research has
shown that in young people, social context measures are superior to both
alcohol expectancies (Thombs, Beck, & Pleace, 1993) and the sensation-
seeking trait (Thombs, Beck, Mahoney, Bromley, & Bezon, 1994) in
explaining drinking behaviors.

Results from these factor-analytic studies show that each social context consists of psychological, situational, and temporal features (Beck,
Thombs, & Summons, 1993; Thombs & Beck, 1994). Importantly, the
same set of factors emerged from samples of youth residing in different geographic regions. The five identified contexts of adolescent drinking are (1)
social facilitation, (2) stress control, (3) school defiance, (4) peer acceptance, (5) and parental control. Among these five factors, social facilitation
is the contextual pattern that accounts for most of variance in alcohol consumption (Thombs & Beck, 1994; Thombs et al., 1994). This pattern
involves drinking in a convivial setting with friends, away from adults, on
weekends, at parties, and at friends' homes when the parents are away.
Stress control (done alone for self-medication) and school defiance (a rebellious pattern) are the contextual patterns of drinking that best discriminate
between problem and nonproblem drinkers. Peer acceptance is a pattern of
drinking done to conform to group expectations. Interestingly, drinking in
this context (as well as that of parental control) tends to be linked with the
maintenance of lighter and nonproblematic drinking patterns. This finding
raises questions about the emphasis placed on peer resistance skill training
currently in prevention programming. It may be an erroneous assumption
to conclude that teenagers abuse alcohol because they "cave in" to peer
pressure (May, 1993). To the contrary, most adolescents appear to maintain
drinking habits because it enhances their social interaction; in problematic

patterns, drinking in contexts of self-medication and rebellion tend to be more pronounced.

"TIME OUT" FROM SOCIAL OBLIGATIONS

The Basic Hypothesis

The time-out hypothesis applies to both alcohol and drug abuse. It maintains that the abuse of intoxicants serves to release individuals temporarily from their ordinary social obligations. By becoming intoxicated, they are excused from their obligations as parents, spouses, students, employees, and so forth. MacAndrew and Edgerton (1969) came upon this notion by observing that many cultures exhibit a certain flexibility in norms that allows for suspension of certain role obligations during times of drunkenness. They were careful to point out that the option of "time out" does not suspend all the rules. In all cultures, certain behavior, even while intoxicated, is considered inexcusable; thus, intoxicated persons are viewed as less responsible rather than as totally unresponsible (Heath, 1988). According to MacAndrew and Edgerton (1969), "the option of drunken time-out affords people the opportunity to 'get it out of their systems' with a minimum of adverse consequences" (p. 169). Heath (1988) notes that the concept is more of a descriptive tool than an analytic one. However, he adds that it may be useful as an early sign of alcoholism. Young people who get intoxicated to avoid, or escape from, social role expectations may be susceptible to developing more serious drinking problems.

Achievement Anxiety Theory

The time-out hypothesis essentially describes "escapist drinking"—that is, drinking to escape role obligations of any sort. Misra (1980) has outlined a model that describes substance abuse as an effort to escape a specific class of role obligations. As Misra (1980) sees it, the substance abuser is attempting to evade the pressures placed on him/her to achieve and produce income. Blame is not placed on the individual who abuses drugs but, rather, on U.S. culture and its obsession with materialism, financial success, and personal achievement.

Achievement anxiety theory maintains that drug abuse is a response to a "fear of failure" (Misra, 1980). It allows the abuser to withdraw from the pressures placed on the individual to achieve. At the same time, substance abuse induces and maintains a sense of apathy toward standards of excellence that U.S. culture defines as important. According to Misra (1980), one of the chief characteristics of technologically advanced countries such as the United States is anxiety about achievement. Obtaining or reaching socially prescribed goals can become a compulsion in itself (i.e., "work-aholism"). Many Americans have a dire need to "be somebody." Such competitive conditions cause people to feel anxious, fearful, inadequate, and self-doubting. As a result of these modern pressures, many Americans, in Misra's view, are likely to rely on alcohol and drugs as a way to cope.

According to achievement anxiety theory, drugs are initially used to seek relief from the pressures of achievement and productivity (Misra, 1980). In effect, they provide a quick "chemical vacation" from the stresses of contemporary life. This conceptualization is quite similar to that of "time out." However, Misra (1980) further develops the concept by noting that continued abuse of drugs tends to reduce the difference between "work life" and leisure-time activities. In essence, the chemical vacations gradually change from being infrequent, temporary respites to full-time pursuits (i.e., addiction).

In addiction, the primary goal becomes freedom from productivity. Misra (1980) applied the label "antiachievement." In this state, relief from achievement anxiety is no longer the goal. Instead, the goal is to maintain a sense of apathy or even hostility toward recognized and socially prescribed standards of excellence. This is the work ethic in reverse. According to Misra (1980):

> Drug abuse is, in a sense, a silent protest against the achieving society. It protects us from a sense of failure: "I may not be achieving what my neighbors and colleagues are, but I do attain a unique feeling of relaxed carelessness." Addictions form the nucleus of a subculture of people who all have the same feeling of nonachievement, and friendships evolve around this theme as efforts are made to create and maintain fellowship among the addicts. (p. 368)

In achievement anxiety theory, leisure, as pursued in technologically advanced countries, has a special relationship. Misra (1980) noted that Americans have to *plan* to relax. This plan is typified by arranging well in advance, elaborate, action-packed vacations. Each day is planned out, including hectic travel itineraries. This situation is exacerbated by the fact that U.S. holidays are relatively short in duration and rigidly defined.

Misra (1980) was critical of this approach to leisure. Doing "something" rather than "nothing" has become the hallmark of relaxation in the United States. As Americans creatively jam their leisure time with activity, they become as anxious about their vacations as they are about work. According to Misra (1980), people often come to believe that relaxation must be achieved, here and now. This sense of immediacy for relaxation encourages the adoption of time-saving techniques. Of course, substance abuse fills this perceived need. Alcohol or drug abuse becomes a quick, easy procedure for "getting away from it all" (Misra, 1980).

PROMOTING GROUP SOLIDARITY/
ESTABLISHING SOCIAL BOUNDARIES

For hundreds of years, the use of alcohol and drugs has been an important feature of identification with one's ethnic or racial group. With the mainstreaming of various sociodemographic groups into U.S. culture, drinking and drug use practices have served to promote solidarity and cohesion within groups (Heath, 1988). The use of substances also demarcates the boundaries between ethnic and racial groups. It is one source of identity. It solidifies a person's social identity and helps the person define him/herself in reference to others. The use of alcohol or drugs also shapes the images that individuals want or expect others to have of them (Heath, 1988).

Alcohol as a Boundary Marker

Anthropologists have identified numerous examples of how drinking has functioned to separate social groups and to promote cohesion within themselves. The American temperance movement (1827–1919) is one such example. During the 19th century, temperance groups were widespread in the United States. Initially, temperance groups sought to reduce the consumption of hard liquor and to promote drinking at home, as opposed to saloon drinking. This emphasis on temperance gradually gave way to one demanding abstinence. As could be expected, this led to quarrelsome disputes between "wets" and "drys," and eventually to Prohibition (1919–1933). However, the dispute actually represented deeper ethnic and social class conflict. According to Ray and Ksir (1999):

> Prohibition was not just a matter of "wets" versus "drys," or a matter of political conviction or health concerns. Intricately interwoven with these factors was a middle-class, rural, Protestant, evangelical concern that the good and true life was being undermined by ethnic groups with a different religion and different standard of living and morality. One way to strike back at these groups was through Prohibition. (p. 154)

For those involved in the temperance movement, abstaining (vs. drinking) was a social boundary marker. It served to promote a self-righteous pride within movement workers and was taken as proof that they were morally superior to those who did drink.

For the temperance movement, abstinence was the source of group identification. In other social/ethnic groups, drunkenness was and is the social boundary marker. Heath (1988), in a description of drunkenness among Native Americans, notes that "some Indians embrace the stereotype and use it as a way of asserting their ethnicity, differentiating themselves from others, and offending sensibilities of those whites who decry such behavior" (p. 269). Lurie (1971) has suggested that alcohol abuse by Native Americans is one of the last ways that they can strike back or rebel against white America. He referred to their drinking as "the world's oldest on-going protest demonstration" (p. 311).

Situated between the extreme conditions of abstinence and drunkenness are a variety of culturally distinct drinking practices. Again, these practices serve to facilitate group identification and boundary marking. One widely recognized example, as mentioned earlier, is the Jewish tradition of moderation (Heath, 1988). Alcohol plays a significant role in Jewish family rituals (Lawson & Lawson, 1998); however, excessive consumption, particularly drunkenness, is viewed as inexcusable behavior. Within the Jewish culture, conduct norms allow for frequent but sensible use. According to Glassner and Berg (1980), these beliefs and conduct norms "protect" Jews from developing problems with alcohol. The Yiddish expression "Schikker ist ein Goy," translates to "drunkenness is a vice of Gentiles" (Glassner & Berg, 1980). The Jewish tradition of moderation and sobriety reflects basic values emphasizing rationality and self-control (Keller, 1970). Thus, Jews perceive drunkenness as being irrational and "out of control."

It is generally accepted that Irish Catholics have relatively high rates of alcoholism (Lawson & Lawson, 1998). For example, Vaillant (1983) found that Irish subjects in his sample were more likely to develop alcohol problems than those of other ethnic backgrounds; in fact, they were seven times more likely to be alcoholic than those of Mediterranean descent. In the same study, Irish subjects were found to be more likely to abstain in an effort to manage a drinking problem. Vaillant (1983) observed: "It is consistent with Irish culture to see the use of alcohol in terms of black and white, good or evil, drunkenness or complete abstinence, while in Italian culture it is the distinction between moderate drinking and drunkenness that is most important" (p. 226). It has been suggested that the Irish have distinctly ambivalent feelings about the use of alcohol (Lawson & Lawson 1998). Viewing alcohol use dichotomously, as either good or bad, eliminates the middle possibility (i.e., moderate, sensible drinking).

Drinking has never been healthfully integrated into Irish family rituals (e.g., drinking at family wakes) or religious traditions (Lawson & Lawson, 1998). Rather, in Irish tradition, drinking has been viewed as a means of coping with oppression and hard times. In the 19th century, the oppression was largely political in nature and came at the hands of the British. Poverty and famine were widespread, and many an Irishman turned to alcohol in an effort to cope (Bales, 1980). At this time, the terms "Irishman" and "drunkard" became synonymous (Bales, 1980).

What appears to have evolved in Irish culture is the shared norm that "alcohol is an effective way to deal with our hard times that so commonly befall us." Bales (1980) has proposed that cultures such as the Irish, which are characterized by suppression of aggression, guilt, and sexual feelings and which condone the use of alcohol to cope with these impulses, will probably have high rates of alcoholism. Alcohol use is seen by the Irish as their way of coping with personal distress. Although on one hand drinking is viewed as the "curse of the Irish," on the other it is seen as the quintessential Irish act, one embodying all that is "Irish." In a symbolic way, drunkenness connects the Irish to all of their similarly anguished ancestors. Though this is probably an overly sentimental portrayal of Irish drinking customs, to some degree it captures the socially unifying aspects of drinking within the culture.

Misperceived Peer Norms: Explaining Alcohol Abuse among Young People

Alcohol abuse is a serious problem on college campuses in the United States (Wechsler et al., 2002). Binge drinking, blackouts, drinking and driving, and an assortment of other alcohol-related problems are more prevalent in this group than in society at large. Though these are not new problems, frequent media reports of unintentional alcohol-related deaths, fraternity-hazing incidents involving alcohol, and celebratory rioting in college towns maintain a high level of public concern about the problem. Why is it a severe problem?

One explanation that is commonly relied on today is the "misperceived norms hypothesis" (Baer, Stacy, & Larimer, 1991; Perkins & Berkowitz, 1986; Thombs, Wokott, & Farkash, 1997). This model maintains that excessive drinking among young people is maintained by misperceptions of peers' drinking practices. Biased drinking norms tend to develop in relatively insular social environments, such as schools and colleges (Baer et al., 1991). The perceptions of peer drinking norms tend to become biased or *exaggerated* because students interact mostly with other students, and less with older adults, and because in these situations, stories about recent drinking episodes tend to be embellished and bragged about in social conversations (see Berkowitz, 1997).

As a result, a large majority of students develop exaggerated perceptions of the extent to which their fellow students are drinking and engaging in related misbehavior. The belief develops that "everybody is drunk on Thursday, Friday, and Saturday nights," or "if I'm not drinking—I'll miss out on the fun." In other words, students come to perceive that their campus environment is very *permissive*. Students who hold norms that are more conservative tend to increase their drinking over time to conform to the false norm (Prentice & Miller, 1993). These perceptual biases fuel alcohol abuse. Students begin to think "heavy drinking is what we do at _____ University" and "everybody at _____ University knows how to party."

Research conducted by this author with middle school, high school, and college students, found that perceived norms are highly correlated not only with alcohol consumption but with drinking and driving and riding with alcohol-impaired drivers (Thombs et al., 1997). Young people who perceived that these behaviors were prevalent among their peers tended to drink heavily as well as engage in drinking and driving and riding with impaired drivers. Interestingly, relatively large majorities of students (66–79%) perceived that other students at their school engaged in these alcohol behaviors more than they did (Thombs et al., 1997). Only a handful of students thought they engaged more frequently in these behaviors than did their peers. Another recent study found that among middle school and high school youth who had not yet initiated use of a drug (tobacco, alcohol, or marijuana), elevated scores on peer norm measures were associated with holding intentions to begin using these substances within the next 6 months (Olds et al., 2005).

Illicit Drugs as Boundary Markers

Illicit drugs have also been used to promote group identity and to establish ethnic boundaries. One frequently described example involves the Chinese laborers who were brought to the western United States in the last half of the 19th century to build the railroad system. Large numbers of Chinese were imported at this time to complete the arduous task of constructing new track; they brought with them their practice of opium smoking. Opium dens were created as places to spend nonworking hours.

The practice of opium smoking never spread to other social groups. Local community leaders in many jurisdictions (who, of course, were white) passed legislation to forbid the practice. In general, most Americans viewed the use of opium by the Chinese with distaste and repugnance. Thus, for the white majority, opium smoking served as a significant social boundary. It was useful to them as a means of identifying who "we" (the good people) were and who "they" (the Chinese, the bad people) were.

Furthermore, the drug experience (opium smoking) itself made apparent the distinctive value structures of the Chinese versus the white Americans. As noted by Ray and Ksir (1999):

> The opium smoking the Chinese brought to this country never became widely popular, although around the turn of the century about one-fourth of the

opium imported was smoking opium. Perhaps it was because the smoking itself occupies only about a minute and is then followed by a dreamlike reverie that may last two or three hours—hardly conducive to a continuation of daily activities or consonant with the outward, active orientation of most Americans in that period. Another reason why opium smoking did not spread was that it originated with Asians, who were scorned by whites (p. 341)

Opium smoking was consistent with the Chinese emphasis on reflection and introspection. It was at odds with the American orientation toward productivity, action, and settling the West.

DRUG SUBCULTURES: REPUDIATION OF MIDDLE-CLASS VALUES

Prior to the 1960s, illicit drug abuse was primarily concentrated among minority ghetto populations. Thus, explaining illicit drug abuse within a subculture framework made a great deal of sense. However, during the 1970s illicit drug abuse became more diffuse among social classes (Oetting & Beauvis, 1988). The availability and use of such substances as marijuana and heroin were not narrowly limited to lower socioeconomic groups, as they were in the 1950s. Thus, sociologists and anthropologists paid somewhat less attention to the subculture concept in the 1970s and 1980s.

There is still value to analyzing drug abuse within a subculture context, however. This is particularly true for examining substance abuse among teens and younger adults. The framework offers insight into how substance abuse is initiated and maintained, and how drug subcultures are related to the youth culture, to the parent culture, and to broad U.S. middle-class culture.

Definitions

Middle-class U.S. culture is characterized by a broad set of rather diverse values and conduct norms for adults. It is essentially a parent culture that includes expectations for what youths can and cannot do. In general, parents expect young people to avoid tobacco, alcohol, and illicit drug use. This is reflected in laws that prohibit youths from purchasing cigarettes and alcohol before the ages of 18 and 21, respectively. To various degrees, the values and conduct norms of the parent culture are internalized by youths. Of course, the extent of this socialization varies from youth to youth, and across particular classes of values as well.

The youth culture defines what peers or friends expect each other to do or not to do (Gans, 1962). In its attempt to control and influence young people, the parent culture competes with the youth culture. This competition is an ongoing, dynamic process. The parent culture usually attempts to defend traditional values, while the youth culture encourages experimentation with new or novel forms of expression. According to B. D. Johnson (1980), the youth culture emphasizes the following conduct norms:

1. The person must be loyal to friends and attempt to maintain group association.
2. Social interaction with the peer group should occur in locations where adult controls are relatively absent.
3. Within such peer groups, a veiled competition exists for status and prestige among group participants and leads to new forms of behavior or operating innovations. (p. 111)

"Youth culture" and "peer group" are closely related but distinct concepts. A young person's close circle of friends is his/her peer group. The term "youth culture" refers to a much broader influence—one that touches all peer groups via community, school, church, and media messages. The pervasive influence of the youth culture explains the great similarity among distant peer groups. This is particularly the case today with so many national media targeting youth (e.g., MTV).

A "subculture" consists of a culture within a larger culture (B. D. Johnson, 1980). It is characterized by values, conduct norms, social situations, and roles that are distinct from and often at odds with those of the middle class. The term "drug subculture" refers to these same components as they pertain to *nonmedical* drug use (B. D. Johnson, 1980).

Excluded from this conceptualization are the values and conduct norms associated with medical and most legal drug use. Thus, psychoactive drugs prescribed by a physician are not included, nor is use of over-the-counter medications or cigarettes. The moderate social use of alcohol is also excluded from a drug subculture analysis, because such drinking practices are clearly part of middle-class culture. However, in the subsequent discussion, the values and conduct norms of the alcohol *abuse* subculture are explored.

A relatively unique constellation of values define a subculture. According to B. D. Johnson (1980), "the most important elements of a subculture are its values and conduct norms. Values are here understood to be shared ideas about what the subgroup believes to be true or what is wants (desires) or ought to want" (p. 113). The most significant value of a drug subculture is the intention or desire to alter consciousness, or to get "high." This value (i.e., the wish to get high) is the organizing theme of all drug subcultures and their activities. The corresponding conduct norm is an expectation that all subculture participants will partake in the use of a drug, or at least express a desire to do so.

Within subcultures, certain behavior is expected of persons in particular social positions. These performances are referred to as "roles." In drug subcultures, there are three primary roles: seller, buyer, and user (B. D. Johnson, 1980). Performance of these roles is almost always illegal, so the execution of them is generally covert, or hidden from the public at large. Thus, the public is generally ignorant of the behavior needed to carry out the role of seller, buyer, or user (B. D. Johnson, 1980), which in part, explains the great fascination and curiosity nonsubculture members often express about these activities.

Also characteristic of drug subcultures are rituals involving highly valued objects. The objects are usually instruments for self-administration of drugs. For example, the heroin subculture favors the use of the hypodermic syringe and incorporates it into rituals in which several addicts may share the same needle (e.g., in "shooting galleries"). The cocaine subculture has several ritualized practices, depending on the route of administration. Objects include mirrors, spoons, special pipes, vials, and straws or rolled-up dollar bills for snorting. The marijuana subculture values such objects as "roach clips," water pipes, and rolling papers. These symbolic objects and drug rituals are rarely known outside the subculture but are widely known within it. They serve to bolster group identity and solidarity.

By the time most illicit drug addicts have reached their mid-20s, they have developed a preference for one drug over others. This preference may simply be a function of their participation in a particular drug subculture. The addicts may have an elaborate set of reasons for why their drug is superior to others. Heavily influencing their attachment to one drug are their bonds and identification with their peer group. B. D. Johnson (1980) has noted that subculture participants tend to ignore great similarities in the behavior of drug addicts and tend to emphasize the importance of differences that seem very small to outsiders. For example, many cocaine addicts "put down" PCP addicts; they believe that cocaine helps one think more clearly, while PCP just makes one "dumb." Alcoholics and heroin addicts take similar views of each other: Alcoholics may perceive heroin addicts as "lowlifes," while many heroin addicts view alcoholics as "wimps" and "crybabies."

Drug Laws as a Means of Striking Back at Low-Status Groups

Drug subcultures are dynamic. Historical, political, economic, and sociocultural factors influence their formation and dissolution. However, some of trends are quite predictable. Johnson (1980) noted with insight:

> When patterns of drug use are limited to low-income and low-status groups, societal reaction tends to be punitive, and government pursues a prohibitionist policy. When drug use becomes common in many segments of the youth population, public reaction is one of temporary alarm with later adjustment and easing of enforcement effects and legal punishments. (p. 115)

A good example of how public perception can shape U.S. drug laws involves the legal distinction between crack cocaine and powder cocaine (Caulkins et al., 1997). Under current federal law, a person convicted of possessing just 1½ grams of crack is subject to a 5-year minimum sentence, whereas 150 grams of powder cocaine are needed for the same sentence (U.S. Sentencing Commission, 1998). Thus, depending on the form of the cocaine, the mandatory minimum sentence for cocaine varies by a factor of 100!

Who tends to be arrested on crack cocaine charges? According to Forst (1995), more than 90% of those arrested on crack cocaine charges are African American. In powder cocaine cases, African Americans comprised only 25% of the arrestees. Thus, critics have charged that the differential sentencing guidelines are racist. The situation illustrates how drug laws are sometimes used to strike back at groups that the dominant culture fear.

Changes in drug use, shifts in public opinion and public debate, and new government initiatives are among the dynamic social forces that spur the development of drug subcultures. Therefore, they are not static social groups; subcultures are always changing. Though identification of their chief features can become quickly dated, key aspects of five of today's drug subcultures can be delineated and are described next.

The Alcohol Abuse Subculture

Alcohol is a powerful mood-altering drug. Yet it is legally available and its use is widespread, even expected, in U.S. middle-class culture. Alcohol is viewed as both a beverage and an intoxicant—one that is principally used to facilitate social interaction and relief from stress. There is significant social pressure in this society to drink, at least in moderation. Abstention from alcohol is considered almost as deviant as binge drinking.

In contrast to the sensible, "social" use of alcohol stands the alcohol *abuse* subculture. The conduct norms of this subculture expect participants to get "wasted," "totaled," "smashed," or "bombed." The emphasis is on excessive consumption. Alcohol is not used as a beverage but as a drug; that is, drunkenness is intentional or purposely sought. Such drinking contrasts sharply with that of the larger middle class, where drunkenness is viewed with embarrassment and met with social disgrace. Many high school and college students become participants of the alcohol abuse subculture, although a sizable proportion seem to "mature out" of it as they assume full-time jobs, get married, and/or have children.

Certain reciprocity conduct norms exist in the alcohol abuse subculture. It is expected that participants will share in the pooling of money to buy relatively large quantities of alcohol (e.g., a case or keg of beer). There is the expectation that one member will buy drinks for other members, and that the favor will later be reciprocated. In some social groups, bottle passing is expected. In others, drinking games (e.g., "quarters," "pass out," and others) or reliance on special paraphernalia (e.g., beer funnels) is encouraged. Again, these rituals and objects serve to promote group identity and solidarity.

These social functions become clear when one considers the very high rate of alcohol abuse in college fraternities and sororities (Cashin, Presley, & Meilman, 1998). These Greek-letter organizations are at the center of the alcohol abuse subculture on campus. It is well established by research that members of fraternities and sororities consume substantially more alcohol than their non-Greek students (e.g., Cashin et al., 1998).

Greek student conduct norms for drinking appear to be established to a great extent by the fraternity/sorority *leaders* (Cashin et al., 1998). Thus, on many campuses, some fraternities come to resemble alcohol-dispensing outlets—particularly for underage drinkers. Drinking games are significant features (Engs & Hanson, 1993). They organize binge drinking and ensure participant intoxication. Current campus rituals include the practice of "keg standing" and consuming "jello shots."

Participants of the alcohol abuse subculture are not always young people. Older adults may also be participants of this subculture. The middle class tends to label such adults "alcoholics." Their drinking may also be ritualized (e.g., three drinks before dinner, never drinking before noon, and stopping at a bar each day after work). Elaborate liquor cabinets or even full-size bars may be set up at home. Large quantities of alcohol may be kept in reserve (e.g., a keg of beer on tap in the refrigerator or a dozen or more cases of beer bought at wholesale prices stored in the garage). Decorative mirrors, pictures, posters, clocks, ashtrays, and other "knickknacks" from alcohol retailers may adorn their homes. Heavy drinking is clearly a central activity in their lives (Fingarette, 1988). That is, they organize their lives around the consumption of alcohol.

The Marijuana Abuse Subculture

Among young adults, the marijuana subculture thrived in the 1960s and 1970s. The sharing of marijuana was promoted. Rock music lyrics reinforced this conduct norm (e.g., Bob Dylan emphasized in one song that "everybody must get stoned"). It should be understood, though, that the predominant values were not ones of aggression and pressure; rather, values emphasized peace, love, understanding, and social harmony. Yet a subtle form of peer pressure did exist within the subculture to use the drug.

Usually, no money was exchanged in the sharing of marijuana. Group participants were trusted to reciprocate at some future date. Those who bought relatively large amounts of "pot" were expected to share small amounts with friends and to sell to friends at cost. There was an expectation that marijuana buyers and sellers were not supposed to turn large profits. Typically, buyers and sellers within this subculture were expected to socialize and smoke together. The business aspects of the transactions were deemphasized.

In this era, there was the naive but persistent belief that marijuana use could correct many of the social ills of the United States. The middle class, particularly the parent culture, was perceived as obsessed with material things as well as racist, sexist, corrupt, and hypocritical. Marijuana use was naively thought to be the single answer to all social problems. This conviction (among others) helped to forge the youth–parent culture conflict (i.e., the "generation gap") of the 1960s and 1970s.

These social values promoted the acceptance of marijuana and its use was relatively high among youth (B. D. Johnson, 1980). However, the 1980s saw a reversal in this trend with fewer and fewer young people experimenting with it or using it regularly (Johnston, O'Malley, & Bachman, 1989). By 1992, marijuana use among youth had fallen to its lowest level in the 23 years of the national Monitoring the Future Study; about 22% of high school seniors reported using marijuana one or more times in the previous 12 months (Johnston, O'Malley, Bachman, & Schulenberg, 2005). Then, in 1993, there appeared a second reversal in the trend. Marijuana use among youth increased each year: 1993–1997. By 1997, the annual prevalence of marijuana use among high school seniors reached a rate of about 39%. This peak was followed by small steady declines until 2004 when about 34% of seniors reported use of the drug in the past year (Johnston et al. 2005). The reasons behind these 5- to 7-year fluctuations are not known.

The Polydrug Abuse Subculture

B. D. Johnson (1980) identified a drug subculture characterized by polydrug abuse. Front-line practitioners working in the field today are keenly aware of the use of multiple substances, either simultaneously or on different occasions. Although polydrug abuse is prevalent among young adults, this is not a new problem. These patterns have been well documented in the research literature for some time (Chen & Kandel, 1995).

According to B. D. Johnson (1980), the polydrug abuse subculture is an outgrowth of the marijuana subculture. One distinguishing conduct norm of this subculture is that participants are expected to use almost any chemical in an effort to alter consciousness. In addition to alcohol and marijuana, the use of cocaine, crack cocaine, tranquilizers, sedatives, narcotics, ketamine ("Special K"), inhalants, methamphetamine, hallucinogenic mushrooms, MDMA ("Ecstasy"), and other designer drugs is encouraged. Conduct norms also require that members be willing to smoke and inhale (snort) a drug, as well as administer it orally. Usually, conduct norms do not expect participants to inject a drug; this is a boundary marker that distinguishes this group from the heroin abuse subculture. Polydrug abuse subculture participants frequently perceive self-administered injection as "going one step too far." They may be heard to say, "That [injection] is the one thing that I would never do."

Sharing drugs (B. D. Johnson, 1980) and using combinations of drugs are important in this subculture. A participant who has pills is expected to share with someone who has cocaine, for example. Some drugs are more highly coveted than others; typically, crack cocaine is more highly valued than than a drug like PCP (Thombs, 1989). Drug sellers (dealers) are not necessarily expected to socialize with buyers in the polydrug abuse subculture.

The popularity of drug combinations are always in flux. For example, in the late 1990s, one drug combination involved the use of nitrite inhalants ("poppers"), Viagra—the medication used to treat erectile dysfunction, and possibly methamphetamine as well (Zamora, 1998). This potentially lethal combination was reported in some circles in the gay community in California. Apparently, users believe that Viagra can improve sexual performance while under the influence of other substances.

The "rave" party scene is one of the more recent manifestations of the polydrug abuse subculture (NIDA, 2005). These are all-night dance parties typically attended by older teens and those in their early 20s. Sometimes they are called underground or afterhours parties. Loud "technomusic" is accompanied by laser and light shows. Raves are considered a forum for so-called Generation X. Participants typically wear 1960s- and 1970s-style clothing (bell bottoms, platform shoes) featuring psychedelic colors.

Rave parties are promoted on the Internet, by flyers, private mailing lists, e-mail, and word of mouth. Clubs that hold rave parties usually check identification at the door, but fake IDs are reported widely used by underage "ravers." Some rave parties promote themselves as alcohol free, but others serve alcohol, and some allow participants to bring their own. Nonalcoholic drinks are typically sold, including "smart drinks" comprised of fruit juice, vitamins, amino acids, and caffeine. The "club drugs" most commonly associated with raves and dance parties are LSD, Ecstasy, GHB, methamphetamine, ketamine, and Rohypnol (Maxwell, 2004), though the use of other drugs has been reported as well. Participants are reported to freely share drugs with one another, and use of multiple substances is common. Media reports have alleged that at some large parties, organizers have distributed substances with the claim that they are legal herbal preparations. One such incident at a New Year's Eve event led to 31 partiers being taken to hospital emergency rooms because they reported difficulty breathing (Canto, 1997).

The Heroin Injection Subculture

Although users may share heroin from time to time, they have strong expectations that peers will reciprocate at a later time (B. D. Johnson, 1980). In addition, participants in this subculture are expected to carry out all three drug subculture roles: buyer, user, and seller (B. D. Johnson, 1980). Participants provide other participants with information ("connections") regarding where to secure more of the drug. Most participants of the heroin injection subculture were previously involved in the polydrug abuse subculture, and they may continue their contacts with this network on a more limited basis.

The heroin *injection* subculture expects participants to self-administer heroin via hypodermic injection (B. D. Johnson, 1980). Heroin can be inhaled or snorted, but in this subculture the conduct norms generally discourage these routes of administration. *Heroin inhalation is more typical of the polydrug abuse subculture.* Snorting (inhalation) is not thought by heroin subculture participants to provide the same "rush" as injection.

Today, conduct norms for injecting heroin vary considerably. Three to four injections a day are typical. However, according to Ray and Ksir (1999), in addition to the 500,000 heroin addicts in the United States, there may be more than 1 million citizens who use the drug on an *occasional* basis. Many of these so-called chippers are needle users.

Even occasional needle use increases the individual's risk for contracting HIV, the virus that causes AIDS. Heroin is typically the drug being injected, but other drug use is implicated in HIV transmission as well, including other opiates, cocaine, and methamphetamine. Of course, it should be recognized that HIV infection does not result from the action of illicit drugs. Rather, infection is a consequence of using a contaminated needle (i.e., the sharing of needles). Many injection drug users are known to obtain syringes from the street and use them several times. Use of contaminated needles has become the greatest risk factor for contracting HIV in high seroprevalence cities (Friedman, Jose, Deren, Des Jarlais, & Neaigus, 1995).

In many of the world's largest cities, it was estimated that as many as 40–50% of the injection drug users had become HIV positive by the early 1990s (Des Jarlais et al., 1995). In the United States today, a substantial number of individuals continue to be exposed to HIV by injection drug use or by having sex with an injection drug user (Centers for Disease Control and Prevention, 2004c). The data in Table 9.1 show the magnitude of this problem in the United States since the beginning of the HIV/AIDS epidemic.

As can be seen in Table 9.1, injection drug use risks for HIV/AIDS have varied across groups defined by race and sex during the epidemic. Among white women, and African Americans and Hispanics of both sexes, injection drug use has been associated with more than one-third of the AIDS cases. In contrast, white men tend to be exposed to HIV through sexual contact with other men (Centers for Disease Control and Prevention, 2004c). The data in Table 9.1 also show that across racial groups, women were more likely to be exposed to HIV through sex with an injection drug user than were men.

The Crack Cocaine Subculture

The crack cocaine subculture emerged in the United States during the mid-1980s. According to data collected by the National Institute of Justice (NIJ) in 1987, crack use had become prevalent by this time in most major U.S. cities (NIJ, 1988). By 1997, the crack cocaine epidemic has slowed. According to the NIJ (1998),

> 1997 data indicate that many communities are dealing with stable or slowly changing cocaine problems. Almost without exception, older age cohorts are testing positive for cocaine at 2 to 10 times the rate of the younger cohorts . . . cocaine use is increasingly a problem of a group of long-term users who developed their habits in the early stage of the epidemic. (p. 1)

TABLE 9.1 Cumulative U.S. AIDS Cases by Drug Injection Exposure Category, Race, and Sex, 2003

Exposure category	White		African American		Hispanic	
	M	F	M	F	M	F
Injection drug use	18%	41%	40%	37%	40%	37%
Sex with an injection drug user	1%	16%	3%	13%	2%	19%
Risk not associated with injection drug use	81%	43%	57%	50%	58%	44%

Note. By 2003, a total of 881,547 AIDS cases among whites, African Americans, and Hispanics had been reported to the Centers for Disease Control and Prevention since the beginning of the epidemic. The percentages in Table 9.1 are based only on adolescent and adult cases within each racial group. Pediatric cases ($n = 9,419$) and cases among Asian/Pacific Islanders ($n = 6,791$) and American Indian/ Alaska Natives ($n = 2,882$) are not reported. M, male; F, female. Data from the Centers for Disease Control and Prevention (2004c).

Though the drug is used by a diverse group of people, the typical crack cocaine subculture participant is a 30- to 40-year-old African American male, often from an impoverished urban neighborhood, that faces significant social and economic barriers to achieving middle-class status.

In the crack cocaine subculture, various conduct norms have developed. It is expected that participants will smoke the drug daily in a binge-like fashion over an 8-, 10-, 12-, or even 24-hour period (NIDA, 1987). The binge or "run" will stop when the addict has run out of money or is too exhausted to continue. The user may "fall out"—that is, have a seizure—and be taken to an emergency room.

Sharing is typically not a conduct norm in this subculture; however, trading a commodity in exchange for crack is common. Participants may swap jewelry, stereos, guns, or even sex for crack. The exchange of sex is particularly true for female addicts, who may engage in prostitution for another "hit."

In many urban settings, crack subculture participants gather in a house, apartment, or other site where the drug can be used in private. In "crack houses," use of the drug may go on 24 hours a day. If the participants come under the scrutiny of police or neighborhood groups, they will probably move to another location. In essence, a crack house is the modern-day version of the "speakeasy" of the Prohibition era.

The distribution conduct norms of the crack subculture are highly secretive. This is hardly surprising, given the harsh legal sanctions that exist for cocaine sale and distribution. However, it appears that the business aspects of the transaction are emphasized. If sellers are cheated in a deal, conduct norms call for retaliation, often involving shootings. Violence and the threat of violence are pervasive in the subculture. In this way, the participants resemble the bootleggers (e.g., Al Capone) of the 1920s. Similar to gangsters of yesteryear, the sellers in this subculture are part of a structured hierarchy in which higher-level distributors attempt to shield themselves from arrest by relying on subordinates. In open-air drug markets, subordinates or "runners" may be young teens who are not subject to the same legal penalties as adults.

IMPLICATIONS FOR COUNSELING

Sociocultural perspectives suggest that prevention and treatment practitioners must be aware of basic human values in working with individuals and communities. Though sociologists and anthropologists are subject to personal biases and value judgments, as Light and Keller (1975) noted some time ago, "For generations sociologists have labored under the eleventh commandment, 'Thou shalt not commit a value judgement'" (p. 36).

Sociocultural analyses do not pass judgment on the "correctness" of addicts' values; instead, they serve as relatively impartial analyses of the social phenomena under scrutiny. If sociologists describe a drug subculture as placing a low priority on economic productivity, they are not insisting that addicts are "lazy." They are simply pointing out that their value structure emphasizes other pursuits, and that this structure deviates from that of the larger middle-class culture.

Many times the "resistance" demonstrated by persons with substance abuse problems reflects conflicts between their value structure and those proposed by helping professionals (Rappaport, 1997). From a social interaction perspective, this may not be as much an unconscious defense as a refusal to adopt the values of the mainstream culture. For instance, a client who indicates that he/she "cannot" attend 90 AA meetings in 90 days is revealing a preference for spontaneity over structure in organizing day-to-day life. A client who will not make a commitment to abstinence may be demonstrating a preference for short-term gratification and excitement over long-term gains (e.g., economic security and family stability) and improved health. Peele (1985), in particular, noted that many addicts place relatively little value on their personal health. The old maxim, "Eat, drink, and be merry, for tomorrow we may die," seems to apply here.

Substance abusers may balk at attempts to encourage serious introspection and self-assessment of their behavior. This may reflect a value structure that elevates social relations, fun, and amusement over rational self-control and serious self-understanding. These conflicts are crucial issues to be uncovered, clarified, and discussed when attempting to help a person with a substance abuse problem. Many, perhaps most, clients are unaware of their value priorities and of how these relate to their substance abuse. Though it may be painful, practitioners should help clients bring these issues to the foreground of consciousness while maintaining an objective attitude toward the clients' value structure.

LIMITATIONS

As a basis for prevention programming or treatment planning, there are two major limitations to sociocultural concepts. First, many of these concepts lack precision and do not seem salient to contemporary helping strategies. In particular, this may be true of such concepts as social boundary markers, subcultures, conduct norms, "time out," and so on. Critics have occasionally charged that sociocultural theorists are the sideline observers of the drug scene. Their concepts provide intellectual insight but are not helpful in enhancing the direct delivery of treatment services.

The second limitation pertains to the relative inability of prevention and treatment practitioners to significantly alter the social, cultural, and environmental factors that cause substance use and abuse. In this vein, sociocultural perspectives may be viewed as interesting but of little practical value because these social variables cannot be readily addressed. This lack of practicality is likely to prevent sociocultural perspectives from gaining more prominent status among theories on addictive behavior.

REVIEW QUESTIONS

1. What is meant by the "medicalization" of addiction? How do cultural factors influence diagnostic determinations?

2. What are the four basic sociological functions of substance abuse? How do they support substance abuse?

3. What are the five social contexts of adolescent drinking? How are these differentially related to alcohol consumption and problems?

4. What is "time out"?

5. How are alcohol and drugs used as social boundary markers?

6. What is the misperceived norms hypothesis?

7. What is a drug subculture? How is it distinct from middle-class culture?

8. When do government drug policies and laws become especially punitive? What groups tend to be targets?

9. What particular values and conduct norms characterize a drug subculture?

10. What are some of the unique aspects of the alcohol abuse subculture, the marijuana abuse subculture, the polydrug abuse subculture, the heroin injection subculture, and the crack cocaine subculture?

11. What are "raves"?

12. To what extent is drug injection an HIV/AIDS risk in the United States today?

13. How should values be dealt with in substance abuse counseling?

14. What are the limitations of the sociocultural concepts in substance abuse counseling?

CHAPTER 10

Conditions That Facilitate and Inhibit Change in Addictive Behavior

This volume has provided an in-depth review and critique of contemporary theories of addictive behavior and supporting research and applications in each area. Each perspective has offered concepts that can be used in substance prevention and treatment. Some of the theories focus on individuals, whereas others concentrate on populations or other social units such as families. Regardless of the focus, there has been increasing emphasis in recent years to attend to the problem of *motivation to change* when analyzing substance abuse problems. Often, alcohol and drug abuse continues because there is either individual or collective ambivalence about change.

In the treatment environment, clinicians traditionally found fault with substance-abusing clients for being "unmotivated" to change. When a client prematurely terminated treatment, there was the tendency to blame the client—not the treatment model. More recently, there has been growing recognition that inflexible treatment models contribute to this problem, and that an explicit goal of psychosocial treatment should be motivation enhancement (Rappaport, 1997). This recognition also should be extended to prevention efforts that seek to change community conditions. In this chapter, we review the stages-of-change model (Prochaska, DiClemente, & Norcross, 1992) and discuss contemporary intervention strategies and related issues (i.e., coercion and managed care pressures) that facilitate and inhibit motivation to change behaviors that support alcohol and drug abuse.

STAGES OF CHANGE IN ADDICTIVE BEHAVIOR

Motivation is a particularly critical issue in helping clients (or even communities) to change. Prochaska et al. (1992) developed a *transtheoretical, stage model* to explain how individuals change unwanted behavior as well as maintain new habits. The stages-of-change model is not another theory but a framework that can organize existing theories to help explain the process people use to change themselves—with or without professional assistance. Within each stage, constructs from various theories can be used to explain movement. It is important to note that the model does not explain *why* people change but, rather, *how* they do so.

Practitioners and researchers have shown much interest in the model because it provides a structure for understanding readiness to change problem behavior. The model has been applied to a variety of health behavior problems characterized by relapse. These have included medication adherence in AIDS treatment (Bradley-Springer, 1996), smoking cessation (DiClemente et al., 1991), recovery from alcohol/drug addiction (DiClemente, 1991), weight control (Prochaska & DiClemente, 1985), and psychological distress (Prochaska & Norcross, 1983).

Research has shown that the stages-of-change model is particularly useful for matching patients with treatments based on their readiness for change. Prochaska and DiClemente (1992) noted that many psychosocial and medical treatment programs have poor outcomes because they assume that new clients (or patients) are highly motivated to participate in their own treatment. In reality, across a broad range of behavioral and medical disorders, clients often do not possess a high level of readiness for change at the onset of treatment. Prochaska and DiClemente (1992) estimated that across populations with active health problems, roughly 10–15% are prepared to take action to improve their condition upon entering treatment.

The stages-of-change model consists of five stages (Prochaska & DiClemente, 1992). Each stage and its implications for helping individuals with substance-abusing problems are described here. It is important to point out that progression through these stages does not usually occur in a linear fashion. Clients who reach the latter three stages often recycle to the first two. However, research does indicate that for most individuals, relapsing is not an endless process (Prochaska & DiClemente, 1992). Most of the time, individuals do not regress all the way back to where they began. It appears that many learn from their mistakes and relapses become less frequent over time.

Precontemplation

Precontemplation describes a stage in which there is no intention to change behavior in the foreseeable future. Often, precontemplators do not define the behavior as a problem (DiClemente, 1991). Bell and Rollnick (1996) described them as "happy users." However, external observers such as their friends, families, employers, and so on identify their behavior as problematic.

DiClemente (1991) argued that there is more to precontemplation than just "denial" and "resistance." Some precontemplators simply lack knowledge about the risks associated with their behavior. Others are rebellious because they have a heavy investment in maintaining the problem behavior. On the other hand, some precontemplators are characterized by resignation. They are overwhelmed by the problem and see themselves as incapable of change; they have no hope and believe it is too late to modify their behavior. Finally, some precontemplators involve themselves in rationalizing away the problem (e.g., "what's the use of going through all the hassle of treatment, you only live once").

DiClemente (1991) argued that there is a pervasive myth in the helping professions pertaining to precontemplators. The myth maintains that the more serious the health or behavior problem, the more intense the education, treatment, or confrontation must be to help the person. With precontemplators, "more" help may actually be harmful or, more commonly, just ignored. Research on brief interventions indicate that they are as effective as more intensive treatment and more effective than no treatment (Miller & Rollnick, 2002; NIAAA, 1997; Bernstein et al., 2005). This may be particularly the case when the focus of the brief intervention is to motivate the client to make a commitment to change.

Contemplation

Contemplation is a stage at which many substance abusers stay for an extended period. Typically, this stage involves an extended "risk–reward analysis" (DiClemente, 1991). Patients are involved in the frequent weighing of the costs and benefits of change. They mull over cost and benefits again and again. In contrast to the precontemplator, the contemplator is willing to consider change, but his/her ambivalence often makes this state chronic. For instance, DiClemente and Prochaska (1985) followed a group of 200 cigarette smokers in the contemplation stage for 2 years and found that the group's modal or most common response was unchanged during this period.

Contemplators have an interest in change but little *commitment*. They demonstrate this by asking about treatment options but not following through, or by scheduling appointments only to fail to show up for them. DiClemente (1991) indicated that contemplators often offer reasons for why "now is not the right time" to begin a program (p. 195).

In working with contemplators, the challenge for practitioners is to facilitate movement toward the next stage: preparation. The content of the information given to contemplators is important. First, it should be *personally relevant* to the individual; a cocaine-dependent person considering treatment may not be swayed by information about Alcoholics Anonymous or long-term sobriety. Second, there is a need to emphasize the *benefits of change* (e.g., "You can stop wasting money on crack), rather than attempting to arouse fear (e.g., "You're damaging your heart and lungs," or "You are going to end up in prison"). A focus on the benefits of change can create incentives for contemplator. Fear arousal messages (scare tactics) generally should be avoided because they serve to undermine self-efficacy; that is, they destroy optimism about the prospects for change by implying "it may already be too late for me."

Preparation (or Determination)

In the preparation stage, persons form an intention to change a behavior in the near future (Prochaska & DiClemente, 1992). Their determination is often demonstrated by small behavior changes. People are typically in this stage for only brief periods. Their experimenting does not necessarily propel them into the next stage: action (DiClemente, 1991). Experiencing barriers to change may result in a return to contemplation.

DiClemente (1991) noted that an important task in helping the client in preparation is to encourage the development of a *realistic* plan of action. Many determined clients fail to recognize or dismiss the difficulties they will encounter when they take action (e.g., entering treatment). A realistic plan will anticipate these barriers and have identified solutions or responses for them.

Action

The next stage, action, involves implementing a plan. Here, people modify their behavior and/or their environment to overcome a problem. However, as Prochaska and DiClemente (1992) noted:

> Modifications of the addictive behavior made in the action stage tend to be most visible and receive the greatest external recognition. People, including professionals, often erroneously equate action with change. As a consequence, they overlook the requisite work that prepares changers for action and

the important efforts necessary to maintain the changes following action. (p. 1104)

Individuals who seek out professional help sometimes have already initiated behavioral changes in their lives; obtaining substance abuse treatment may be just one part of their change efforts. Studies have found that it is not unusual for clients to initiate abstinence days or even weeks before entering treatment (Maisto, Sobell, Sobell, Lei, & Sypora, 1988; Tucker, Vuchinich, & Pukish, 1995). According to DiClemente (1991), these are the clients who make therapists feel good about themselves; these are the "easy clients," and the "miracle cures" (p. 199). Clients already in action sometimes enter counseling to (1) make a public commitment to action, (2) obtain external confirmation of the plan, (3) seek support and confidence, and (4) create external monitors of their activity (DiClemente, 1991).

DiClemente (1991) maintained that the primary tasks of treatment personnel for helping clients in action is to identify ways to enhance their self-efficacy (e.g., introducing them to peer support networks) and, if possible, to remove any bureaucratic barriers that may impede their progress. Individuals are classified as in "action" if they successfully alter their behavior for a period of 1 day to 6 months. After 6 months of success, they are considered to have moved to the next stage (Prochaska & DiClemente, 1992).

Maintenance

In maintenance, people continue their efforts to prevent relapse and to consolidate gains made in treatment. Prochaska and DiClemente (1992) do not view maintenance as a static state but, rather, as a continuation of change. The threat of relapse becomes less and less intense with the passage of time. However, relapse to another stage remains a possibility.

Here, an important task for practitioners is to develop, with the client, a relapse prevention plan that anticipates, and protects against, "abstinence violation effects." As discussed in Chapter 7, these are the intense, negative, emotional reactions, often involving self-downing, that many patients experience when they have a small setback or "lapse." The significance of a lapse is exaggerated and leads to feelings of doom. In turn, these emotional reactions undermine self-efficacy and typically result in a more severe relapse than otherwise would be the case. One particularly deleterious consequence of abstinence violation effects is that out of embarrassment or shame, clients may conceal their return to drinking and/or drug use, or even worse, drop out of treatment. Relapse prevention plans must be realistic in educating clients about setbacks or "backsliding" and prescribe health-enhancing response options.

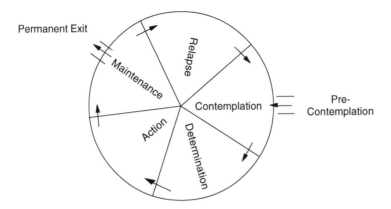

FIGURE 10.1. Prochaska and DiClemente's six stages of change.

Figure 10.1 is the "wheel of change," which shows how people cycle through the stages. Notice that precontemplation is not part of the motion of the wheel, which represents a static state. Most people who attempt change will move around the wheel several times before achieving permanent change (Miller & Rollnick, 2002).

If we conceptualize treatment as an effort to facilitate movement through the stages of change, then it becomes necessary to examine both our helping strategies and the social ecology in which these services are delivered to the client; treatment services are not provided in a social vacuum. Issues such as legal coercion affect client motivation as well. Further complicating this mix are dramatic shifts in thinking about how to help difficult to reach clients (e.g., harm reduction approaches) and new ways to finance treatment services (managed care). Next we look at some of the most pressing issues in treatment today and examine their impact on client motivation.

COERCION

There is disagreement about how to define coercion (Marlowe et al., 1996). For the purpose of this discussion, it is defined as the "imposition of an aversive stimulus to deter further substance use." In substance abuse treatment, many clients are subject to multiple coercive pressures. Legal coercion is not the only source. Other domains of coercion are social, familial, and medical (Marlowe et al., 1996). Often, coercion is used as a "lever" to push clients into treatment. Sometimes these pressures are applied by treatment personnel or programs. However, a mix of pressures can be exerted on an individual client when applied by some combination of the family, employer, criminal justice system, and so on. There is limited research on the use of coercion (Marlowe et al., 1996), and where such research does exist it usually focuses on the most extreme methods, such as compulsory residential treatment (Leukefeld & Tims, 1988).

Coercion is thought to operate on an escape or avoidance reinforcement schedule in which an aversive stimulus precedes the desired event or behavior (entering treatment, providing a "clean" urine, etc.). The client can avoid the aversive stimulus by engaging in the target conduct (Crowley, 1984). A rationale for using coercion in mental health care has been put forth by the Group for the Advancement of Psychiatry (1994). This group postulates that under optimal conditions, clients appropriately forced into treatment will eventually make the following transitions: initial defiance to reluctant compliance to a therapeutic alliance to a successful outcome.

Only a few coercive practices are mentioned briefly here. A historical example is the civil commitment of narcotic addicts in the United States. From about 1965 to 1975, some states, most notably California and New York, operated compulsory treatment programs—primarily for intravenous heroin users involved in criminal activity. In the California Civil Addict Program (CAP), addicts were forced into inpatient treatment, for an average of 18 months, and subsequently released to supervised community follow-up programs that relied on urine drug testing (Anglin, 1988). The full civil commitment procedure was 7 years in duration. At the end of this period, the CAP appeared to reduce nondrug arrests by 40% and daily drug use by 7%. A number of other positive outcomes were observed, but these were of modest magnitude (Anglin, 1988). According to Inciardi (1988) and Inciardi, McBride, and Rivers (1996), other states and the federal government also operated civil commitment programs for narcotic addicts from 1965 to 1975, but these were often poorly managed and when they were evaluated, the outcomes were quite poor.

The civil commitment programs of the 1960s and 1970s were the forerunners of today's "drug courts." The more official name for these units is "court-enforced drug treatment program." Though the structure and operation of these programs vary, there are some common features (Inciardi et al., 1996):

1. Nonviolent drug offenders are either diverted to treatment or sentenced to treatment as a part of probation.
2. Treatment is court supervised—drug court judges essentially act as case managers.
3. Urine testing is relied on to monitor compliance.
4. There is an emphasis on processing a large number of cases as efficiently as possible.

In a review of drug court evaluation studies, Inciardi et al. (1996) concluded that these programs substantially reduce justice system *costs* (decreased time from arraignment to disposition and sentencing, fewer jury trials, reduced days spent in jail, etc.). However, it remains an open question as to whether these diversion programs are effective at significantly reducing *drug use* among offenders over an extended period of time. Two more recent studies have found significant reductions in rearrest rates at 1-year (Fielding, Tye, & Ogawa, 2002) and 2-year (National Center on Addiction and Substance Abuse, 2003) follow-ups. More long-term research is needed in this area.

Another example of a coercive strategy involves requiring convicted drinking drivers to install ignition–interlock devices in their cars as a condition of probation (Elliott, Morse, & Mihalic, 1993). These devices require the operator of a motor vehicle to provide an alcohol-free breath sample in order to start a car, as well as to continue to operate it. Preliminary studies suggest that ignition–interlock technology has some deterrence effect (Baker & Beck, 1991; Elliott et al., 1993). However, some offenders do attempt to thwart the system.

Other coercive methods exist (drug testing, referrals by employee assistance programs), although they are not reviewed here. In general, it appears that coercive methods, when properly applied, do motivate some individuals to change their behavior. *However, the magnitude of the impact does not seem great over an extended period of time*; when the aversive stimulus is removed it might be expected that substance use and related risk behavior will return to previous levels.

When are coercive methods likely to produce *internal motivation* to reduce or eliminate substance use? The stages-of-change model suggests that coercion may best influence the contemplator (i.e., the substancer abuser who has been wrestling with whether to change but is waiting for a compelling reason to do so). External pressure in the form of a mandate from the court or an employer may provide the needed rationale to change oneself. The external control may bolster what the psychoanalyst refers to as "weak ego strength" or the social cognitive therapist may identify as "low self-efficacy." Cognitively, exposure to coercive requirements may be accompanied by heightened negative expectancies. Thus, in the risk–reward analysis of the contemplator, the balance between positive drug expectancies and negative social consequences could shift toward the latter.

In contrast, the response of the precontemplator to legal or worksite directives to change likely will be met with rebellious acting out, attempts at evasion, or even absconding in some cases. When coercive methods are poorly managed as a result of inadequate monitoring and inconsistent enforcement, precontemplators will likely attempt to evade the external control. Theory then suggests that coercive methods are best used selectively in the addictive behaviors. How this would be accomplished within the boundaries of civil rights and the bureaucracy of the criminal justice system is an open question.

CONFRONTATIVE TREATMENT

The use of confrontation has long been associated with substance abuse counseling (Fisher & Harrison 1997; Lightfoot, 1993; Lewis, Dana, & Blevins, 1994). The conventional view has been that substance abusers are "manipulative" and in "denial." Therefore, confrontation is necessary to break down this pattern of conduct and accompanying psychological defenses. This view is still prevalent today, especially in criminal justice settings. Torres (1997), a professor of criminal justice, writes:

> For the probation officer, the most effective approach in supervising the substance-abusing offender is to set explicit limits, to inform the probationer/parolee of the consequences for noncompliance, and to be prepared to enforce the limits in case of violations. The preferred course of action for many, if not most, users is placement in a therapeutic community, with credible threats and coercion if necessary (p. 38).

Such views are common in settings in which there is an emphasis on external controls and a concern about appearing strong or "credible." In the past, some addiction treatment programs, such as therapeutic communities, shared this philosophy (Fisher & Harrison, 1997); many addictions practitioners believed that confrontation was the only counseling skill needed to work with people who have alcohol and other drug problems (Doweiko, 1993; Lewis et al., 1994).

Views about confrontative counseling have changed during the past decade or so, and concerns have been raised that there has been an overreliance on these methods in the past. Two of the negative outcomes that have been identified are counselor disillusionment or "burnout," and clients avoiding or dropping out of treatment (Brown, 1995). *Increasingly, it is recognized that much of what has been described as denial and resistance is actually a consequence of the therapist's style* (Bell & Rollnick, 1996; Lightfoot, 1993; Miller, Zweben, DiClemente, & Rychtarik, 1992). For example, one study randomly assigned problem drinkers to two different therapist styles: confrontational/directive versus motivational/reflective (Miller, Benefield, & Tonigan, 1993). Clients who received the confrontational/directive therapy showed more resistance, were less likely to acknowledge their problems, and less often voiced the need to change. Furthermore, these patterns were predictive of less long-term change (Miller et al., 1993).

Why does client motivation appear to be dampened by confrontation? Several of the theories reviewed in this volume offer explanations. From a psychoanalytic perspective, being confronted evokes anxiety, particularly among clients with weak ego strength, and this triggers psychological defenses necessary for coping. Thus, resistance actually may be an attempt to protect the self from threat; leaving treatment prematurely should be expected in such situations. In behavior-analytic terms, confrontation creates an aversive condition that the person will usually attempt to escape. Self-efficacy theory would predict that confrontation does little to increase client optimism about treatment success or to enhance coping with stress. If the client was raised in an addictive family, confrontation and conflict may well be threatening experiences that they associate with substance use rather than abstinence. In short, there does not appear to be much theoretical basis for using confrontational therapy to help persons with substance abuse problems.

MOTIVATION ENHANCEMENT

William Miller, Stephen Rollnick, and colleagues developed motivation enhancement therapy (MET) to work with substance abusers that are ambivalent about change. MET (also known as "motivational interviewing") is a departure from traditional methods in that the purpose of counseling is to enhance the client's readiness for change. According to Miller et al. (1992):

> In sum, people with alcohol problems do not, in general, walk through the therapist's door already possessing high levels of denial and resistance. These important client behaviors are more a function of the interpersonal interactions that occur during treatment. An important goal in MET, then, is to avoid evoking client resistance (antimotivational statements). Said more bluntly, *client resistance is a therapist problem.* How you *respond* to resistant behaviors is one of the defining characteristics of MET. (p. 22)

The theoretical basis for MET is the stages-of-change model (Miller et al., 1992; Rollnick & Morgan, 1995).To a great extent, MET focuses on helping clients move from contemplation to preparation. In contemplation, the client is *unsure* about change. The preparation stage involves getting *ready* for change. Rollnick and Morgan (1995) described this movement as passing through a "decision gate." There are five important clinical implications of this model (Rollnick & Morgan, 1995):

1. Clients approach and move away from the decision gate.
2. Confrontation by the counselor about moving away from the gate can prompt greater backward movement.
3. Ambivalence about change increases as the client moves toward the decision gate.
4. When the counselor jumps ahead of the client, the client is perceived as resistant.
5. Resistance results when the counselor indicates the client *should* change.

An important strategy of MET is eliciting self-motivational statements from the client (Miller et al., 1992). In other words, MET is working when the client, rather than the counselor, provides reasons for change. The basic principles that guide this effort are as follows (Miller & Rollnick, 2002; Miller et al., 1992):

1. Express empathy for the client.
2. Develop and amplify a discrepancy, in the client's mind, between their substance use and their broader life goals.
3. Avoid argumentation about these issues.
4. "Roll with" the client's resistance.
5. Support the client's self-efficacy.

An interesting question is whether MET constitutes "treatment" in the traditional sense or is more appropriately considered an attempt to facilitate *self-change* among clients who are ambivalent? In the medical model, treatment involves procedures that are designed to somehow alter the patient. With its grounding in the stages-of-change model, MET seems to follow the client's movement, hoping to facilitate change among contemplators, at the same time respecting the reluctance of precontemplators. This is not a criticism of MET but, rather, to point out that it may be capitalizing on self-change (or natural recovery) processes in the addictions that are not completely understood (see Sobell, Sobell, & Tonneato, 1992; Sobell, Cunningham, Sobell, & Tonneato, 1993).

HARM REDUCTION APPROACHES

The previous discussion might suggest that there is little that can be done to help the precontemplator. Coercion may have only a modest impact on this group—that is, if it can be applied at all. Furthermore, there is not much reason to expect that precontemplators will benefit from confrontational therapy, and MET may be best suited for those who have moved beyond precontemplation.

A controversial intervention strategy known as "harm reduction" offers help to those who are resistant to conventional treatment options (Erickson, Riley, Cheung, & O'Hare, 1997). The goal of harm reduction strategies is to minimize personal risks among chronic or recalcitrant users based on the recognition that abstinence is not always realistic for all segments of the addicted population (Rotgers, 1996). Harm reduction programs do not view substance use as intrinsically immoral and the user is not viewed to be abnormal. The focus is mostly on the *problems* caused by the substance use rather than the substance use itself. Furthermore, these programs are "user-centered," meaning they encourage users to make their own choices about how to protect themselves, and they avoid marginalizing or stigmatizing participants (Erickson et al., 1997). Thus, harm reduction can be defined as "policies and programs which attempt primarily to reduce the adverse health, social, and economic consequences of mood-altering substances to individual drug users, their families, and their communities" (Bewley-Taylor, 2004, p. 283).

Harm reduction programs tolerate some level of substance use and are primarily concerned with extending help to high-risk groups. As a public policy, the harm reduction concept represents a middle ground between the harsh "zero tolerance" stance and the extremely permissive drug legalization position. According to Erickson et al. (1997), the harm reduction movement avoids unnecessary constraints imposed by moral, legal, and standard medical interpretations of substance use. The public health community usually advocates for harm reduction programs, whereas the criminal justice system often opposes such efforts when they extend help to illicit drug users (Marlatt & Tapert, 1993).

This approach is quite congruent with Prochaska and DiClemente's stages-of-change model. In stage-of-change jargon, harm reduction aims to provide some level of protection to those who are in precontemplation and contemplation about their risk behavior, as well as to offer an alternative form of "action" and "maintenance" to those who reject abstinence. Some of these strategies are more controversial than others. Those that seek to reduce harm associated with illicit drug use usually draw the most vocal opposition. Some examples of harm reduction strategies for substance abuse include (1) syringe-exchange programs for injection drug users, (2) methadone and heroin maintenance, (3) addict registration programs, (4) nicotine replacement therapies, (5) controlled drinking training, and (6) designated driver and safe-ride programs. These strategies provide a way to reach individuals who are not interested in abstinence. Participation in these types of programs can prompt contemplation about the risk behavior, particularly where the service has an educational or coping skills component. Thus, harm reduction strategies show much promise for reducing risk and increasing readiness to change in a broader spectrum of people than that served by abstinence-oriented prevention and treatment programs.

THE IMPACT OF MANAGED CARE

The rapid development of managed care organizations (MCOs) in the United States has produced dramatic changes in virtually all aspects of health care delivery, including public and private addiction treatment services (Miller, 1999; Morey, 1996; NIAAA, 1997). Managed care can be defined as a strategy for controlling access to care, including types of care, and to constrain the overall costs of care (Wells, Astrachan, Tischler, & Unutzer, 1995). Cost containment is accomplished through utilization reviews that rely on preadmission approval for care as well as in-treatment review to determine the necessity of continuing care. The review process typically relies on placement criteria that specify the type of care a person can receive from his/her MCO. According to Morey (1996), MCO use of placement criteria has "significantly challenged the alcohol field" (p. 38). Many addiction practitioners may consider this to be an understatement.

The primary impact of managed care pressures on addiction treatment has been to severely restrict access to inpatient care, shift clients to outpatient settings, and increase use of nonmedical approaches, such as halfway houses and nonmedical residential programs (National Institute on Alcohol Abuse and Alcoholism, 1997). It might be expected that the decreased utilization of inpatient services would be accompanied by an increase in use of outpatient services. Unfortunately, this has not been the case. *The use of outpatient services decreased during the period that access to inpatient services was restricted as well* (Mechanic, Schlesinger, & McAlpine, 1995).

As a result of these changes, addictions practitioners have turned to brief therapy models, and placed greater emphasis on helping clients use Twelve-Step programs such as Alcoholics Anonymous (Miller, 1999). Skill building to prevent relapse must start at the beginning of treatment. Under these conditions, assessment of client readiness for change becomes critical. The time constraints compel practitioners to focus on client motivation at the onset of treatment and to make decisions based on these initial judgments.

Unfortunately, at this time, there is little empirical basis for making decisions about client placement and level of care. The American Society of Addiction Medicine (ASAM) has developed a set of criteria for this purpose, but it has been not validated to determine whether it improves treatment outcomes (Morey, 1996). Nevertheless, the criteria are an important starting point and they do attempt to account for the role of client motivation in making these critical decisions about care.

Under the ASAM guidelines, there are four levels of care ranging from outpatient to partial inpatient to nonmedical inpatient to medical inpatient. The client's level of care should be determined by six dimensions that reflect the severity of the client's problems. The ASAM dimensions include (1) acute intoxication at admission and/or potential for withdrawal, (2) the possible presence of biomedical conditions and complications, (3) emotional and behavioral conditions and complications, (4) treatment acceptance/resistance (i.e., readiness for change), (5) relapse potential, and (6) recovery environment. Morey (1996) noted that criticisms of the ASAM guidelines abound. They have not been uniformly accepted in the private or public sectors; in fact, MCO placement criteria tend to be more restrictive. Thus, more research is needed to develop tools that will improve treatment outcomes and thereby justify the provision of services in the managed care environment.

There is little doubt that managed care has had a dramatic impact on the delivery of substance abuse treatment in the United States. Services of all types have decreased significantly with the advent of MCOs. The irony of the situation is that the health care industry has justified its cost-containent practices on the grounds that findings from outcome research do not support a higher level of service delivery. In essence, past efforts to improve clinical practice through research have been used against the treatment community. Out of necessity, the substance abuse prevention and treatment communities will now have to work more closely with one another, as well as with the research community, to develop more effective intervention tools.

REVIEW QUESTIONS

1. What was the traditional view of the unmotivated client?

2. What are the stages of change that clients cycle through in an effort to change addictive behavior?

3. What is the role of the practitioner at each change stage?

4. Under what conditions might coercion be effective?

5. Based on theory and research, is confrontational treatment effective?

6. What are the features of motivation enhancement therapy?

7. What is the "harm reduction" concept? What are examples of harm reduction strategies?

8. In what ways has managed care affected addictions treatment in recent years?

References

Abrams, D. B., & Niaura, R. S. (1987). Social learning theory. In H. T. Blane & K. E. Leonard (Eds.), *Psychological theories of drinking and alcoholism*. New York: Guilford Press.

Agosti, V., Nunes, E., & Levin, F. (2002). Rates of psychiatric comorbidity among U.S. residents with lifetime cannabis dependence. *American Journal of Drug and Alcohol Abuse, 28*, 643–652.

Agrawal, A., Neale, M. C., Prescott, C. A., & Kendler, K. S. (2004). Cannabis and other illicit drugs: Comorbid use and abuse/dependence in males and females. *Behavioral Genetics, 34*(3), 217–228.

Alcoholics Anonymous. (1976). *The story of how many thousands of men and women have recovered from alcoholism* [the "Big Book"]. New York: AA World Services.

Alcoholics Anonymous. (1981). *Twelve steps and twelve traditions*. New York: AA World Services.

Alexander, B. K. (1988). The disease and adaptive models of addiction: A framework evaluation. In S. Peele (Ed.), *Visions of addiction: Major contemporary perspectives on addiction and alcoholism*. Lexington, MA: D.C. Heath.

Alexander, J., & Barton, C. (1995). Family therapy research. In R. H. Mikesell, D.D. Lusterman, & S. H. McDaniel (Eds.), *Integrating family therapy: Handbook of family psychology and systems theory*. Washington, DC: American Psychological Association.

Alterman, A. I., Searles, J. S., & Hall, J. G. (1989). Failure to find differences in drinking behavior as a function of familial risk for alcoholism: A replication. *Journal of Abnormal Psychology, 98*, 50–53.

American Hospital Association. (1995). *AHA hospital statistics* (1994–1995 ed.). Chicago: Author.

American Psychiatric Association. (1980). *Diagnostic and statistical manual of mental disorders* (3rd ed.). Washington, DC: Author.

American Psychiatric Association. (1994). *Diagnostic and statistical manual of mental disorders*. (4th ed.). Washington, DC: Author.

American Psychiatric Association. (2000). *Diagnostic and statistical manual of mental disorders* (4th ed., text rev.). Washington, DC: Author.

Anglin, M.D. (1988). The efficacy of civil commitment in treating narcotic addiction. In C. G. Leukefeld & F. M. Tims (Eds.), *Compulsory treatment of drug abuse: Research and clinical practice* (NIDA Research Monograph 86; DHHS Publication No. ADM 88–1578). Washington, DC: U.S. Government Printing Office.

Anglin, M. D., Brecht, M. L., Woodward, J. A., & Bonett, D. G. (1986). An empirical study of maturing out: Conditional factors. *International Journal of the Addictions, 21*(2), 233–246.

Anthenelli, R. M., & Tabakoff, B. (1995). Hypothesized subtypes of alcoholism. *Alcohol Health and Research World, 19*(3), 178.

Armstrong, T. D., & Costello, E. J. (2002). Community studies on adolescent substance use, abuse, or dependence and psychiatric comorbidity. *Journal of Consulting and Clinical Psychology, 70*, 1224–1239.

Azrin, N.H. (1976). Improvements in the community-reinforcement approach to alcoholism. *Behaviour Research and Therapy, 14*, 3 39–348.

Backer, T. E., David, S. L., & Soucy, G. (1995). *Reviewing the behavioral science knowledge base on technology transfer* (NIDA Research Monograph 155; NIH Publication No. 95-4035). Rockville, MD: National Clearinghouse on Alcohol and Drug Information.

Baer, J. S., Stacy, A., & Larimer, M. (1991). Biases in the perception of drinking norms among college students. *Journal of Studies on Alcohol, 52*(6), 580–586.

Baker, E .A., & Beck, K. (1991). Ignition interlocks for DWI offenders: A useful tool. *Alcohol, Drugs and Driving, 7*(2), 107–115.

Bales, F. (1980). Cultural differences in roles of alcoholism. In D. Ward (Ed.), *Alcholism: Introduction to theory and treatment.* Dubuque, IA: Kendall/Hunt.

Bandura, A. (1971). Analysis of modelling processes. In A. Bandura (Ed.), *Psychological modelling: Conflicting models.* Chicago: Aldine-Atherton.

Bandura, A. (1977). *Social learning theory.* Englewood Cliffs, NJ: Prentice-Hall.

Bandura, A. (1995). Exercise of personal and collective efficacy in changing societies. In A. Bandura (Ed.), *Self-efficacy in changing societies.* New York: Cambridge University Press.

Bandura, A. (1997). *Self-efficacy: The exercise of control.* New York: Freeman.

Barnard, C. P. (1981). *Families, alcoholism, and therapy.* Springfield, IL: Charles C. Thomas.

Barnes, G. M. (1990). Impact of the family on adolescent drinking patterns. In R. L. Collins, K. E. Leonard, B. A. Miller, & JS. Searles (Eds.), *Alcohol and the family: Research and clinical perspectives.* New York: Guilford Press.

Barnes, G. M., Farrell, M. P., & Cairns, A. L. (1986). Parental socialization factors and adolescent drinking behaviors. *Journal of Marriage and the Family, 48*, 27–36.

Barnes, G. M., & Windle, M. (1987). Family factors in adolescent alcohol and drug abuse. *Pediatrician: International Journal of Child and Adolescent Health, 14*, 13–18.

Beattie, M. (1987). *Co-dependent no more.* Center City, MN: Hazelden.

Beck, K. H., Thombs, D. L., & Summons, T. G. (1993). The social context of drinking scales: Construct validation and relationship to indicants of abuse in an adolescent population. *Addictive Behaviors, 18,* 159–163.

Begleiter, H., Porjesz, B., Bihari, B., & Kissin, B. (1984). Event-related potentials in boys at risk for alcoholism. *Science, 225,* 1493–1496.

Begleiter, H., Porjesz, B., Reich, T., Edenberg, H.J., Goate, A., Blangero, J., et al. (1998). Quantitative trait loci analysis of human event-related brain potentials: P3 voltage. *Electroencephalography and Clinical Neurophysiology, 108,* 244–250.

Begleiter, H., Reich, T., Hesselbrock, V., Porjesz, B., Li, T., Schuckit, M. A., et al. (1995). The collaborative study on the genetics of alcoholism. *Alcohol Health and Research World, 19*(3), 228–236.

Bell, A., & Rollnick, S. (1996). Motivational interviewing in practice: A structured approach. In F. Rotgers, D. S. Keller, & J. Morgenstern (Eds.), *Treating substance abuse: Theory and technique.* New York: Guilford Press.

Bennett, L. A., Wolin, S. J., & Reiss, D. (1988). Cognitive, behavioral, and emotional problems among school-age children of alcoholic parents. *American Journal of Psychiatry, 145*(2), 185–190.

Berkowitz, A. D. (1997). From reactive to proactive prevention: Promoting an ecology of health on campus. In P. C. Rivers & E. R. Shore (Eds.), *Substance abuse on campus: A handbook for college and university personnel.* Westport, CT: Greenwood Press.

Bernstein, J., Bernstein, E., Tassiopoulos, K., Heeren, T., Levenson, S., & Hingson, R. (2005). Brief motivational interview at a clinic visit reduces cocaine and heroin use. *Drug and Alcohol Dependence, 77,* 49–59.

Bewley-Taylor, D. R. (2004). Harm reduction and the global drug control regime: Contemporary problems and future prospects. *Drug and Alcohol Review, 23,* 483–489.

Bickel, W. K., & Marsch, L. A. (2001). Toward a behavioral economic understanding of drug dependence: Delay discounting processes. *Addiction, 96,* 73–86.

Bierut, L. J., Dinwiddie, S. H., Begleiter, H., Crowe, R. R., Hesselbrock, V., Nurnberger, J. I., et al. (1998). Familial transmission of substance dependence: Alcohol, marijuana, cocaine, and habitual smoking. A report from the Collaborative Study on the Genetics of Alcoholism. *Archives of General Psychiatry, 55,* 982–988.

Bigelow, W., & Liebson, J. (1972). Cost factors controlling alcoholic drinking. *Psychological Record, 22,* 305–314.

Bolles, R. C. (1972). Reinforcement, expectancy, and learning. *Psychological Review, 79,* 394–409.

Botvin, G. J. (2004). Advancing prevention science and practice: Challenges, critical issues, and future directions. *Prevention Science, 5*(1), 69–72.

Botvin, G. J., Baker, E., Botvin, E. M., Filazzola, A. D., & Millman, R. B. (1984). Prevention of alcohol misuse through the development of personal and social competence: A pilot study. *Journal of Studies on Alcohol, 45,* 550–552.

Botvin, G. J., Baker, E., Dusenbury, L., Botvin, E. M., & Diaz, T. (1995). Long-term follow-up results of a randomized drug abuse prevention trial in a white middle-class population. *Journal of the American Medical Association, 273*(14), 1106–1112.

Botvin, G. J., Baker, E., Dusenbury, L., Tortu, S., & Botvin, E. M. (1990). Preventing adolescent drug abuse through a multimodal cognitive-behavioral approach: Results of a three-year study. *Journal of Consulting and Clinical Psychology, 58,* 437–446.

Botvin, G. J., Dusenbury, L., Baker, E., James-Ortiz, S., Botvin, E. M., & Kerner, J. (1992). Smoking prevention among urban minority youth: Assessing effects on outcome and mediating variables. *Health Psychology, 11,* 290–299.

Botvin, G. J., & Eng, A. (1982). The efficacy of a multi-component approach to the prevention of cigarette smoking. *Preventive Medicine, 11,* 199–211.

Botvin, G. J., Eng, A., & Williams C. L. (1980). Preventing the onset of cigarette smoking through life skills training. *Preventive Medicine, 9,* 135–143.

Botvin, G. J., Griffin, K. W., Diaz, T., & Ifill-Williams, M. (2001). Drug abuse prevention among minority adolescents: Posttest and one-year follow-up of a school-based preventive intervention. *Prevention Science, 2,* 1–13.

Botvin, G. J., Griffin, K. W., Paul, E., & Macaulay, A. P. (2003). Preventing tobacco and alcohol use among elementary school students through Life Skills Training. *Journal of Child and Adolescent Substance Abuse, 12,* 1–18.

Botvin, G. J., Renick, N. L., & Baker, E. (1983). The effects of scheduling format and booster sessions on a broad-spectrum psychosocial smoking prevention program. *Journal of Behavioral Medicine, 6,* 359–379.

Bowen, M. (1976). Theory in the practice of psychotherapy. In P. J. Guerin (Ed.), *Family therapy: Theory and practice.* New York: Gardner Press.

Bradley-Springer, L. (1996). Patient education for behavior change: Help from the transtheoretical and harm reduction models. *Journal of the Association of Nurses in AIDS Care, 7,* 23–33.

Brecht, M. L., & Anglin, M. D. (1990). Conditional factors of maturing out: Legal supervision and treatment. *International Journal of the Addictions, 25*(4), 393–407.

Brecht, M. L., Anglin, M. D., Woodward, J. A., & Bonett, D. G. (1987). Conditional factors of maturing out: Personal resources and preaddiction sociopathy. *International Journal of the Addictions, 22*(1), 55–69.

Brick, J. (1990). Learning and motivational factors in alcohol consumption. In W. M. Cox (Ed.), *Why people drink: Parameters of alcohol as a reinforcer.* New York: Gardner Press.

Brickman, B. (1988). Psychoanalysis and substance abuse: Toward a more effective approach. *Journal of the American Academy of Psychoanalysis, 16*(3), 359–379.

Brook, J. S., Whiteman, M., Gordon, A. S., & Brenden, C. (1983). Older brother's influence on younger sibling's drug use. *Journal of Psychology, 114,* 83–90.

Brown, B. S. (1995). Reducing impediments to technology transfer in drug abuse programming. In T. E. Backer, S. L. David, & G. Soucy (Eds.), *Reviewing the behavioral science knowledge base on technology transfer* (NIDA Research Monograph 155; NIH Publication No. 95-4035). Rockville, MD: National Clearinghouse on Alcohol and Drug Information.

Brown, S. A. (1985). Expectancies versus background in the prediction of college drinking patterns. *Journal of Consulting and Clinical Psychology, 53*(1), 123–130.

Brown, S. A. (1995). *Treating alcoholism.* San Francisco: Jossey-Bass.

Brown, S. A., Christiansen, B. A., & Goldman, M. S. (1987a). The Alcohol Expectancy Questionnaire: An instrument for the assessment of adolescent and adult alcohol expectancies. *Journal of Studies on Alcohol, 48*(5), 483–491.

Brown, S. A., Creamer, V. A., & Stetson, B. A. (1987b). Adolescent alcohol expectancies as a function of personal and parental drinking patterns. *Journal of Abnormal Psychology, 96,* 177–121.

Brownson, R. C., Baker, E. A., & Kreuter, M. W. (2001). Prevention research partnerships in community settings: What are we learning? *Journal of Public Health Management and Practice, 7*(2), vii–ix.

Brunette, M. F., Drake, R. E., Woods, M., & Hartnett, T. (2001). A comparison of long-term and short-term residential treatment programs for dual diagnosis patients. *Psychiatric Services, 52,* 526–528.

Brunette, M. F., Mueser, K. T., & Drake, R. E. (2004). A review of research on residential programs for people with severe mental illness and co-occurring substance use disorders. *Drug and Alcohol Review, 23,* 471–481.

Bryant, A. I., Schulenberg, J., Bachman, J. G., O'Malley, P. M., & Johnston, L. D. (2000). Understanding the links among school misbehavior, academic achievement, and cigarette use: A national panel study of adolescents. *Prevention Science, 1,* 71–87.

Bunker, J. P., Frazier, H. S., & Mosteller, F. (1994). Improving health: Measuring effects of medical care. *Milbank Quarterly, 72,* 225–258.

Burling, T. A., Reilly, P. M., Moltzen, J. O., & Ziff, D. C. (1989). Self-efficacy and relapse among inpatient drug and alcohol abusers: A predictor of outcome. *Journal of Studies on Alcohol, 50,* 354–360.

Burnside, M. A., Baer, P. E., McLaughlin, R. J., & Pokorny, A. D. (1986). Alcohol use by adolescents in disrupted families. *Alcoholism, Clinical and Experimental Research, 10,* 274–278.

Cameron, D., & Spence, M. (1976). Recruitment of problem drinkers. *British Journal of Psychiatry, 11,* 544–546.

Canto, M. (1997, January 2). Drink sickens concertgoers in L.A.; 31 go to hospitals. *Associated Press.*

Cappell, H., & Greeley, J. (1987). Alcohol and tension reduction: An update on research and theory. In H. T. Blane & K. E. Leonard (Eds.), *Psychological theories of drinking and alcoholism.* New York: Guilford Press.

Carey, K. B. (1995). Treatment of substance use disorders and schizophrenia. In A.F. Lehman & L. B. Dixon (Eds.), *Double jeopardy: Chronic mental illness and substance use disorders.* Chur, Switzerland: Harwood Academic.

Carmelli, D., Swan, G. E., Robinette, D., & Fabsitz, R. (1992). Genetic influence on smoking—A study of male twins. *New England Journal of Medicine, 327*(12), 829–833.

Cashin, J. R., Presley, C. A., & Meilman, P. W. (1998). Alcohol use in the greek system: Follow the leader? *Journal of Studies on Alcohol, 59,* 63–70.

Catalano, R. F., Berglund, M. L., Ryan, J. A. M., Lonczak, H. S., & Hawkins, J. D. (1998a). *Positive youth development in the United States: Research findings on evaluations of positive youth development programs.* Paper funded by and submitted to U.S. Department of Health and Human Services, Office of the

Assistant Secretary for Planning and Evaluation and National Institute for Child Health and Human Development. Available: at aspe.os.dhhs.gov/hsp/PositiveYouthDev99. Accessed on December 14, 2004.

Catalano, R. F., & Hawkins, J. D. (1996). The social development model: A theory of antisocial behavior. In J. D. Hawkins (Ed.), *Delinquency and crime: Current theories.* New York: Cambridge University Press.

Catalano, R. F., Kosterman, R., Haggerty, K., Hawkins, J. D., & Spoth, R. L. (1998b). A universal intervention for the prevention of substance abuse: Preparing for the drug-free years. In R. S. Ashery, E. B. Robertson, & K. L. Kumpfer (Eds.), *Drug abuse prevention through family interventions* (NIDA Research Monograph 177; NIH Publication No. 97-4135). Rockville, MD: National Institutes of Health, U.S. Department of Health and Human Services.

Caudill, B., & Hoffman, J.A. (1994, August). *Cocaine expectancies and treatment outcomes among crack users.* Paper presented at the annual meeting of the American Psychological Association, Los Angeles.

Caudill, B. D., & Marlatt, G. A. (1975). Modeling influences in social drinking: An experimental analogue. *Journal of Consulting and Clinical Psychology, 43*(3), 405–415.

Caulkins, J. P., Rydell, C. P., Schwabe, W. L., & Chiesa, J. (1997). *Mandatory minimum sentences: Throwing away the key or the taxpayers' money?* Santa Monica, CA: Rand Drug Policy Research Center.

Center for Substance Abuse Treatment. (1997). *The national treatment improvement evaluation study* (DHHS Publication No. SMA 97-3154). Rockville, MD: Substance Abuse and Mental Health Services Administration.

Centers for Disease Control and Prevention. (1987). Progress in chronic disease prevention cigarette smoking in the United States, 1986, September 11. *Morbidity and Mortality Weekly Report, 36*(12), 581–585.

Centers for Disease Control and Prevention. (1994). *Preventing tobacco use among young people: A report of the Surgeon General.* Atlanta: U.S. Department of Health and Human Services. Available at www.cdc.gov/tobacco/sgr. Accessed on January 4, 2005.

Centers for Disease Control and Prevention. (1999). Ten great public health achievements—United States, 1990–1999, April 2. *Morbidity and Mortality Weekly Report, 48*(12), 241–243.

Centers for Disease Control and Prevention. (2004a). Methodology of the Youth Risk Behavior Surveillance System. *Morbidity and Mortality Weekly Report, 53*(RR-12), 1–12.

Centers for Disease Control and Prevention. (2004b). Surveillance summaries, May 21. *Morbidity and Mortality Weekly Report, 53*(SS-2), 51, 57, 59, 61.

Centers for Disease Control and Prevention. (2004c). *HIV/AIDS Surveillance Report, 2003* (Vol. 15). Atlanta: U.S. Department of Health and Human Services, Centers for Disease Control and Prevention. Available at www.cdc.gov/hiv/stats/hasrlink.htm. Accessed on May 7, 2005.

Channing Bete Company. (2005). *Positive youth development.* Available at www.channing-bete.com/positiveyouth. Accessed on January 3, 2005.

Chassin, L., Rogosch, F., & Barrera, M. (1991). Substance use and symptomatology among adolescent children of alcoholics. *Journal of Abnormal Psychology,* *100,* 449–463.

Chen, K., & Kandel, D. B. (1995). The natural history of drug use from adolescence to the mid-thirties in a general population sample. *American Journal of Public Health, 85*(1), 41–47.

Chou, C. P., Montgomery, S., Pentz, M., Rohrbach, L. A., Johnson, C. A., Flay, B. R., et al. (1998). Effects of a community-based prevention program on decreasing drug use in high-risk adolescents. *American Journal of Public Health, 88,* 944–948.

Christian, C. M., Dufour, M., & Bertolucci, D. (1989). Differential alcohol-related mortality among American Indian tribes in Oklahoma. *Social Science and Medicine, 28,* 275–284.

Christiansen, B. A., Roehling, P. V., Smith, G. T., & Goldman, M. S. (1989). Using alcohol expectancies to predict adolescent drinking behavior after one year. *Journal of Consulting and Clinical Psychology, 57*(1), 93–99.

Clayton, R. R., Leukefeld, C. G., Harrington, N. G., & Cattarello, A. (1996). DARE (Drug Abuse Resistance Education): Very popular but not very effective. In C.B. McCoy, L.R. Metsch, & J.A. Inciardi (Eds.), *Intervening with drug involved youth.* Beverly Hills, CA: Sage.

Cloninger, C. R. (1987). Neurogenetic adaptive mechanisms in alcoholism. *Science, 236,* 410–416.

Cohen, H. L., Wang, W., Porjesz, B., & Begleiter, H. (1995). Auditory P300 in young alcoholics: Regional response characteristics. *Alcoholism, Clinical and Experimental Research, 19*(2),469–475.

Cohen, M., Liebson, J., Fallace, L., & Allen, R. (1971a). Moderate drinking by chronic alcoholics: A schedule-dependent phenomenon. *Journal of Nervous and Mental Disease, 153,* 434–444.

Cohen, M., Liebson, J., Fallace, L., & Speers, W. (1971b). Alcoholism: Controlled drinking and incentives for abstinence. *Psychological Reports, 28,* 575–580.

Coleman, J. C., Butcher, J. N., & Carson, R. C. (1980). *Abnormal psychology and modern life* (6th ed.). Glenview, IL: Scott, Foresman.

Collins, F. S., & Fink L. (1995). Tools of genetic research: The human genome project. *Alcohol Health and Research World, 19,* 190–195.

Collins, R. L. (1990). Family treatment of alcohol abuse: Behavioral and systems perspectives. In R. L. Collins, K. E. Leonard, B. A. Miller, & J. S. Searles (Eds.), *Alcohol and the family: Research and clinical perspectives.* New York: Guilford Press.

Collins, R. L., Parks, G. A., & Marlatt, G. A. (1985). Social determinants of alcohol consumption: The effects of social interaction and model status on the self-administration of alcohol. *Journal of Consulting and Clinical Psychology, 53*(2), 189–200.

COMMIT Research Group. (1995a). Community intervention trial for smoking cessation (COMMIT): I. Cohort results from a four-year community intervention. *American Journal of Public Health, 85*(2), 183–192.

COMMIT Research Group. (1995b). Community intervention trial for smoking cessation (COMMIT): I. Changes in adult cigarette smoking prevalence. *American Journal of Public Health, 85*(2), 193–200.

Conger, J. J. (1951). The effects of alcohol on conflict and avoidance behavior. *Quarterly Journal of Studies on Alcohol, 12,* 1–29.

Conger, J. J. (1956). Alcoholism: Theory, problem, and challenge. II. Reinforcement theory and the dynamics of alcoholism. *Quarterly Journal of Studies on Alcohol, 13,* 296–305.

Connors, G. R., & Tarbox, A. R. (1985). Macroenvironmental factors as determinants of substance use and abuse. In M. Galizio & S. A. Maisto (Eds.), *Determinants of substance abuse: Biological, psychological, and environmental factors.* New York: Plenum Press.

Conrad, K. M., Flay, B. R., & Hill, D. (1992). Why children start smoking: Predictors of onset. *British Journal of Addiction, 87,* 1711–1724.

Conrad, P. (1992). Medicalization and social control. *Annual Review of Sociology, 18,* 209–232.

Conrad, P., & Schneider, J. W. (1992). *Deviance and medicalization: From badness to sickness.* Philadelphia: Temple University Press.

Cox, W. M. (1985). Personality correlates of substance abuse. In M. Galizio & S. A. Maisto (Eds.), *Determinants of substance abuse.* New York: Plenum Press.

Critchlow, B. (1987). Brief report: A utility analysis of drinking. *Addictive Behaviors, 12,* 269–273.

Crowley, T. J. (1984). Contingency contracting treatment of drug-abusing physicians, nurses, and dentists. In J. Grabowski, M.L. Stitzer, & J. E. Henningfield (Eds.), *Behavioral intervention techniques in drug abuse* (NIDA Research Monograph 46; DHHS Publication No. ADM 86-1282). Washington, DC: U.S. Government Printing Office.

Croyle, R. T., & Lerman C. (1995). Psychological impact of genetic testing. In R. T. Croyle (Ed.), *Psychosocial effects of screening for disease prevention and detection.* New York: Oxford University Press.

Cummings, K. M., Hyland, A., Saunders-Martin, T., Perla, J., Coppola, P. R., & Pechacek, T. F. (1998). Evoluation of an enforcement program to reduce tobacco sales to minors. *American Journal of Public Health, 88,* 932–936.

Dent, C. W., Sussman, S., & Stacy, A. W. (2001). Project Towards No Drug Abuse: Generalizability to a general high school sample. *Preventive Medicine, 32,* 514–520.

Dermen, K. H., Cooper, M. L., & Agocha, V. B. (1998). Sex-related alcohol expectancies as moderators of the relationship between alcohol use and risky sex in adolescents. *Journal of Studies on Alcohol, 59,* 71–77.

Des Jarlais, D. C. (2000). Prospects for a public health perspective on psychoactive drug use. *American Journal of Public Health, 90*(3), 335–337.

Des Jarlais, D. C., Hagan, H., Friedman, S. R., Goldberg, D., Frischer, M., Green, S., et al. (1995). Maintaining low HIV seroprevalence in populations of injecting drug users. *Journal of the American Medical Association, 274,* 1226–1231.

Deutsch, C. (1982). *Broken bottles, broken dreams: Understanding and helping the children of alcoholics.* New York: Teachers College Press.

Diamond, M. A. (1995). Organizational change as human process, not technique. In T.E. Backer, S. L. David, & G. Soucy (Eds.), *Reviewing the behavioral science knowledge base on technology transfer* (NIDA Research Monograph

155; NIH Publication No. 95-4035). Rockville, MD: National Clearinghouse on Alcohol and Drug Information.

Dickey, B., & Azeni, H. (1996). Persons with dual diagnoses of substance abuse and major mental illness: Their excess costs of psychiatric care. *American Journal of Public Health, 86*, 973–977.

DiClemente C. C. (1991). Motivational interviewing and the stages of change. In W. R. Miller & S. Rollnick (Eds.), *Motivational interviewing: Preparing people to change addictive behavior.* New York: Guilford Press.

DiClemente C. C., & Prochaska JO. (1985). Processes and stages of change: Coping and competence in smoking behavior change. In S. Shiffman & T. A. Wills (Eds.), *Coping and substance abuse.* New York: Academic Press.

DiClemente, C. C., Prochaska, J. O., Fairhurst, S. K., Velicer, W. F., Velasquez, M. M., & Rossi, J. S. (1991). The process of smoking cessation: An analysis of precontemplation, contemplation, and preparation stages of change. *Journal of Consulting and Clinical Psychology, 59*(2), 295–304.

Dishion, T. J., & Loeber, R. (1985). Adolescent marijuana and alcohol use: The role of parents and peers revisited. *American Journal of Drug and Alcohol Abuse, 11*, 11–25.

Dolan, M. P., Black, J. L., Penk, W. E., Robinowitz, R., & DeFord, H. A. (1985). Contracting for treatment termination to reduce illicit drug use among methadone maintenance treatment failures. *Journal of Consulting and Clinical Psychology, 53*(4), 549–551.

Donchin, E., & Coles, M G. (1988). Is the P300 component a manifestation of context updating? *Behavioral & Brain Sciences, 11*(3), 357–427.

Doweiko, H. E. (1993). *Concepts of chemical dependency* (2nd ed.). Pacific Grove, CA: Brooks/Cole.

Drake, R. E., Essock, S. M., Shaner, A., Carey, K. B., Minkoff, K., Kola, L., et al. (2001). Implementing dual diagnosis services for clients with severe mental illness. *Psychiatric Services, 52*, 469–476.

Drake, R. E., Mercer-McFadden, C., Mueser, K. T., McHugo, G. J., & Bond, G. R. (1998). Review of integrated mental health and substance abuse treatment for patients with dual disorders. *Schizophrenia Bulletin, 24*, 589–608.

Drake, R. E., & Mueser, K. T. (2000). Psychosocial approaches to dual diagnosis. *Schizophrenia Bulletin, 26*, 105–118.

Drake, R. E., & Mueser, K. T. (2001). Managing comorbid schizophrenia and substance abuse. *Current Psychiatry Reports, 3*, 418–422.

Drake, R. E., Osher, F. C., & Wallach, M. A. (1991). Homelessness and dual diagnosis. *American Psychologist, 46*, 1149–1159.

Drake, R. E., & Wallach, M. A. (1999). Homelessness and mental illness: A story of failure. *Psychiatric Services, 50*, 589.

Drake, R. E., Wallach, M. A., Alverson, H. S., & Mueser, K. T. (2002). Psychosocial aspects of substance abuse by clients with severe mental illness. *Journal of Nervous and Mental Disease, 190*, 100–106.

Drake, R. E., Xie, H., McHugo, G. J., & Green, A. I. (2000). The effects of clozapine on alcohol and drug use disorders among patients with schizophrenia. *Schizophrenia Bulletin, 26*, 441–449.

Duffy, J. (1992). *The sanitarians: A history of American public health*. Urbana: University of Illinois Press.

Dunn, M. E., & Goldman, M. S. (1996). Empirical modeling of an alcohol expectancy memory network in elementary school children as a function of grade. *Experimental and Clinical Psychopharmacology, 4*(1), 1–9.

Dunn, N. J., Jacob, T., Hummon, N., & Seilhammer, R. A. (1987). Marital stability in alcoholic-spouse relationships as a function of drinking pattern and location. *Journal of Abnormal Psychology, 96*(2), 99–107.

Dustin, R., & George, R. (1973). *Action counseling for behavior change*. New York: Intext Press.

Egami, Y., Ford, D. E., Greenfield, S. F., & Crum, R. M. (1996). Psychiatric profile and sociodemographic characteristics of adults who report physically abusing or neglecting children. *American Journal of Psychiatry, 153*(7), 921–928.

Ellickson, P. L., Bell, R. M., & McGuigan, K. (1993). Preventing adolescent drug use: Long-term results of a junior high program. *American Journal of Public Health, 83*, 856–861.

Elliot, J. (1995, March). Drug prevention placebo: How DARE wastes time money, and police. *Reason, 26*, 14–21.

Elliott, D. S., Morse, B. J., & Mihalic, S. W. (1993). *In-vehicle BAC test devices as a deterrent to DUI, final Report*. Rockville, MD: National Institute on Alcohol Abuse and Alcoholism.

Ellis, A., McInerney, J. J., DiGiuseppe, R., & Yeager, R. J. (1988). *Rational-emotive therapy with alcoholics and substance abusers*. Elmsford, NY: Pergamon Press.

Ellis, D. A., Zucker, R. A., & Fitzgerald, H. E. (1997). The role of family influences in development and risk. *Alcohol Health and Research World, 21*(3), 218–226.

Emery, S., Gilpin, E. A., Ake, C., Farkas, A. J., & Pierce, J. P. (2000). Characterizing and identifying "hard-core" smokers: Implications for further reducing smoking prevalence. *American Journal of Public Health, 90*(3), 387–394.

Engs, R. C., & Hanson, D. J. (1993). Drinking games and problems related to drinking among moderate and heavy drinkers. *Psychological Reports, 73*, 115–120.

Ennett, S. T., Ringwalt, C. L., Thorne, J., Rohrbach, L. A., Vincus, A., Simons-Rudolph, A., et al. (2003). A comparison of current practice in school-based substance use prevention programs with meta-analytic findings. *Prevention Science, 4*, 1–14.

Ennett, S. T., Tobler, N. S., Ringwalt, C. L., & Flewelling, R. L. (1994). How effective is drug abuse resistance education? A meta-analysis of Project DARE outcome evaluations. *American Journal of Public Health, 84*, 1394–1401.

Epping-Jordan, M. P., Watkins, S. S., Koob, G. F., & Markou, A. (1998). Dramatic decreases in brain reward function during nicotine withdrawal. *Nature, 393*, 76–79.

Erickson, P. A., Riley, D. M., Cheung, Y. W., & O'Hare, P. A. (1997). *Harm reduction: A new direction for drug policies and programs*. Toronto: University of Toronto Press.

Eysenck, H. J. (1981). *A model for personality*. Berlin: Springer-Verlag.

Faraone, S. V., Tsuang, M. T., & Tsuang, D. W. (1999). *Genetics of mental disorders: A guide for students, clinicians, and researchers.* New York: Guilford Press.

Fielding, J. E., Tye, G., & Ogawa, M. (2002). Los Angeles County Drug Court Programs: Initial results. *Journal of Substance Abuse Treatment, 23,* 217–224.

Fields, R. (1995). *Drugs in perspective* (2nd ed.). Madison, WI: WCB/Brown & Benchmark.

Fillmore, K. M. (1987a). Prevalence, incidence and chronicity of drinking patterns and problems among men as a function of age: A longitudinal and cohort analysis. *British Journal of Addiction, 82,* 77–83.

Fillmore, K. M. (1987b). Women's drinking across the adult life course as compared to men's. *British Journal of Addiction, 82,* 801–811.

Fillmore, K. M., & Midanik, L. (1984). Chronicity of drinking problems among men: A longitudinal study. *Journal of Studies on Alcohol, 45,* 228–236.

Fingarette, H. (1988). *Heavy drinking: The myth of alcoholism as a disease.* Berkeley: University of California Press.

Fisher, E. B., Auslander, W. F., Munro, J. F., Arfken, C. L., Brownson, R. C., & Owens, N. W. (1998). Neighbors for a smoke-free north side: Evaluation of a community organization approach to promoting smoking cessation among African-Americans. *American Journal of Public Health, 88,* 1658–1663.

Fisher, G. L., & Harrison, T. C. (1997). *Substance abuse: Information for school counselors, social workers, therapists, and counselors.* Boston: Allyn & Bacon.

Flay, B. R., & Allred, C. G. (2003). Long-term effects of the Positive Action Program. *American Journal of Health Behavior, 27*(Suppl. 1), S6–S21.

Fogarty, T. (1976). Marital crisis. In P. J. Guerin (Ed.), *Family therapy: Theory and practice.* New York: Gardner Press.

Ford, J. M., White, P., Lim, K. O., & Pfefferbaum, A. (1994). Schizophrenics have fewer and smaller P300's: A single trial analysis. *Biological Psychiatry, 35,* 96–103.

Forst, B. (1995). Prosecution and sentencing. In J.Q. Wilson & J. Petersilia (Eds.), *Crime.* San Francisco: Institute for Contemporary Studies.

Forster, J. L., Murray, D. M., Wolfson, M., Blaine, T. M., Wagenaar, A. C., & Hennrikus, D. J. (1998). The effects of community policies to reduce youth access to tobacco. *American Journal of Public Health, 88*(8), 1193–1198.

Framo, J. L. (1976). Family of origin as a therapeutic resource for adults in marital and family therapy: You can and should go home again. *Family Process, 15,* 193-209.

Frankish, C. J., George, A., Daniel, M., Doyle-Waters, M., Walker, M., & Members of the BC Consortium for Health Promotion Research. (1997). *Participatory health promotion research in Canada: A community guidebook.* Ottawa, Ontario, Canada: Minister of Public Works and Government Services.

Freud, S. (1953). The interpretation of dreams. In J. Strachey (Ed. and trans.), *The standard edition of the complete psychological works of Sigmund Freud* (Vols. 4 and 5). London: Hogarth Press. (Original work published 1900)

Friedman, G. D. (1987). *Primer of epidemiology* (3rd ed.). New York: McGraw-Hill.

Friedman, S. R., Jose, B., Deren, S., Des Jarlais, D. C., & Neaigus, A. (1995). Risk factors for human immunodeficiency virus seroconversion among out-of-treat-ment drug injectors in high and low seroprevalence cities. The National AIDS Research Consortium. *American Journal of Epidemiology, 142,* 864–874.

Gabbard, G. O. (1999). Psychodynamic therapy in an age of neuroscience. *The Harvard Mental Health Letter, 15*(7), 4–5.

Gans, H. J. (1962). *The urban villagers.* New York: Free Press.

Gardner, E. L. (1992). Brain reward mechanisms. In J. H. Lowinson, P. Ruiz, R. B. Millman, & J. G. Langrod (Eds.), *Substance abuse: A comprehensive textbook* (2nd ed.). Baltimore: Williams & Wilkins.

Gay, P. (1988). *Freud: A life for our time.* New York: Norton.

Gemson, D. H., Moats, H. L., Watkins, B. X., Ganz, M. L., Robinson, S., & Healton, E. (1998). Laying down the law: Reducing illegal tobacco sales to minors in central Harlem. *American Journal of Public Health, 88,* 936–939.

George, R. L. (1990). *Counseling the chemically dependent: Theory and practice.* Englewood Cliffs, NJ: Prentice-Hall.

George, R. L., & Cristiani, T. S. (1995). *Counseling: Theory and practice.* Needham Heights, MA: Allyn & Bacon.

Glassner, B., & Berg, B. (1980). How Jews avoid drinking problems. *American Sociological Review, 45,* 647–664.

Goldman, D., & Bergen, A. (1998). General and specific inheritance of substance abuse and alcoholism. *Archives of General Psychiatry, 55,* 964–965.

Goldman, M. S., Brown, S .A., & Christiansen, B.A. (1987). Expectancy theory: Thinking about drinking. In H. T. Blane & K. E. Leonard (Eds.), *Psychological theories of drinking and alcoholism.* New York: Guilford Press.

Goode, E. (1993). *Drugs in American society* (4th ed.). New York: McGraw-Hill.

Goodman, R. W. (1987). Adult children of alcoholics. *Journal of Counseling and Development, 66,* 162–163.

Goodwin, D. W. (1990). Genetic determinants of reinforcements from alcohol. In W.M. Cox (Ed.), *Why people drink: Parameters of alcohol as a reinforcer.* New York: Gardner Press.

Gotham, H. J., & Sher, K. J. (1996). Do codependent traits involve more than just basic dimensions of personality and psychopathology? *Journal of Studies on Alcohol, 57,* 34–39.

Gotham, H. J., Sher, K. J., & Wood, P. K. (1997). Predicting stability and change in frequency of intoxication from the college years to beyond: Individual-differ-ence and role transition variables. *Journal of Abnormal Psychology, 106*(4), 619–629.

Gough, J. B. (1881). *Sunlight and shadow.* Hartford, CT: Worthington.

Grant, B. F., & Dawson, D. A. (1997). Age of onset of alcohol use and its associa-tion with DSM-IV Alcohol Abuse and Dependence: Results from the National Longitudinal Alcohol Epidemiologic Survey. *Journal of Substance Abuse, 9,* 103–110.

Grant, B. F., Hasin, D. S., Chou, S. P., Stinson, F. S., & Dawson, D. A. (2004a). Nic-otine dependence and psychiatric disorders in the United States: Results from the National Epidemiologic Survey on Alcohol and Related Conditions. *Archives of General Psychiatry, 61,* 1107–1115.

Grant, B. F., Stinson, F. S., Dawson, D. A., Chou, S. P., Dufour, M. C., Compton, W., et al. (2004b). Prevalence and co-occurrence of substance use disorders and independent mood and anxiety disorders: Results from the National Epidemiologic Survey on Alcohol and Related Conditions. *Archives of General Psychiatry, 61,* 807–816.

Grant, B. F., Stinson, F. S., Dawson, D. A., Chou, S. P., Ruan, W. J., & Pickering, R. P. (2004c). Co-occurrence of 12-month alcohol and drug use disorders and personality disorders in the United States: Results from the National Epidemiologic Survey on Alcohol and Related Conditions. *Archives of General Psychiatry, 61,* 361–368.

Green, L. W. (1992). Promoting comprehensive interventions. In H. D. Holder & J. M. Howard (Eds.), *Community prevention trials for alcohol problems: Methodological issues* (pp. 247–250). Westport, CT: Praeger.

Green, L. W., George, M. A., Daniel, M., Frankish, C. J., Herbert, C. J., Bowie, W.R., et al. (1995). *Study of participatory research in health promotion: Review and recommendations for the development of participatory research in health promotion in Canada.* Ottawa, Ontario: Royal Society of Canada.

Green, L. W., & Kreuter, M. W. (2002). Fighting back or fighting themselves? Community coalitions against substance abuse and their use of best practices. *American Journal of Preventive Medicine, 23,* 303–306.

Green, L. W., & Mercer, S. L. (2001). Can public health researchers and agencies reconcile the push from funding bodies and the pull from communities? *American Journal of Public Health, 91*(12), 1926–1929.

Greenblatt, J.C. (1998). Practitioners should be aware of co-occurring marijuana use and delinquent/depressive behaviors among youth. (Data from the Substance Abuse and Mental Health Services Administration, Office of Applied Studies). University of Maryland–Center for Substance Abuse Research. *CESAR FAX, 7*(45), 1.

Griffin, K. W., Botvin, G. J., Nichols, T. R., & Doyle, M. (2003). Effectiveness of a universal drug abuse prevention approach for youth at high risk for substance use initiation. *Preventive Medicine, 36,* 1–7.

Group for the Advancement of Psychiatry. (1994). *Forced into treatment: The role of coercion in clinical practice.* Washington, DC: American Psychiatric Press.

Haaga, J. G., & Reuter, P. H. (1995). Prevention: The (lauded) orphan of drug policy. In R. H. Coombs & D. M. Ziedonis (Eds.), *Handbook on drug abuse prevention: A comprehensive strategy to prevent the abuse of alcohol and other drugs.* Boston: Allyn & Bacon.

Haber, J. R., & Jacob, T. (1997). Marital interactions of male versus female alcoholics. *Family Process, 36,* 385–402.

Hackett, G. (1995). Self-efficacy in career choice and development. In A. Bandura (Ed.), *Self-efficacy in changing societies.* New York: Cambridge University Press.

Hall, C. S., & Lindzey, G. (1978). *Theories of personality* (3rd ed.). New York: Wiley.

Hallfors, D., Cho, H., Livert, D., & Kadushin, C. (2002). Fighting back against substance abuse—Are community coalitions winning? *American Journal of Preventive Medicine, 23,* 237–45.

Hansen, W. B., & Graham, J. W. (1991). Preventing alcohol, marijuana, and cigarette use among adolescents: Peer pressure resistance training versus establishing conservative norms. *Preventive Medicine, 20,* 414–430.

Harburg, E., Davis, D. R., & Caplan, R. (1982). Parent and offspring alcohol use. *Journal of Studies on Alcohol, 43,* 497–516.

Harris, K. B., & Miller, W. R. (1990). Behavioral self-control training for problem drinkers: Components of efficacy. *Psychology of Addictive Behaviors, 4*(2), 82–90.

Hawkins, J. D., Catalano, R. F., & Kent, L. A. (1991). Combining broadcast media and parent education to prevent teenage drug abuse. In I. Donohew, H. E. Sypher, & W. J. Bukowski (Eds.), *Persuasive communication and drug abuse prevention.* Hillsdale, NJ: Erlbaum.

Heath, A. C., Jardine, R., & Martin, N. G. (1989). Interactive effects of genotype and social environment of alcohol consumption in female twins. *Journal of Studies on Alcohol, 50*(1), 38–48.

Heath, D. B. (1988). Emerging anthropological theory and models of alcohol use and alcoholism. In C. D. Chaudron & D. A. Wilkinson (Eds.), *Theories on alcoholism.* Toronto, Ontario, Canada: Addiction Research Foundation.

Heather, N., & Robertson, I. (1983). *Controlled drinking.* London: Methuen.

Helzer, J. E., Canino, G. J., Yeh, E. K., Bland, R. C., Lee, C. K., Hwu, H. G., et al. (1990). Alcoholism: North America and Asia. *Archives of General Psychiatry, 47*(4), 313–319.

Heuser, J. P. (1990). *A preliminary evaluation of short-term impact of the Preparing for Drug-Free Years community service program in Oregon.* Salem: Oregon Department of Justice, Crime Analysis Center.

Higgins, S. T., Alessi, S. M., & Dantona, R. L. (2002). Voucher-based incentives: A substance abuse treatment innovation. *Addictive Behaviors, 27,* 887–910.

Higgins, S. T., Budney, A. J., Bickel, W. K., Foerg, F. E., Donham, R., & Badger, G. J. (1994). Incentives improve treatment retention and cocaine abstinence in ambulatory cocaine-dependent patients. *Archives of General Psychiatry, 51,* 568–576.

Higgins, S. T., Budney, A. J., Bickel, W. K., Foerg, F. E., Ogden, D., & Badger, G. J. (1995). Outpatient behavioral treatment for cocaine dependence. *Experimental and Clinical Psychopharmacology, 3,* 205–212.

Higgins, S. T., Budney, A. J., Bickel, W. K., Hughes, J. R., Foerg, F., & Badger, G. (1993). Achieving cocaine abstinence with a behavioral approach. *American Journal of Psychiatry, 150,* 763–769.

Higgins, S. T., Delaney, D. D., Budney, A. J., Bickel, W. K., Hughes, J. R., Foerg, F., et al. (1991). A behavioral approach to achieving initial cocaine abstinence. *American Journal of Psychiatry, 148*(9), 1218–1224.

Higgins, S. T., Heil, S. H., & Lussier, J. P. (2004). Clinical implications of reinforcement as a determinant of substance use disorders. *Annual Review of Psychology, 55,* 431–461.

Higgins, S. T., Sigmon, S. C., Wong, C. J., Heil, S. H., Badger, G. J., Donham, R., et al. (2003). Community reinforcement therapy for cocaine-dependent outpatients. *Archives of General Psychiatry, 60,* 1043–1052.

Higgins, S. T., Wong, C. J., Badger, G. J., Haug-Ogden, D. E., & Dantona, R. L. (2000). Contingent reinforcement increases cocaine abstinence during outpatient treatment and one year of follow-up. *Journal of Consulting and Clinical Psychology, 68,* 64–72.

Hingson, R. W., & Howland, J. (2002). Comprehensive community interventions to promote health: Implications for college-age drinking problems. *Journal of Studies on Alcohol,* (Suppl. 14), 226–240.

Hingson, R., McGovern, T., Howland, J., & Hereen, T. (1996). Reducing alcohol-impaired driving in Massachusetts. *American Journal of Public Health, 86,* 791–797.

Holdcraft, L. C., Iacono, W. G., & McGue, M. K. (1998). Antisocial personality disorder and depression in relation to alcoholism: A community-based sample. *Journal of Studies on Alcohol, 59,* 222–226.

Holder, H. (Ed.). (1997). A community prevention trial to reduce alcohol-involved trauma. *Addiction, 92* (Suppl. No. 2), S155–S301.

Holder, H., Gruenewald, P. J., Ponicki, W. R., Treno, A. J., Grube, J. W., Saltz, R. F., et al. (2000). Effects of community-based interventions on high-risk driving and alcohol-related injuries. *Journal of the American Medical Association, 284,* 2341–2347.

Hunt, G. H., & Azrin, N. H. (1973). The community-reinforcement approach to alcoholism. *Behaviour Research and Therapy, 11,* 91–104.

Hunter, T. A., & Salmone, P. R. (1986). Dry drunk syndrome and alcoholic relapse. *Journal of Applied Rehabilitation Counseling, 18,* 22–25.

Inciardi, J. A. (1988). Some considerations on the efficacy of compulsory treatment: Reviewing the New York experience. In C. G. Leukefeld & F. M. Tims (Eds.), *Compulsory treatment of drug abuse: Research and clinical practice* (NIDA Research Monograph 86; DHHS Publication No. ADM 88-1578). Washington, DC: U.S. Government Printing Office.

Inciardi, J. A., McBride, D. C., & Rivers, J. E. (1996). *Drug control and the courts.* Thousand Oaks, CA: Sage

Ingvar, M., Ghatan, P. H., Wirsén-Meurling, A., Risberg, J., Von Heijne, G., Stone-Elander, S., et al. (1998). Alcohol activates the cerebral reward system in man. *Journal of Studies on Alcohol, 59,* 258–269.

Institute of Medicine. (1994). *Reducing risks for mental disorders: Frontiers for preventive intervention research.* Washington, DC: National Academy Press.

Jacob, T., & Leonard, K. (1986). Psychological functioning in children and alcoholic fathers, depressed fathers and control fathers. *Journal of Studies on Alcohol, 47,* 373–380.

Jang, K. J., Livesley, W. J., & Vernon, P. A. (1995). Alcohol and drug problems: A multivariate behavioural genetic analysis of co-morbidity. *Addiction, 90(9),* 1213–1221.

Jellinek, E. M. (1945). The problem of alcohol. In Yale Studies on Alcohol (Ed.), *Alcohol, science, and society.* Westport, CT: Greenwood Press.

Jellinek, E. M. (1955). The "craving" for alcohol. *Quarterly Journal of Studies on Alcohol, 16,* 35–38.

Jerusalem, M., & Mittag, W. (1995). In A. Bandura (Ed.), *Self-efficacy in changing societies.* New York: Cambridge University Press.

Jessor, R., Donovan, J. E., & Costa, F. M. (1991). *Beyond adolescence: Problem behavior and young adult development.* New York: Cambridge University Press.

Jessor, R., & Jessor, S. L. (1977). *Problem behavior and psychosocial development: A longitudinal study of youth.* New York: Academic Press.

Johnson, B. D. (1980). Toward a theory of drug subcultures. In D.J. Lettieri, M. Bayers, & H. W. Pearson (Eds.), *Theories on drug abuse: Selected contemporary perspectives* (DHHS Publication No. ADM 84-967). Washington, DC: U.S. Government Printing Office.

Johnson, V. E. (1980). *I'll quit tomorrow* (rev. ed.). San Francisco: Harper & Row.

Johnston, L. D., O'Malley, P. M., & Bachman, J. G. (1989). *Drug use, drinking, and smoking: National survey results from high school, college, and young adult populations* (DHHS Publication No. ADM 89-1638). Washington, DC: U.S. Government Printing Office.

Johnston, L. D., O'Malley, P. M., & Bachman, J. G., & Schulenberg, J. E. (2005). *Monitoring the Future national results on adolescent drug use: Overview of key findings, 2004* (NIH Publication No. 05-5726). Bethesda, MD: National Institute on Drug Abuse. Available at www.monitoringthefuture.org. Accessed on May 6, 2005.

Join Together. (1996). *Fixing a failed system.* Boston: Author.

Join Together. (1998). *Treatment for addiction: Advancing the common good.* Boston: Author.

Jones, B. T., & McMahon, J. (1994). Negative and positive alcohol expectancies as predictors of abstinence after discharge from a residential treatment program: A one-month and three-month follow-up study in men. *Journal of Studies on Alcohol, 55,* 543–548.

Jowett, B. (Trans.). (1931). *The dialogues of Plato* (3rd ed., Vol. 5). London: Oxford University Press.

Judd, P. H., Thomas, N., Schwartz, T., Outcalt, A., & Hough, R. (2003). A dual diagnosis demonstration project: Treatment outcomes and costs analysis. *Journal of Psychoactive Drugs* (SARC Suppl. 1), 181–192.

Julien, R. M. (1998). *A primer of drug action* (8th ed.). New York: Freeman.

Kandel, D. B. (2003). Does marijuana use cause use of other drugs? *Journal of the American Medical Association, 289,* 482–483.

Kandel, D. B., & Andrews, K. (1987). Processes of adolescent socialization by parents and peers. *International Journal of the Addictions, 22,* 319–342.

Kandel, D., & Faust, R. (1975). Sequence and stages in patterns of adolescent drug use. *Archives of General Psychiatry, 32*(7), 923–932.

Kandel, D. B., Huang, F. Y., & Davies, M. (2001). Comorbidity between patterns of substance dependence and psychiatric syndromes. *Drug and Alcohol Dependence, 64,* 233–241.

Kandel, D. B., Kessler, R. C., & Marguiles, R. Z. (1978). Antecedents of adolescent initiation into stages of drug use: A developmental analysis. In D. B. Kandel (Ed.), *Longitudinal research on drug use.* Washington, DC: Hemisphere.

Kandel, D. B., Yamaguchi, K., & Chen, K. (1992). Stages of progression in drug involvement from adolescence to adulthood: Further evidence for the gateway theory. *Journal of Studies on Alcohol, 53*(5), 447–457.

Kaprio, J., Koskenvuo, M., Langinvainio, H., Romanov, K., Sarna, S., & Rose, R. J. (1987). Genetic influences on use and abuse of alcohol: A study of 5638 adult Finnish twin brothers. *Alcoholism, Clinical and Experimental Research 11*(4), 349–356.

Keller, M. (1970). The great Jewish drink mystery. *British Journal of Addictions, 64,* 287–295.

Kendler, K. (1997). Social support: A genetic–epidemiologic analysis. *American Journal of Psychiatry, 154,* 1398–1404.

Kendler, K. S., Heath, A. C., Neale, M. C., Kessler, R. C., & Eaves, L. J. (1992). A population-based twin study of alcoholism in women. *Journal of the American Medical Association, 268*(14), 1877–1882.

Khantzian, E. J. (1980). An ego/self theory of substance dependence: A contemporary psychoanalytic perspective. In D. J. Lettieri, M. Sayers, & H. W. Pearson (Eds.), *Theories on drug abuse: Selected contemporary perspectives* (DHHS Publication No. ADM8-967). Washington, DC: U.S. Government Printing Office.

Khantzian, E. J., Halliday, K. S., & McAuliffe, W. E. (1990). *Addiction and the vulnerable self: Modified dynamic group therapy for substance abusers.* New York: Guilford Press.

Khoury, M. J., & Genetics Work Group. (1996). From genes to public health: The applications of genetic technology in disease prevention. *American Journal of Public Health, 86,* 1717–1722.

Kidorf, M., & Stitzer, M.L. (1993). Contingent access to methadone maintenance treatment: Effects on cocaine use of mixed opiate-cocaine abusers. *Experimental and Clinical Psychopharmacology, 1*(1–4), 200–206.

Kidorf, M., & Stitzer, M. L. (1996). Contingent use of take-homes and split-dosing to reduce illicit drug use of methadone patients. *Behavior Therapy, 27,* 41–51.

Klein, D. N., & Riso, L. P. (1993). Psychiatric disorders: problems of boundaries and comorbidity. In C. G. Costello (Ed.), *Basic issues in psychopathology.* New York: Guilford Press.

Klorman, R., Salzman, L., Pass, H., Borgstedt, A. D., & Dainer, K. B. (1979). Effects of methylphenidate on hyperactive children's evoked responses during passive and active attention. *Psychophysiology, 16*(1), 23–29.

Koepp, M. J., Gunn, R. N., Lawrence, A. D., Cunningham, V. J., Dagher, A., Jones, T., et al. (1998). Evidence of striatal dopamine release during a video game. *Nature, 393,* 266–268.

Koffinke, C. (1991). Family recovery issues and treatment resources. In D.C. Daley & M. S. Raskin (Eds.), *Treating the chemically dependent and their families.* Newbury Park, CA: Sage.

Koob, G. F. (1992). Drugs of abuse: Anatomy, pharmacology, and function of reward pathways. *Trends in Pharmacologic Sciences, 13,* 177–182.

Kreuter, M. W., Lezin, N. A., & Young, L. A. (2000). Evaluating community-based collaborative mechanisms: Implications for practitioners. *Health Promotion Practice, 1,* 49–63.

Lamb, S., Greenlick, M. R., & McCarty, D. (1998). *Bridging the gap between prac-*

tice and research: Forging partnerships with community-based drug and alcohol treatment. Washington, DC: National Academy Press.

Langenbucher, J. W., & Nathan, P. E. (1990). The tension-reduction hypothesis: A reanalysis of some early crucial data. In W. M. Cox (Ed.), *Why people drink: Parameters of alcohol as a reinforcer.* New York: Gardner Press.

Langton, P. A. (Ed.). (1995). *The challenge of participatory research: Preventing alcohol-related problems in ethnic communities.* Washington, DC: Center for Substance Abuse Prevention, U.S. Department of Health and Human Services.

Laundergan, J. C., & Williams, T. (1993). The Hazelden residential family program: A combined systems and disease model approach. In T. J. O'Farrell (Ed.), *Treating alcohol problems: Marital and family interventions.* New York: Guilford Press.

Lawson, A., & Lawson, G. A. (1998). *Alcoholism and the family: A guide to treatment and prevention* (2nd ed.). Gaithersburg, MD: Aspen.

Lawson, G., Peterson, J. S., & Lawson, A. (1983). *Alcoholism and the family: A guide to treatment and prevention.* Rockville, MD: Aspen.

Lee, W. V., & Weinstein, S. P. (1997). How far have we come? A critical review of the research on men who batter. *Recent Developments in Alcoholism, 13,* 337–356.

Leeds, J., & Morgenstern, J. (1996). Psychoanalytic theories of substance abuse. In F. Rotgers, D. S. Keller, & J. Morgenstern (Eds.), *Treating substance abuse: Theory and technique.* New York: Guilford Press.

Lerman, C., Cuporaso, N. E., Audrain, J., Main, D., Bowman, E. D., Lockshin, B., et al. (1999). Evidence suggesting the role of specific genetic factors in cigarette smoking. *Health Psychology, 18,* 14–20.

Leshner, A. I. (1996). Molecular mechanisms of cocaine addiction. *New England Journal of Medicine, 335*(2), 128–129.

Lester, D. (1988). Genetic theory: An assessment of the heritability of alcoholism. In C.D. Chaudron & D. A. Wilkinson (Eds.), *Theories on alcoholism.* Toronto, Ontario, Canada: Addiction Research Foundation.

Leukefeld, C. G., & Tims, F. M. (Eds.) (1988). *Compulsory treatment of drug abuse: Research and clinical practice* (NIDA Research Monograph 86; DHHS Publication No. ADM 88-1578). Washington, DC: U.S. Government Printing Office.

Levenson, R. W., Sher, K. J., Grossman, L. M., Newman, J., & Newlin, D. B. (1980). Alcohol and stress response dampening: Pharmacological effects, expectancy, and tension reduction. *Journal of Abnormal Psychology, 89,* 528–538.

Levine, H. G. (1978). The discovery of addiction: Changing conceptions of habitual drunkenness in America. *Journal of Studies on Alcohol, 39*(1), 143–174.

Lewis, J. A., Dana, R. Q., & Blevins, G. A. (1988). *Substance abuse counseling: An individualized approach.* Pacific Grove, CA: Brooks/Cole.

Lewis, J. A., Dana, R. Q., & Blevins, G. A. (1994). *Substance abuse counseling: An individualized approach* (2nd ed.). Pacific Grove, CA: Brooks/Cole.

Li, T. K. (2000). Pharmacogenetics of responses to alcohol and genes that influence drinking. *Journal of Studies on Alcohol, 61,* 5–12.

Light, D., & Keller, S. (1975). *Sociology.* New York: Knopf.

Lightfoot, L. O. (1993). The offender substance abuse pre-release program: An empirically based model of treatment for offenders. In J. S. Baer, G. A. Marlatt, & R. J. McMahon (Eds.), *Addictive behaviors across the life span: Prevention, treatment, and policy issues.* Newbury Park, CA: Sage.

Lurie, N. (1971). The World's oldest on-going protest demonstration: North American Indian drinking patterns. *Pacific Historical Review, 40,* 311–332.

Lynam, D. R., Milich, R., Zimmerman, R., Novak, S. P., Logan, T. K., Martin, C., et al. (1999). Project DARE: No effects at 10-year follow-up. *Journal of Consulting and Clinical Psychology, 67,* 590–593.

Lynskey, M. T., Heath, A. C., Bucholz, K. K., Slutske, W. S., Madden, P. A. F., Nelson, E. C., et al. (2003). Escalation of drug use in early-onset cannabis users vs co-twin controls. *Journal of the American Medical Association, 289,* 427–433.

MacAndrew, C., & Edgerton, R.B. (1969). *Drunken comportment: A social explanation.* Chicago: Aldine.

MacCoun, R. (1998). *In what sense (if any) is marijuana a gateway drug?* Federation of American Scientists Drug Policy Analysis Bulletin, Issue #4. Available at www.fas.org/drugs/issue4.htm#gateway. Accessed on January 5, 2005.

Maisto, S. A., Sobell, L. C., Sobell, M. B., Lei, H., & Sykora, K. (1988). Profiles of drinking patterns before and after outpatient treatment for alcohol abuse. In T. Baker & D. Cannon (Eds.), *Assessment and treatment of addictive behaviors.* New York: Praeger.

Mann, C. C. (1994). Behavioral genetics in transition. *Science, 264,* 1686–1689.

Marion, T. R., & Coleman, K. (1990). Recovery issues and treatment resources. In D.C. Daley & M. S. Raskin (Eds.), *Treating the chemically dependent and their families.* Newbury Park, CA: Sage.

Marlatt, G. A. (1985). Cognitive factors in the relapse process. In G. A. Marlatt & J. R. Gordon (Eds.), *Relapse prevention* (pp. 128–200). New York: Guilford Press.

Marlatt, G. A., Baer, J. S., & Quigley, L. A. (1995). Self-efficacy and addictive behavior. In A. Bandura (Ed.), *Self-efficacy in changing societies.* New York: Cambridge University Press.

Marlatt, G. A., Demming, B., & Reid, J. B. (1973). Loss of control drinking in alcoholics: An experimental analogue. *Journal of Abnormal Psychology, 81,* 233–241.

Marlatt, G. A., & Gordon, J. R. (1979). Determinants of relapse: Implications for the maintenance of behavior change. In P. A. Davidson & S. M. Davidson (Eds.), *Behavioral medicine: Changing health lifestyles.* New York: Brunner/Mazel.

Marlatt, G. A., & Gordon, J. R. (Eds.). (1985). *Relapse prevention.* New York: Guilford Press.

Marlatt, G. A., & Tapert, S. F. (1993). Harm reduction: Reducing the risks of addictive behaviors. In J. S. Baer, G. A. Marlatt, & R. J. McMahon (Eds.), *Addictive behaviors across the life span: Prevention, treatment, and policy issues.* Newbury Park, CA: Sage.

Marlowe, D. B., Kirby, K. C., Bonieskie, L. M., Glass, D. J., Dodds, L. D., Husband, S. D., et al. (1996). Assessment of coercive and noncoercive pressures to enter drug abuse treatment. *Drug and Alcohol Dependence, 42*(2), 77–84.

Massella, J. D. (1990). Intervention: Breaking the addiction cycle. In D. C. Daley & M. S. Raskin (Eds.), *Treating the chemically dependent and their families*. Newbury Park, CA: Sage.

Masserman, J. H., Jacques, M. G., & Nicholson, M. R. (1945). Alcohol as a preventive of experimental neurosis. *Quarterly Journal of Studies on Alcohol, 6,* 281–299.

Mather, C. (1708). *Sober considerations on a growing flood of iniquity*. Boston.

Maxwell, J. C. (2004). *Patterns of club drug use in the U.S., 2004*. The Center for Excellence in Drug Epidemiology, The Gulf Coast Addiction Technology Transfer Center. Austin: University of Texas. Available at www.utexas.edu/research/cswr/gcattc/Trends/ClubDrug-2004-web.pdf. Accessed on May 8, 2005.

May, C. (1993). Resistance to peer group pressure: An inadequate basis for alcohol education. *Health Education Research*, 8(2), 159–165.

Maynard, S. (1997). Growing up in an alcoholic family: The effect on anxiety and differentiation of self. *Journal of Substance Abuse, 9,* 161–170.

McAuliffe, W. E., & Gordon, R. A. (1980). Reinforcement and the combination of effects: Summary of a theory of opiate addiction. In D. J. Lettieri, M. Sayers, & H. Wallenstein-Pearson (Eds.), *Theories on drug abuse: Selected contemporary perspectives* (DHHS Publication No. ADM 84-967). Washington, DC: U.S. Government Printing Office.

McCrady, B. S., Moreau, J., Paolino, T. J., & Longabaugh, R. (1982). Joint hospitalization and couples therapy for alcoholism: A four year follow-up. *Journal of Studies on Alcohol, 43,* 1244–1250.

McCrady, B. S., Paolino, T. J., Longabaugh, R., & Rossi, J. (1979). Effects of joint hospital admission and couples' treatment for hospitalized alcoholics: A pilot study. *Addictive Behaviors, 4,* 155–165.

McGue, M., Pickens, R. W., & Svikis, D. S. (1992). Sex and age effects on the inheritance of alcohol problems: A twin study. *Journal of Abnormal Psychology, 101,* 3–17.

McKim, W. A. (1986). *Drugs and behavior: An introduction to behavioral pharmacology*. Englewood Cliffs, NJ: Prentice-Hall.

McKinlay, J. B., & Marceau, L. D. (2000). To boldly go . . . *American Journal of Public Health, 90*(1), 25–33.

Mechanic, D., Schlesinger, M., & McAlpine, D. D. (1995). Management of mental health and substance abuse services: State of the art and early results. *Milbank Quarterly, 73,* 19–55.

Mehr, J. (1988). *Human services: Concepts and intervention strategies*. Boston: Allyn & Bacon.

Mercer, C. G., Mueser, K. T., & Drake, R. E. (1998). Organizational guidelines for dual disorders programs. *Psychiatric Quarterly, 69,* 145–168.

Mercer, S. L., MacDonald, G., & Green, L. W. (2004). Participatory research and evaluation: From best practices for all states to achievable practices within each state in the context of the Master Settlement Agreement. *Health Promotion Practice, 5*(3, July Supp.), 167S–178S.

Merikangas, K. R., Stolar, M., Stevens, D. E., Goulet, J., Preisig, M. A., Fenton, B., et al. (1998). Familial transmission of substance use disorders. *Archives of General Psychiatry, 55,* 973–979.

Merry, J. (1966). The "loss of control" myth. *Lancet, I,* 1257–1258.

Messing, F. A., & Hazelwood, B. A. (2005). *U.S. drug control policy and international operations.* Alexandria, VA: The National Defense Council Foundation. Available at www.ndcf.org Accessed on August 4, 2005.

Milam, J. R., & Ketcham, K. (1983). *Under the influence.* New York: Bantam.

Milkman, H. B., & Sunderwirth, S. G. (1987). *Craving for ecstasy: The consciousness and chemistry of escape.* Lexington, MA: D.C. Heath.

Milkman, H., Weiner, S. E., & Sunderwirth, S. (1984). Addiction relapse. *Addictive Behaviors, 3,* 119–134.

Miller, G. A. (1999). *Learning the language of addiction counseling.* Boston: Allyn & Bacon.

Miller, L. K. (1980). *Principles of everyday behavior analysis.* Monterey, CA: Brooks/Cole.

Miller, P. M., Smith, G. T., & Goldman, M. S. (1990). Emergence of alcohol expectancies in childhood: A possible critical period. *Journal of Studies on Alcohol, 51*(4), 343–349.

Miller, W. R. (1982). Treating problem drinkers: What works. *The Behavior Therapist, 5,* 15–19.

Miller, W. R., Benefield, R., & Tonigan, S. (1993). Enhancing motivation for change in problem drinking: A controlled comparison of two therapist styles. *Journal of Consulting and Clinical Psychology, 61,* 455–461.

Miller, W. R., & Hester, R. K. (1980). Treating the problem drinker. In W. R. Miller (Ed.), *The addictive behaviors: Treatment of alcoholism, drug abuse, smoking, and obesity.* Elmsford, NY: Pergamon Press.

Miller, W. R., & Rollnick, S. (2002). *Motivational interviewing (2nd ed.): Preparing people for change.* New York: Guilford Press.

Miller, W. R., Zweben, A., DiClemente, C. C., & Rychtarik, R. G. (1992). *Motivational enhancement therapy manual: A clinical research guide for therapists treating individuals with alcohol abuse and dependence* (DHHS Publication No. ADM 92-1894). Washington, DC: U.S. Government Printing Office.

Miller-Tutzauer, C., Leonard, K. E., & Windle, M. (1991). Marriage and alcohol use: A longitudinal study of "maturing out." *Journal of Studies on Alcohol, 52*(5), 434–440.

Minkler, M., & Wallerstein, N. (Eds.). (2003). *Community-based participatory research in health.* San Francisco: Jossey-Bass.

Misra, R. K. (1980). Achievement, anxiety, and addiction. In D. J. Lettieri, M. Sayers, & H. W. Pearson (Eds.), *Theories on drug abuse: Selected contemporary perspectives* (DHHS Publication No. ADM 84-967). Washington, DC: U.S. Government Printing Office.

Monette, D. R., Sullivan, T. J., & DeJong, C. R. (1990). *Applied social research: Tool for the human services.* Fort Worth, TX: Holt, Rinehart & Winston.

Monte, C. F. (1980). *Beneath the mask: An introduction to theories of personality.* New York: Holt, Rinehart & Winston.

Montgomery, H. E., Marshall, R., Hemingway, H., Myerson, S., Clarkson, P.,

Dollery, C., et al. (1998). Human gene for physical performance. *Nature, 393,* 221.

Morey, L. C. (1996). Patient placement criteria: Linking typologies to managed care. *Alcohol Health and Research World, 20,* 36–44.

Mueller, M. D., & Wyman, J. R. (1997). Study sheds light on the state of drug abuse treatment nationwide. *NIDA Notes, 12*(5), 1, 4–8.

Mueser, K. T., Drake, R. E., & Wallach, M. A. (1998). Dual diagnosis: A review of etiological theories. *Addictive Behaviors, 23,* 717–734.

Mueser, K. T., Noordsy, D. L., Drake, R. E., & Fox, L. (2003). *Integrated treatment for dual disorders.* New York: Guilford Press.

Murphy, S. L., & Khantzian, E. J. (1995). Addiction as a "self-medication" disorder: Application of ego psychology to the treatment of substance abuse. In A. M. Washton (Ed.), *Psychotherapy and substance abuse: A practitioner's handbook.* New York: Guilford Press.

National Center on Addiction and Substance Abuse. (2003). *Crossing the bridge: An evaluation of the drug treatment alternative-to-prison (DATP) program.* New York: Columbia University. Available at www.casacolumbia.org/pdshopprov/shop/item.asp?itemid=8. Accessed on May 8, 2005.

National Health Promotion Associates. (2004). *LifeSkills® Training.* White Plains, NY. Available at www.lifeskillstraining.com. Accessed on December 14, 2004.

National Institute on Alcohol Abuse and Alcoholism. (1987). *Alcohol and health: Sixth special report to the U.S. Congress* (DHHS Publication No. ADM 87-1519). Washington, DC: U.S. Government Printing Office.

National Institute on Alcohol Abuse and Alcoholism. (1990). *Alcohol and health: Seventh special report to the U.S. Congress* (DHHS Publication No. ADM 90-1656). Washington, DC: U.S. Government Printing Office.

National Institute on Alcohol Abuse and Alcoholism. (1994). *Alcohol and health: Eighth special report to the U.S. Congress* (NIH Publication No. 94-3699). Bethesda, MD: National Institutes of Health.

National Institute on Alcohol Abuse and Alcoholism. (1997). *Alcohol and health: Ninth special report to the U.S. Congress* (NIH Publication No. 97-4017). Bethesda, MD: National Institutes of Health.

National Institute on Alcohol Abuse and Alcoholism. (2003, July). *Alcohol Alert, 60,* 1-4. Available at www.niaaa.nih.gov. Accessed on April 28, 2005.

National Institute on Drug Abuse (NIDA). (2005). *Club drugs.* Available at www.clubdrugs.org. Accessed on May 5, 2005.

National Institute on Drug Abuse. (1987). *Drug abuse and drug abuse research: The second triennial report to Congress* (DHHS Publication No. ADM 87-1486). Rockville, MD: Author.

National Institute on Drug Abuse. (2003). *Preventing drug use among children and adolescents: A research-based guide for parents, educators, and community leaders* (2nd ed.) (NIH Publication No. 04-4212(A)). Bethesda, MD: National Institutes of Health.

National Institutes of Health. (1998). COGA suggests genetic loci for P3 brain wave activity. *NIH News Release,* (May 20). Bethesda, MD: National Institutes of Health.

National Institute of Justice. (1988, January). *Drug use forecasting (DUF)*. Washington, DC: U.S. Department of Justice.

National Institute of Justice. (1998). *Arrestee drug abuse monitoring program: 1997 annual report on adult and juvenile arrestees*. Washington, DC: U.S. Department of Justice.

Neale, M. C., & Kendler, K. S. (1995). Models of comorbidity for multifactorial disorders. *American Journal of Human Genetics, 57*, 935–953.

Needle, R., McCubbin, H., Wilson, M., Reineck, R., Lazar, A., & Mederer, H. (1986). Interpersonal influences in adolescent drug use: The role of older siblings, parents, and peers. *International Journal of the Addictions, 21*, 739–766.

Nijhuis, H. G. J., & van der Maesen, L. J. G. (1994). The philosophical foundations of public health: An invitation to debate. *Journal of Epidemiology and Community Health, 48*, 1–3.

Noel, N. E., & McGrady, B. S. (1993). Alcohol-focused spouse involvement with behavioral marital therapy. In T. J. O'Farrell (Ed.), *Treating alcohol problems: Marital and family interventions*. New York: Guilford Press.

Norwood, R. (1985). *Women who love too much*. New York: Simon & Schuster.

Oetting, E. R., & Beauvis, F. (1988). Common elements in youth drug abuse: Peer clusters and other psychosocial factors. In S. Peele (Ed.), *Visions of addiction: Major contemporary perspectives on addiction and alcoholism*. Lexington, MA: Lexington Books.

O'Farrell, T. J., Cutter, H. S., & Floyd, F.J. (1985). Evaluating behavioral marital therapy for male alcoholics: Effects of marital adjustment and communication from before to after treatment. *Behavior Therapy, 16*, 147–167.

Office of Applied Studies. (2004a). *Results from the 2003 National Survey on Drug Use and Health: National findings* (NSDUH Series H-25; DHHS Publication No. SMA 04-3964). Rockville, MD: Substance Abuse and Mental Health Services Administration. Available at www.oas.samhsa.gov/. Accessed on June 17, 2005.

Office of Applied Studies. (2004b). *Drug Abuse Warning Network, 2003: Interim National Estimates of Drug-Related Emergency Department Visits* (DAWN Series: D-26; DHHS Publication No. (SMA) 04-3972). Rockville, MD: Substance Abuse and Mental Health Services Administration. Available at www.oas.samhsa.gov/. Accessed on June 17, 2005.

Office of Applied Studies. (2004c). *The NSDUH Report: Alcohol dependence or abuse and age at first use* (October 22). Rockville, MD: Substance Abuse and Mental Health Services Administration. Available at www.oas.samhsa.gov/. Accessed on June 17, 2005.

Okada, T., & Mizoi, Y. (1982). Studies on the problem of blood acetaldehyde determination in man and level after alcohol intake. *Japanese Journal of Alcohol and Drug Dependence, 17*, 141–159.

Olds, R. S., Thombs, D. L., & Ray-Tomasek, J. (2005). Relations between normative beliefs and initiation intentions toward cigarettes, alcohol and marijuana. *Journal of Adolescent Health, 37*, 75.e7–75e.13.

Palfai, T., & Jankiewicz, H. (1997). *Drugs and human behavior* (2nd ed.). Madison, WI: Brown and Benchmark.

Patterson, G. R. (1982). *Coercive family process*. Eugene, OR: Castalia.

Patterson, G. R. (1986). Performance models for antisocial boys. *American Psychologist, 41*(4), 432–444.

Patterson, G. R. (1996). Some characteristics of a developmental theory for early-onset delinquency. In M. F. Lenzenweger & J. J. Haugaard (Eds.), *Frontiers of developmental psychopathology*. New York: Oxford University Press.

Pattison, E. M., Sobell, M. B., & Sobell, L. C. (1977). *Emerging concepts of alcohol dependence*. New York: Springer.

Pearlman, S. (1988). Systems theory and alcoholism. In C. D. Chaudron & D. A. Wilkinson (Eds.), *Theories on alcoholism*. Toronto, Ontario, Canada: Addiction Research Foundation.

Peele, S. (1985). *The meaning of addiction: Compulsive experience and its interpretation*. Lexington, MA: D.C. Heath.

Peele, S. (1996). Assumptions about drugs and the marketing of drug policies. In W. K. Bickel & R. J. DeGrandpre (Eds.), *Drug policy and human nature: Psychological perspectives on the prevention, management, and treatment of illicit drug abuse*. New York: Plenum Press.

Pentz, M. A., Dwyer, J. H., MacKinnon, D. P., Flay, B. R., Hansen, W. B., Wang, E. Y. I., et al. (1989). Multicommunity trial for primary prevention of adolescent drug abuse. *Journal of the American Medical Association, 261*(22), 3259–3266.

Perkins, H. W., & Berkowitz, A. D. (1986). Perceiving the community norms of alcohol use among students: Some research implications for campus alcohol education programming. *International Journal of the Addictions, 21*, 961–976.

Perry, C. L., Williams, C. L., Veblen-Mortenson, S., Toomey, T. L., Komro, K. A., Anstine, P. S., et al. (1996). Project Northland: Outcomes of a communitywide alcohol use prevention program during early adolescence. *American Journal of Public Health, 86*, 956–965.

Petry, N. M. (2002). Discounting of delayed rewards in substance abusers: Relationship to antisocial personality disorder. *Psychopharmacology, 162*, 425–432.

Petry, N. M., & Casarella, T. (1999). Excessive discounting of delayed rewards in substance abusers with gambling problems. *Drug and Alcohol Dependence, 56*, 25–32.

Pfefferbaum, A., Ford, J. M., White, P. M., & Mathalon, D. (1991). Event-related potentials in alcoholic men: P3 amplitude reflects family history but not alcohol consumption. *Alcoholism, Clinical and Experimental Research, 15*, 839–850.

Pianezza, M. L., Sellers, E. M., & Tyndale, R. F. (1998). Nicotine metabolism defect reduces smoking. *Nature, 393*, 750.

Polich, J., & Bloom, F. E. (1988). Event-related brain potentials in individuals at high and low risk for developing alcoholism: Failure to replicate. *Alcoholism, Clinical and Experimental Research, 12*(3), 368–373.

Polich, J., Pollock, V. E., & Bloom, F. E. (1994). Meta-analysis of P300 amplitude from males at risk for alcoholism. *Psychological Bulletin, 115*(1), 55–73.

Porjesz, B., & Begleiter, H. (1985). Human brain electrophysiology and alcoholism. In R. E. Tartar & D. H. van Thiel (Eds.), *Alcohol and the brain*. New York: Plenum Press.

Powers, R. J., & Kutash, I.L. (1985). Stress and alcohol. *International Journal of the Addictions, 20*, 461–482.

Prentice, D. A., & Miller, D. T. (1993). Pluralistic ignorance and alcohol use on campus: Some consequences of misperceiving the social norm. *Journal of Personality and Social Psychology, 64*(2), 243–256.

Prescott, C. A. (2002). Sex differences in the genetic risk for alcoholism. *Alcohol Research and Health, 26*, 264–273.

Prochaska J. O., & DiClemente C. C. (1985). Common processes of change in smoking, weight control, and psychological distress. In S. Shiffman & T. Wills (Eds.), *Coping and substance abuse*. New York: Academic Press.

Prochaska J. O., & DiClemente C. C. (1992). Stages of change in the modification of problem behaviors. In M. Herson, R. M. Eisler & P. M. Miller (Eds.), *Progress in behavior modification* (Vol. 28). Sycamore, IL: Sycamore.

Prochaska J. O., DiClemente C. C., & Norcross J. C. (1992). In search of how people change: Application to addictive behavior. *American Psychologist, 47*(9), 1102–1114.

Prochaska, J. O., & Norcross J. C. (1983). Psychotherapists' perspectives on treating themselves and their clients for psychic distress. *Professional Psychology: Research and Practice, 14*, 642–655.

Project MATCH Research Group. (1997). Matching alcoholism treatments to client heterogeneity: Project MATCH posttreatment drinking outcomes. *Journal of Studies on Alcohol, 58*, 7–29.

Rand Corporation. (1994). *Controlling cocaine: Supply versus demand programs*. Santa Monica, CA: Author.

Rappaport, R. L. (1997). *Motivating clients in therapy: Values, love, and the real relationship*. New York: Routledge.

Rather, B. C., & Goldman, M. S. (1994). Drinking-related differences in the memory organization of alcohol expectancies. *Experimental and Clinical Psychopharmacology, 2*(2), 167–183.

Rather, B. C., Goldman, M. S., Roehrich, L., & Brannick, M. (1992). Empirical modeling of an alcohol expectancy memory network using multidimensional scaling. *Journal of Abnormal Psychology, 101*(1), 174–183.

Ray, O., & Ksir, C. (1999). *Drugs, society, and human behavior* (8th ed.). Boston: WCB/McGraw-Hill.

Reese, F. L., Chassin, L., & Molina, B. S. (1994). Alcohol expectancies in early adolescence: Predicting drinking behavior from alcohol expectancies and paternal alcoholism. *Journal of Studies on Alcohol, 55*, 276–284.

Reich, T., Edenberg, H. J., Goate, A., Williams, J. T., Rice, J. P., Van Eerdewegh, P., et al. (1998). Genome-wide search for genes affecting the risk for alcohol dependence. *American Journal of Medical Genetics, 81*, 207–215.

Rigotti, N. A., DiFranza, J. R., Chang, Y., Tisdale, T., Kemp, B., & Singer, D.E. (1997). The effect of enforcing tobacco-sales laws on adolescents, access to tobacco and smoking behavior. *New England Journal of Medicine, 337*, 1044–1051.

Risner, M. E., & Goldberg, S. R. (1983). A comparison of nicotine and cocaine self-administration in the dog: Fixed-ratio and progressive-ratio schedules of intravenous drug infusion. *Journal of Pharmacology and Experimental Therapeutics, 224,* 319–326.

Rivara, F. P., Mueller, B. A., Somes, G., Mendoza, C. T., Rushforth, N. B., & Kellermann, A. L. (1997). Alcohol and illicit drug abuse and the risk of violent death in the home. *Journal of the American Medical Association, 278*(7), 569–575.

Robertson, I., Heather, N., Dzialdowski, A., Crawford, J., & Winton, M. (1986). A comparison of minimal versus intensive controlled drinking treatment interventions for problem drinkers. *British Journal of Clinical Psychology, 25,* 185–194.

Rocha, B. A., Scearce-Levie, K., Lucas, J. J., Hiroi, N., Castanon, N., Crabbe, J. C., et al. (1998). Increased vulnerability to cocaine in mice lacking the serotonin-1B receptor. *Nature, 393,* 175–178.

Rogers, E. M. (1995a). Diffusion of drug abuse prevention programs: Spontaneous diffusion, agenda setting, and reinvention. In T. E. Backer, S. L. David, & G. Soucy (Eds.), *Reviewing the behavioral science knowledge base on technology transfer* (NIDA Research Monograph 155; NIH Publication No. 95-4035). Rockville, MD: National Clearinghouse on Alcohol and Drug Information.

Rogers, E.M. (1995b). *Diffusion of innovations* (4th ed.). New York: Free Press.

Rollnick, S., & Morgan, M. (1995). Motivational interviewing: Increasing readiness to change. In A. M. Washton (Ed.), *Psychotherapy and substance abuse: A practioner's handbook.* New York: Guilford Press.

Rorabaugh, W. J. (1976). *The alcoholic republic; America, 1790-1840.* PhD dissertation, University of California, Berkeley.

Rosenberg, H., Melville, J., Levell, D., & Hodge, J. E. (1994). A 10-year follow-up survey of acceptability of controlled drinking in Britain. *Journal of Studies on Alcohol, 53,* 441–446.

Ross, H. E., Glaser, F. B., & Germanson, T. (1988). The prevalence of psychiatric disorders in patients with alcohol and drug problems. *Archives of General Psychiatry, 45*(11), 1023–1031.

Rotgers, F. (1996). Behavioral theory of substance abuse treatment: Bringing science to bear on practice. In F. Rotgers, D. S. Keller, & J. Morgenstern (Eds.), *Treating substance abuse: Theory and technique.* New York: Guilford Press.

Rychtarik, R. G., Prue, D. M., Rapp, S. R., & King, A. C. (1992). Self-efficacy, aftercare and relapse in a treatment program for alcoholics. *Journal of Studies on Alcohol, 53,* 435–440.

Sabol, S. Z., Nelson, M. L., Fisher, C., Marcus, S. E., Gunzerath, L., Brody, C., et al. (1999). A genetic association for cigarette smoking behavior. *Health Psychology, 18,* 7–13.

Saitz, R. (1998). Introduction to alcohol withdrawal. *Alcohol Health and Research World, 22,* 5–12.

Sanchez-Craig, M., & Lei, H. (1986). Disadvantages of imposing the goal of abstinence on problem drinkers: An empirical study. *British Journal of Addiction, 81,* 505–512.

Sayette, M.A. (1993). An appraisal-disruption model of alcohol's effects on stress responses in social drinkers. *Psychological Bulletin, 114,* 459–476.

Sayette, M. A., Breslin, F. C., Wilson, G. T., & Rosenblum, G. D. (1994). Parental history of alcohol abuse and the effects of alcohol and expectations of intoxication on social stress. *Journal of Studies on Alcohol, 55*(2), 214–223.

Schafer, J., & Brown, S. A. (1991). Marijuana and cocaine effect expectancies and drug use patterns. *Journal of Consulting and Clinical Psychology, 59*(4), 558–565.

Schuckit, M. A. (1984). Biochemical markers of a predisposition to alcoholism. In S.B. Rosalki (Ed.), *Clinical biochemistry of alcoholism.* Edinburgh: Churchill Livingstone.

Schuckit, M. A. (1989). Familial alcoholism. *Drug Abuse and Alcoholism Newsletter, 18*(9), 1–3.

Schwartz, H. D., & Kart, C. S. (1978). *Dominant issues in medical sociology.* Reading, MA: Addison-Wesley.

Schwarzer, R., & Fuchs, R. (1995). Changing risk behaviors and adopting health behaviors: The role of self-efficacy beliefs. In A. Bandura (Ed.), *Self-efficacy in changing societies.* New York: Cambridge University Press.

Schwitters, S. Y., Johnson, R. C., McClearn, G. E., & Wilson, J. R. (1982). Alcohol use and the flushing response in different racial–ethnic groups. *Journal of Studies on Alcohol, 43,* 1259–1262.

Searles, J. S. (1988). The role of genetics in the pathogenesis of alcoholism. *Journal of Abnormal Psychology, 97*(2), 153–167.

Searles, J. S., & Windle, M. (1990). Introduction and overview: Salient issues in the children of alcoholics literature. In M. Windle & J. S. Searles (Eds.), *Children of alcoholics: Critical perspectives.* New York: Guilford Press.

Seefeldt, R. W., & Lyon, M. A. (1992). Personality characteristics of adult children of alcoholics. *Journal of Counseling and Development, 70,* 588–593.

Seilhamer, R. A., & Jacob, T. (1990). Family factors and adjustment of children of alcoholics. In M. Windle & J. S. Searles (Eds.), *Children of alcoholics: Critical perspectives.* New York: Guilford Press.

Seilhamer, R. A., Jacob, T., & Dunn, N.J. (1993). The impact of alcohol consumption on parent-child relationships in families of alcoholics. *Journal of Studies on Alcohol, 54,* 1189–1198.

Sher, K. J. (1987). Stress response dampening. In H. T. Blane & K. E. Leonard (Eds.), *Psychological theories of drinking and alcoholism.* New York: Guilford Press.

Sher, K. J. (1991). *Children of alcoholics: A critical appraisal of theory and research.* Chicago: University of Chicago Press.

Sher, K. J. (1997). Psychological characteristics of children of alcoholics. *Alcohol, Health and Research World, 21*(3), 247–254.

Shiffrin, R. M., & Schneider, W. (1977). Controlled and automatic human information processing: II. Perceptual learning, automatic attending, and a general theory. *Psychological Review, 84,* 127–190.

Siegel, S. (1982). Drug dissociation in the nineteenth century. In F. C. Colpaert & J. L. Slangen (Eds.), *Drug discrimination: Applications in CNS pharmacology.* Amsterdam: Elsevier.

Sisson, R. W., & Azrin, N. A. (1986). Family-member involvement to initiate and promote treatment of problem drinkers. *Journal of Behavior Therapy and Experimental Psychiatry, 17,* 15–21.

Sisson, R. W., & Azrin, N. A. (1993). Community reinforcement training for families: A method to get alcoholics into treatment. In T. J. O'Farrell (Ed.), *Treating alcohol problems: Marital and family interventions.* New York: Guilford Press.

Skinner, B. F. (1975). *Beyond freedom and dignity.* New York: Bantam.

Skog, O. J., & Duckert, F. (1993). The development of alcoholics' and heavy drinkers' consumption: A longitudinal study. *Journal of Studies on Alcohol, 54,* 178–188.

Slutske, W. S., Heath, A. C., Madden, P. A. F., Bucholz, K. K., Statham, D. J., & Martin, N. G. 2002). Personality and the genetic risk for alcohol dependence. *Journal of Abnormal Psychology, 111,* 124–133.

Smith, G. T., Goldman, M. S., Greenbaum, P. E., & Christiansen, B. A. (1995). Expectancy for social facilitation from drinking: The divergent paths of high-expectancy and low-expectancy adolescents. *Journal of Studies on Alcohol, 104*(1), 32–40.

Sobell, L. C., Cunningham, J. A., Sobell, M. B., & Toneatto, T. (1993). A life-span perspective on natural recovery (self-change) from alcohol problems. In J. S. Baer, G. A. Marlatt, & R. J. McMahon (Eds.), *Addictive behaviors across the life span: Prevention, treatment, and policy issues.* Newbury Park, CA: Sage.

Sobell, L. C., Sobell, M. B., & Toneatto, T. (1992). Recovery from alcohol problems without treatment. In N. Heather, W. R. Miller, & J. Greeley (Eds.), *Self-control and the addictive behaviors.* Botany Bay, New South Wales, Australia: Maxwell Macmillan.

Sobell, M. B., & Sobell, L. C. (1976). Second year treatment outcome of alcoholics treated by individualized behavior therapy: Results. *Behaviour Research and Therapy, 14,* 195–215.

Sobell, M. B., Wilkinson, D. A., & Sobell, L. C. (1990). Alcohol and drug problems. In A. S. Bellack, M. Hersen, & A. E. Kazdin (Eds.), *International handbook of behavior modification* (2nd ed.). New York: Plenum Press.

Spoth, R. L., Redmond, C., & Shin, C. (2001). Randomized trial of brief family interventions for general populations: Adolescent substance use outcomes 4 years after baseline. *Journal of Consulting and Clinical Psychology, 69,* 627–642.

Stacy, A. W., Newcomb, M. D., & Bentler, P. M. (1991). Cognitive motivation and drug use: A 9-year longitudinal study. *Journal of Abnormal Psychology, 100*(4), 502–515.

Stanton, M. D. (1980). A family theory of drug abuse. In D. J. Lettieri, M. Sayers, & H. W. Pearson (Eds.), *Theories on drug abuse: Selected contemporary perspectives* (DHHS Publication No. ADM 84-967). Washington, DC: U.S. Government Printing Office.

Stanton, M. D., & Heath, A. W. (1995). Family treatment of alcohol and drug abuse. In R. H. Mikesell, D. D. Lusterman, & S.H. McDaniel (Eds.), *Integrating family therapy: Handbook of family psychology and systems theory.* Washington, DC: American Psychological Association.

Stefflre, B., & Burks, H. M. (1979). Function of theory in counseling. In H. M. Burks & B. Stefflre (Eds.), *Theories of counseling*. New York: McGraw-Hill.

Steinglass, P. (1978). The conceptualization of marriage from a systems theory perspective. In T. J. Paolino, Jr., & B. S. McCrady (Eds.), *Marriage and marital therapy*. New York: Brunner/Mazel.

Steinglass, P. (1981). The alcoholic at home: Patterns of interaction in dry, wet, and transitional stages of alcoholism. *Archives of General Psychiatry, 38,* 578–584.

Stitzer, M., & Bigelow, G. (1978). Contingency management in a methadone maintenance program: Availability of reinforcers. *International Journal of the Addictions, 13*(5), 737–746.

Stitzer, M. L., Bigelow, G. E., & Liebson, I. (1980). Reducing drug use among methadone maintenance clients: Contingent reinforcement for morphine-free urines. *Addictive Behaviors, 5,* 333–340.

Stockwell, T. (1985). Stress and alcohol. *Stress Medicine, 1,* 209–215.

Stone, D. B., Armstrong, R. W., Macrina, D. M., & Pankau, J. W. (1996). *Introduction to epidemiology*. Boston: McGraw-Hill.

Subby, R., & Friel, J. (1984). Co-dependency: A paradoxical dependency. In Codependency: An emerging issue. Hollywood, FL: Heath Communications.

Substance Abuse and Mental Health Services Administration. (2002). *Report to Congress on the prevention and treatment of co-occurring substance abuse and mental disorders*. Available at alt.samhsa.gov/reports/congress2002/idex.html. Accessed on June 17, 2005.

Substance Abuse and Mental Health Services Administration. (2004). *SAMHSA model programs: Effective substance abuse and mental health programs for every community*. Washington, DC: U.S. Department of Health and Human Services. Available at www.modelprograms.samhsa.gov. Accessed on December 14, 2004.

Sun, W., Skara, S., Sun, P., Dent, C. W., & Sussman, S. (in press). Project Towards No Drug Abuse: Long-term substance use outcomes evaluation. *Preventive Medicine*.

Sussman, S. (1996). Development of a school-based drug abuse prevention curriculum for high risk youth. *Journal of Psychoactive Drugs, 26,* 214–267.

Sussman, S., Dent, C. W., & Stacy, A. W. (2002). Project Towards No Drug Abuse: A review of the findings and future directions. *American Journal of Health Behavior, 26,* 354–365.

Sussman, S., Dent, C. W., Stacy, A. W., & Craig, S. (1998). One-year outcomes of Project Towards No Drug Abuse. *Preventive Medicine, 27,* 632–642.

Sussman, S., Rohrbach, L. A., Patel, R., & Holiday, K. (2003a). A look at an interactive classroom-based drug abuse prevention program: Interactive contents and suggestions for research. *Journal of Drug Education, 33,* 355–368.

Sussman, S., Sun, P., McCuller, W. J., & Dent, C. W. (2003b). Project Towards No Drug Abuse: Two-year outcomes of a trial that compares health educator delivery to self-instruction. *Preventive Medicine, 37,* 155–162.

Talbott, G. D. (1989). Alcoholism should be treated as a disease. In B. Leone (Ed.), *Chemical dependency: Opposing viewpoints*. San Diego: Greenhaven.

Taleff, M. J. (1997). *A handbook to assess and treat resistance in chemical dependency.* Dubuque, IA: Kendall/Hunt.

Tenkasi, R. V., & Mohrman, S. A. (1995). Technology transfer as collaborative learning. In T. E. Backer, S. L. David, & G. Soucy (Eds.), *Reviewing the behavioral science knowledge base on technology transfer* (NIDA Research Monograph 155; NIH Publication No. 95-4035). Rockville, MD: National Clearinghouse on Alcohol and Drug Information.

Thombs, D. L. (1989). A review of PCP abuse trends and perceptions. *Public Health Reports, 104*(4), 325–328.

Thombs, D. L. (1991). Expectancies versus demographics in discriminating between college drinkers: Implications for alcohol abuse prevention. *Health Education Research, 6*(4), 491–495.

Thombs, D. L. (1993). The differentially discriminating properties of alcohol expectancies for female and male drinkers. *Journal of Counseling and Development, 71*(3), 321–325.

Thombs, D. L., & Beck, K. H. (1994). The social context of four adolescent drinking patterns. *Health Education Research, 9*(1), 13–22.

Thombs, D. L., Beck, K. H., Mahoney, C. A., Bromley, M. D., & Bezon, K. M. (1994). Social context, sensation seeking, and teen-age alcohol abuse. *Journal of School Health, 64*(2), 73–79.

Thombs, D. L., Beck, K. H., & Pleace, D. J. (1993). The relationship of social context and expectancy factors to alcohol use intensity among 18 to 22 year-olds. *Addiction Research, 1,* 59–68.

Thombs, D. L., Mahoney, C. A., & Olds, R. S. (1998). Application of a bogus testing procedure to determine college students' utilization of genetic screening for alcoholism. *Journal of American College Health, 47,* 103–112.

Thombs, D. L., & Ray-Tomasek, J. (2001). Superintendents' intentions toward DARE: Results from a statewide survey. *American Journal of Health Education, 32,* 267–274.

Thombs, D. L., Wolcott, B. J., & Farkash, L. G. E. (1997). Social context, perceived norms, and drinking behavior in young people. *Journal of Substance Abuse, 9,* 257–267.

Tiffany, S. T. (1990). A cognitive model of drug urges and drug-use behavior: Role of automatic and nonautomatic processes. *Psychological Review, 97,* 147–168.

Torres, S. (1997). An effective supervision strategy for substance-abusing offenders. *Federal Probation, 61*(2), 38–44.

Torrey, W. C., Drake, R. E., Cohen, M., Fox, L. B., Lynde, D., Gorman, P., et al. (2002). The challenge of implementing and sustaining integrated dual disorders treatment programs. *Community Mental Health Journal, 38,* 507–521.

Transnational Institute. (2005). *Drugs & Democracy.* Available at www.tni.org/drugs/index.html. Accessed on August 4, 2005.

Tsuang, M. T., Lyons, M. J., Meyer, J. M., Doyle, T., Eisen, S. A., Goldberg, J., et al. (1998). Co-occurrence of abuse of different drugs in men: The role of drug-specific and shared vulnerabilities. *Archives of General Psychiatry, 55,* 967–972.

Tsukamoto, S., Sudo, T., Karasawa, S., Kajiwara, M., & Endo, T. (1982). Quantitative recovery of acetaldehyde in biological samples. *Nihon University Journal of Medicine, 24,* 313–331.

Tucker, J. A., Vuchinich, R. E., & Pukish, M. M. (1995). Molar environmental contexts surrounding recovery from alcohol problems by treated and untreated problem drinkers. *Experimental and Clinical Psychopharmacology, 3,* 195–204.

Ullman, L. P., & Krasner, L. (1965). *Case studies in behavior modification.* New York: Holt, Rinehart & Winston.

U.S. Department of Education. (2001). *Exemplary and promising safe, disciplined, and drug-free schools programs.* Washington, DC: Office of Special Educational Research and Improvement and Office of Reform Assistance and Dissemination. Available at www.ed.gov/admins/lead/safety/exemplary01/exemplary01.pdf. Accessed on December 14, 2004.

U.S. Department of Health and Human Services. (2000). *Healthy people 2010* (2nd ed.). Washington, DC: U.S. Government Printing Office.

U.S. General Accounting Office. (1994). *Foster care: Parental drug abuse has alarming impact on young children.* Washington, DC: Author.

U.S. Office of National Drug Control Policy. (2004). *National drug control strategy 2004.* Available at www.whitehousedrugpolicy.gov/publications/policy/ndcs04/index.html. Accessed on May 11, 2005.

U.S. Sentencing Commission. (1998). *Federal sentencing guidelines (1998).* Washington, DC: Author.

Vaillant, G. E. (1983). *The natural history of alcoholism.* Cambridge, MA: Harvard University Press.

Vaillant, G. E. (1990). We should retain the disease concept of alcoholism. *Harvard Medical School Mental Health Letter, 6(9),* 4–6.

Vaillant, G. E. (1995). *The natural history of alcoholism revisited.* Cambridge, MA: Harvard University Press.

Wagenaar, A. C., Gehan, J. P., Jones-Webb, R., Toomey, T. L., & Forster, J. (1999). Communities mobilizing for change on alcohol: Lessons and results from a 15-community randomized trial. *Journal of Community Psychology, 27,* 315–326.

Wagenaar, A. C., Murray, D. M., Gehan, J. P., Wolfson, M., Forster, J., Toomey, T. L., et al. (2000a). Communities mobilizing for change on alcohol: Outcomes from a randomized community trial. *Journal of Studies on Alcohol, 61,* 85–94.

Wagenaar, A. C., Murray, D. M., & Toomey, T. L. (2000b). Communities mobilizing for change on alcohol (CMCA): Effects of a randomized trial on arrests and traffic crashes. *Addiction, 95,* 209–217.

Walters, G. D. (2002). The heritability of alcohol abuse and dependence: A meta-analysis of behavior genetic research. *American Journal of Drug and Alcohol Abuse, 28,* 557–584.

Wanberg, K. W. (1969). Prevalence of symptoms found among excessive drinkers. *International Journal of the Addictions, 4,* 169–185.

Wang, J. C., Hinrichs, A. L., Stock, H., Budde, J., Allen, R., Bertelsen, S., et al. (2004). Evidence of common and specific genetic effects: Association of the

muscarinic acetylcholine receptor M2 (CHRM2) gene with alcohol dependence and major depressive syndrome. *Human Molecular Genetics, 13,* 1903–
1911.

Washington State Department of Social & Health Services. (1997). *Cost savings in
Medicaid medical expenses: An outcome study of publicly funded chemical
dependency treatment in Washington State.* Briefing paper #4.30 (June).
Olympia, WA: DSHS Division of Research and Data Analysis.

Wechsler, H., Lee, J. E., Kuo, M., Seibring, M., Nelson, T. F., & Lee, H. (2002).
Trends in college binge drinking during a period of increased prevention
efforts. Findings from 4 Harvard School of Public Health College Alcohol Surveys: 1993–2001. *Journal of American College Health, 50,* 203–217.

Wells, K. B., Astrachan, B. M., Tischler, G. L., & Unutzer, J. (1995). Issues and
approaches in evaluating managed mental health care. *Milbank Quarterly, 73,*
57–75.

White, F. J. (1998). Cocaine and the serotonin saga. *Nature, 393,* 118–119.

Wilbanks, W. L. (1989). Drug addiction should be treated as a lack of self-discipline. In B. Leone (Ed.), *Chemical dependency: Opposing viewpoints.* San
Diego: Greenhaven.

Wilson, G. T. (1988). Alcohol use and abuse: A social learning theory analysis. In C.
D. Chaudron & D.A. Wilkinson (Eds.), *Theories on alcoholism.* Toronto,
Ontario, Canada: Addiction Research Foundation.

Winick, C. (1962). Maturing out of narcotic addiction. *Bulletin on Narcotics, 14,*
1–7.

Woititz, J. G. (1983). *Adult children of alcoholics.* Hollywood, FL: Heath Communications.

Wolff, T. (2001a). Community coalition building—Contemporary practice and
research: Introduction. *American Journal of Community Psychology, 29,* 165–
172.

Wolff, T. (2001b). A practitioner's guide to successful coalitions. *American Journal
of Community Psychology, 29,* 173–191.

Wolock, I., & Magura, S. (1996). Parental substance abuse as a predictor of child
maltreatment re-reports. *Child Abuse and Neglect, 20*(12), 1183–1193.

Wong, C. J., Anthony, S., Sigmon, S. C., Mongeon, J. A., Badger, G. J., & Higgins,
S. T. (2004). Examining interrelationships between abstinence and coping self-
efficacy in cocaine-dependent outpatients. *Experimental and Clinical Psychopharmacology, 12,* 190–199.

World Health Organization. (1998). *Health promotion glossary.* Available at
www.wpro.who.int/hpr/docs/glossary.pdf. Accessed on November 3, 2004.

Wurmser, L. (1974). Psychoanalytic considerations of the etiology of compulsive
drug use. *Journal of the American Psychoanalytic Association, 22,* 820–843.

Wurmser, L. (1978). *The hidden dimension: Psychodynamics in compulsive drug
use.* New York: Jason Aronson.

Wurmser, L. (1980). Drug use as a protective system. In D. J. Lettieri, M. Sayers, &
H. W. Pearson, (Eds.), *Theories on drug abuse: Selected contemporary perspectives* (DHHS Publication No. ADM 84-967). Washington, DC: U.S. Government Printing Office.

Yalisove, D. L. (1989). Psychoanalytic approaches to alcoholism and addiction: Treatment and research. *Psychology of Addictive Behaviors, 3*(3), 107–113.

Yalisove, D. (1998). The origins and evolution of the disease concept of treatment. *Journal of Studies on Alcohol, 59,* 469–476.

Young, N. K., Gardner, S. L., & Dennis, K. (1998). *Responding to alcohol and other drug problems in child welfare: Weaving together practice and policy.* Washington, DC: Child Welfare League of America.

Zamora, J. H. (1998, July 29). Viagra a killer when combined with "poppers." *San Francisco Examiner.*

Zimberg, S. (1978). Principles of alcoholism psychotherapy. In S. Zimberg, J. Wallace, & S.B. Blume (Eds.), *Practical approaches to alcoholism psychotherapy.* New York: Plenum Press.

Zimmerman, B. J. (1995). Self-efficacy in career choice and development. In A. Bandura (Ed.), *Self-efficacy in changing societies.* New York: Cambridge University Press.

Zucker, R. (1976). Parental influences on the drinking patterns of their children. In M. Greenblatt & M.A. Schuckit (Eds.), *Alcoholism problems in women and children.* New York: Grune & Stratton.

Zucker, R. A., Ellis, D. A., Bingham, C. R., & Fitzgerald, H. E. (1996). The development of alcoholic subtypes: Risk variation among alcoholic families during the early childhood years. *Alcohol, Health and Research World, 20*(1), 46–54.

Zucker, R. A., Kincaid, S. B., Fitzgerald, H. E., & Bingham, C. R. (1995). Alcohol schema acquisition in preschoolers: Differences between children of alcoholics and children of nonalcoholics. *Alcoholism, Clinical and Experimental Research, 19,* 1011–1017.

Zuckerman, M. (1983). *Biological bases of sensation seeking, impulsivity, and anxiety.* Hillsdale, NJ: Erlbaum.

Author Index

Subject Index